Control of Communicable Diseases in Human and in Animal Populations: 70th Anniversary Year of the Birth of Professor Rick Speare (2 August 1947–5 June 2016)

Control of Communicable Diseases in Human and in Animal Populations: 70th Anniversary Year of the Birth of Professor Rick Speare (2 August 1947–5 June 2016)

Special Issue Editor

Jorg Heukelbach

MDPI • Basel • Beijing • Wuhan • Barcelona • Belgrade

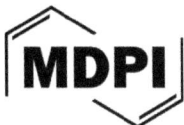

MDPI

Special Issue Editor
Jorg Heukelbach
Federal University of Ceará
Brazil

Editorial Office
MDPI
St. Alban-Anlage 66
Basel, Switzerland

This is a reprint of articles from the Special Issue published online in the open access journal *Tropical Medicine and Infectious Disease* (ISSN 2414-6366) from 2017 to 2018 (available at: https://www.mdpi.com/journal/tropicalmed/special_issues/rick_speare)

For citation purposes, cite each article independently as indicated on the article page online and as indicated below:

LastName, A.A.; LastName, B.B.; LastName, C.C. Article Title. *Journal Name* **Year**, *Article Number, Page Range*.

ISBN 978-3-03897-314-0 (Pbk)
ISBN 978-3-03897-315-7 (PDF)

Cover image courtesy of Jorg Heukelbach.

Contents

About the Special Issue Editor . . . . **vii**

Jorg Heukelbach
Control of Communicable Diseases in Human and in Animal Populations: 70th Anniversary of
the Year of the Birth of Professor Rick Speare (2 August 1947–5 June 2016)
Reprinted from: *Trop. Med. Infect. Dis.* **2018**, 3, 106, doi: 10.3390/tropicalmed3040106 . . . . **1**

Angela Wilson and Deborah Fearon
Paediatric Strongyloidiasis in Central Australia
Reprinted from: *Trop. Med. Infect. Dis.* **2018**, 3, 64, doi: 10.3390/tropicalmed3020064 . . . . **4**

Gemma J. Robertson, Anson V. Koehler, Robin B. Gasser, Matthew Watts, Robert Norton and
Richard S. Bradbury
Application of PCR-Based Tools to Explore *Strongyloides* Infection in People in Parts of
Northern Australia
Reprinted from: *Trop. Med. Infect. Dis.* **2017**, 2, 62, doi: 10.3390/tropicalmed2040062 . . . . **17**

Matthew Paltridge and Aileen Traves
The Health Effects of Strongyloidiasis on Pregnant Women and Children: A Systematic
Literature Review
Reprinted from: *Trop. Med. Infect. Dis.* **2018**, 3, 50, doi: 10.3390/tropicalmed3020050 . . . . **32**

Wendy Page, Jenni A. Judd and Richard S. Bradbury
The Unique Life Cycle of *Strongyloides stercoralis* and Implications for Public Health Action
Reprinted from: *Trop. Med. Infect. Dis.* **2018**, 3, 53, doi: 10.3390/tropicalmed3020053 . . . . **53**

Adrian Miller, Elizebeth L. Young, Valarie Tye, Robert Cody, Melody Muscat,
Vicki Saunders, Michelle L. Smith, Jenni A. Judd and Rick Speare
A Community-Directed Integrated *Strongyloides* Control Program in Queensland, Australia
Reprinted from: *Trop. Med. Infect. Dis.* **2018**, 3, 48, doi: 10.3390/tropicalmed3020048 . . . . **64**

Meruyert Beknazarova, Harriet Whiley, Jenni Judd, Jennifer Shield, Wendy Page,
Adrian Miller, Maxine Whittaker and Kirstin Ross
Argument for Inclusion of Strongyloidiasis in the Australian National Notifiable Disease List
Reprinted from: *Trop. Med. Infect. Dis.* **2018**, 3, 61, doi: 10.3390/tropicalmed3020061 . . . . **75**

Erin Fergus, Richard Speare and Clare Heal
Immunisation Rates of Medical Students at a Tropical Queensland University
Reprinted from: *Trop. Med. Infect. Dis.* **2018**, 3, 52, doi: 10.3390/tropicalmed3020052 . . . . **86**

Catherine A. Gordon, Malcolm K. Jones and Donald P. McManus
The History of Bancroftian Lymphatic Filariasis in Australasia and Oceania: Is There a Threat
of Re-Occurrence in Mainland Australia?
Reprinted from: *Trop. Med. Infect. Dis.* **2018**, 3, 58, doi: 10.3390/tropicalmed3020058 . . . . **93**

Muhammad Zahoor Khan and Muhammad Zahoor
An Overview of Brucellosis in Cattle and Humans, and its Serological and Molecular Diagnosis
in Control Strategies
Reprinted from: *Trop. Med. Infect. Dis.* **2018**, 3, 65, doi: 10.3390/tropicalmed3020065 . . . . **118**

Amy L. Shima, Constantin C. Constantinoiu, Linda K. Johnson and Lee F. Skerratt
Echinococcus Granulosus Infection in Two Free-Ranging Lumholtz's Tree-Kangaroo
(*Dendrolagus lumholtzi*) from the Atherton Tablelands, Queensland
Reprinted from: *Trop. Med. Infect. Dis.* **2018**, *3*, 47, doi: 10.3390/tropicalmed3020047 . . . . **132**

**Uade Samuel Ugbomoiko, Samuel Adeola Oyedeji, Olarewaju Abdulkareem Babamale and
Jorg Heukelbach**
Scabies in Resource-Poor Communities in Nasarawa State, Nigeria: Epidemiology, Clinical
Features and Factors Associated with Infestation
Reprinted from: *Trop. Med. Infect. Dis.* **2018**, *3*, 59, doi: 10.3390/tropicalmed3020059 . . . . **139**

**Jennifer M. Shield, Thérèse M. Kearns, Joanne Garngulkpuy, Lisa Walpulay,
Roslyn Gundjirryirr, Leanne Bundhala, Veronica Djarpanbuluwuy, Ross M. Andrews
and Jenni Judd**
Cross-Cultural, Aboriginal Language, Discovery Education for Health Literacy and Informed
Consent in a Remote Aboriginal Community in the Northern Territory, Australia
Reprinted from: *Trop. Med. Infect. Dis.* **2018**, *3*, 15, doi: 10.3390/tropicalmed3010015 . . . . **149**

R. C. Andrew Thompson
Exotic Parasite Threats to Australia's Biosecurity—Trade, Health, and Conservation
Reprinted from: *Trop. Med. Infect. Dis.* **2018**, *3*, 76, doi: 10.3390/tropicalmed3030076 . . . . **160**

Simone Gillespie and Richard S. Bradbury
A Survey of Intestinal Parasites of Domestic Dogs in Central Queensland
Reprinted from: *Trop. Med. Infect. Dis.* **2017**, *2*, 60, doi: 10.3390/tropicalmed2040060 . . . . **168**

**Mohamed Lemine Cheikh Brahim Ahmed, Abdellahi Weddih, Mohammed Benhafid,
Mohamed Abdellahi Bollahi, Mariem Sidatt, Khattry Makhalla, Ali H. Mokdad,
Jorg Heukelbach and Abdelkarim Filali-Maltouf**
Hospitalizations and Deaths Associated with Diarrhea and Respiratory Diseases among
Children Aged 0–5 Years in a Referral Hospital of Mauritania
Reprinted from: *Trop. Med. Infect. Dis.* **2018**, *3*, 103, doi: 10.3390/tropicalmed3030103 . . . . **178**

Humphrey D. Mazigo and Jorg Heukelbach
Diagnostic Performance of Kato Katz Technique and Point-of-Care Circulating Cathodic
Antigen Rapid Test in Diagnosing *Schistosoma mansoni* Infection in HIV-1 Co-Infected Adults
on the Shoreline of Lake Victoria, Tanzania
Reprinted from: *Trop. Med. Infect. Dis.* **2018**, *3*, 54, doi: 10.3390/tropicalmed3020054 . . . . **186**

**Eliana Amorim de Souza, Anderson Fuentes Ferreira, Jorg Heukelbach,
Reagan Nzundu Boigny, Carlos Henrique Alencar and Alberto Novaes Ramos Jr.**
Epidemiology and Spatiotemporal Patterns of Leprosy Detection in the State of Bahia, Brazilian
Northeast Region, 2001–2014
Reprinted from: *Trop. Med. Infect. Dis.* **2018**, *3*, 79, doi: 10.3390/tropicalmed3030079 . . . . **197**

About the Special Issue Editor

Jorg Heukelbach is an internationally renowned specialist in the area of epidemiology and control of neglected tropical diseases and emerging infectious diseases, with extensive experience in epidemiological methods in many countries worldwide.

Tropical Medicine and Infectious Disease

MDPI

Editorial

Control of Communicable Diseases in Human and in Animal Populations: 70th Anniversary of the Year of the Birth of Professor Rick Speare (2 August 1947–5 June 2016)

Jorg Heukelbach [1,2]

[1] Department of Community Health, School of Medicine, Federal University of Ceará, Fortaleza CE 60430-140, Brazil; heukelbach@web.de

[2] College of Public Health, Medical and Veterinary Sciences, Division of Tropical Health and Medicine, James Cook University, Townsville 4811, Australia

Received: 25 September 2018; Accepted: 26 September 2018; Published: 28 September 2018

This book is dedicated to the memory of Prof. Rick Speare, whose academic contribution included high level research of human and veterinarian medical interest on zoonotic diseases and public health in general, following the One Health approach. He dedicated much of his work to Aboriginal communities. In 2016, Rick was tragically killed in a car crash while driving to a seminar at James Cook University in Queensland, Australia.

This book contains a total of 17 peer-reviewed papers (9 original papers, 1 case report, 7 reviews), many of them published by Rick's former colleagues and co-researchers. Some papers contain material collected together with Rick, which for the first time is published here.

Several papers are on strongyloidiasis—one of Rick's main research focuses. Wilson & Fearon [1] describe high prevalence of pediatric strongyloidiasis in Australia. Different aspects of diagnosis of strongyloidiasis in hyperendemic regions in northern Australia are presented by Robertson et al. [2]. Another review paper on strongyloidiasis focuses on the disease during pregnancy [3]. The authors describe the effects of strongyloidiasis, such as low birth weight and anemia, in children and pregnant women. Page et al. [4] discuss public health issues and intervention measures, considering the particular life cycle of *Strongyloides stercoralis*; and Miller et al. [5] present results from a community-based health promotion and control program in an Aboriginal community in central Queensland, Australia, with impressive community involvement. This is the first community-directed strongyloidiasis control program—a work that had been initiated by Rick during his lifetime. Beknazarova et al. [6] discuss the importance of strongyloidiasis being a notifiable disease in Australia, presenting plausible arguments for their case.

Another study from James Cook University investigated immunization rates of medical students [7]. The idea for this study was given by Rick during a lecture. Despite an attitude of high importance of vaccination for personal protection, immunization rates were astonishingly low in the group at in this high risk for contracting communicable diseases.

Gordon et al. [8] review the history of lymphatic filariasis in Australia and Oceania and discuss the possibility of reintroduction of the disease into Australia. In another review, Khan & Zhador [9] give an overview of brucellosis, an important zoonotic disease, and highlight its importance to both human health and livestock. Shima et al. [10] describe two cases of echinococcosis in Lumholtz's tree-kangaroos. This paper is of particular interest, because Rick Speare was the first person to identify hydatid cysts in a Lumholtz's tree-kangaroo, although he never published his findings.

Two papers include data on scabies. Ugbomoiko et al. [11] performed a field study in rural communities in Nigeria. Scabies was present in almost two-thirds of the population, and associated morbidity was considerable. They also show that even in resource-poor settings, scabies is associated with extreme poverty. Shield et al. [12] present their work on community education about strongyloidiasis and scabies—two highly endemic diseases in remote aboriginal communities. Using a discovery education approach including cultural knowledge in the local language, they achieved impressive results.

Andrew Thompson's review on threats to Australia's biosecurity presents a comprehensive overview on the topic and discusses misconceptions and challenges [13]. A survey on intestinal parasites from dog fecal samples collected in Queensland/Australia detected a variety of parasites, including those with zoonotic potential [14].

Ahmed et al. [15] describe case fatality rates due to diarrhea and respiratory diseases in preschool children in Mauritania. While the rates are shockingly high, this paper fills a knowledge gap from a country where still little evidence is being published. A study from Tanzania assessed the diagnostic performance of an antigen rapid test in diagnosing intestinal schistosomiasis in HIV-1 infected patients, as compared to classical Kato Katz technique [16]. The authors show that in HIV1-infected individuals, Kato Katz technique has a low sensitivity and proposes use of the rapid test in high HIV prevalence settings. A Brazilian paper by de Amorim de Souza et al. [17] describes the epidemiology of leprosy during a period of 14 years. Spatial analyses show that the disease is heterogeneously distributed in a state in Brazil's northeast region, and the authors argue that control actions should be intensified in focal areas.

Taken together, the diversity of papers, depth of the topics, geographical range, and the inclusion of impressive studies from aboriginal and remote communities published in this book perfectly reflect Rick's enthusiasm, scientific spirit, and diversity. I am very much pleased to share the content with the international scientific community. Rick would have loved to see all these papers being published!

Funding: This research received no external funding.

Conflicts of Interest: The author declares no conflict of interest.

References

1. Wilson, A.; Fearon, D. Paediatric Strongyloidiasis in Central Australia. *Trop. Med. Infect. Dis.* **2018**, *3*, 64. [CrossRef]
2. Robertson, G.; Koehler, A.; Gasser, R.; Watts, M.; Norton, R.; Bradbury, R. Application of PCR-Based Tools to Explore Strongyloides Infection in People in Parts of Northern Australia. *Trop. Med. Infect. Dis.* **2017**, *2*, 62. [CrossRef]
3. Paltridge, M.; Traves, A. The Health Effects of Strongyloidiasis on Pregnant Women and Children: A Systematic Literature Review. *Trop. Med. Infect. Dis.* **2018**, *3*, 50. [CrossRef]
4. Page, W.; Judd, J.; Bradbury, R. The Unique Life Cycle of *Strongyloides stercoralis* and Implications for Public Health Action. *Trop. Med. Infect. Dis.* **2018**, *3*, 53. [CrossRef]
5. Miller, A.; Young, E.; Tye, V.; Cody, R.; Muscat, M.; Saunders, V.; Smith, M.; Judd, J.; Speare, R. A Community-Directed Integrated Strongyloides Control Program in Queensland, Australia. *Trop. Med. Infect. Dis.* **2018**, *3*, 48. [CrossRef]
6. Beknazarova, M.; Whiley, H.; Judd, J.; Shield, J.; Page, W.; Miller, A.; Whittaker, M.; Ross, K. Argument for Inclusion of Strongyloidiasis in the Australian National Notifiable Disease List. *Trop. Med. Infect. Dis.* **2018**, *3*, 61. [CrossRef]
7. Fergus, E.; Speare, R.; Heal, C. Immunisation Rates of Medical Students at a Tropical Queensland University. *Trop. Med. Infect. Dis.* **2018**, *3*, 52. [CrossRef]
8. Gordon, C.; Jones, M.; McManus, D. The History of Bancroftian Lymphatic Filariasis in Australasia and Oceania: Is There a Threat of Re-Occurrence in Mainland Australia? *Trop. Med. Infect. Dis.* **2018**, *3*, 58. [CrossRef]
9. Khan, M.; Zahoor, M. An Overview of Brucellosis in Cattle and Humans, and its Serological and Molecular Diagnosis in Control Strategies. *Trop. Med. Infect. Dis.* **2018**, *3*, 65. [CrossRef]

10. Shima, A.; Constantinoiu, C.; Johnson, L.; Skerratt, L. *Echinococcus granulosus* Infection in Two Free-Ranging Lumholtz's Tree-Kangaroo (*Dendrolagus lumholtzi*) from the Atherton Tablelands, Queensland. *Trop. Med. Infect. Dis.* **2018**, 3, 47. [CrossRef]
11. Ugbomoiko, U.; Oyedeji, S.; Babamale, O.; Heukelbach, J. Scabies in Resource-Poor Communities in Nasarawa State, Nigeria: Epidemiology, Clinical Features and Factors Associated with Infestation. *Trop. Med. Infect. Dis.* **2018**, 3, 59. [CrossRef]
12. Shield, J.; Kearns, T.; Garŋgulkpuy, J.; Walpulay, L.; Gundjirryirr, R.; Bundhala, L.; Djarpanbuluwuy, V.; Andrews, R.; Judd, J. Cross-Cultural, Aboriginal Language, Discovery Education for Health Literacy and Informed Consent in a Remote Aboriginal Community in the Northern Territory, Australia. *Trop. Med. Infect. Dis.* **2018**, 3, 15. [CrossRef]
13. Thompson, R. Exotic Parasite Threats to Australia's Biosecurity—Trade, Health, and Conservation. *Trop. Med. Infect. Dis.* **2018**, 3, 76. [CrossRef]
14. Gillespie, S.; Bradbury, R. A Survey of Intestinal Parasites of Domestic Dogs in Central Queensland. *Trop. Med. Infect. Dis.* **2017**, 2, 60. [CrossRef]
15. Ahmed, M.; Weddih, A.; Benhafid, M.; Bollahi, M.; Sidatt, M.; Makhalla, K.; Mokdad, A.; Heukelbach, J.; Filali-Maltouf, A. Hospitalizations and Deaths Associated with Diarrhea and Respiratory Diseases among Children Aged 0–5 Years in a Referral Hospital of Mauritania. *Trop. Med. Infect. Dis.* **2018**, 3, 103. [CrossRef]
16. Mazigo, H.; Heukelbach, J. Diagnostic Performance of Kato Katz Technique and Point-of-Care Circulating Cathodic Antigen Rapid Test in Diagnosing *Schistosoma mansoni* Infection in HIV-1 Co-Infected Adults on the Shoreline of Lake Victoria, Tanzania. *Trop. Med. Infect. Dis.* **2018**, 3, 54. [CrossRef]
17. Amorim de Souza, E.; Fuentes Ferreira, A.; Heukelbach, J.; Nzundu Boigny, R.; Alencar, C.; Novaes Ramos, A. Epidemiology and Spatiotemporal Patterns of Leprosy Detection in the State of Bahia, Brazilian Northeast Region, 2001–2014. *Trop. Med. Infect. Dis.* **2018**, 3, 79. [CrossRef]

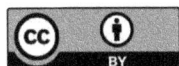

Tropical Medicine and Infectious Disease

MDPI

Article

Paediatric Strongyloidiasis in Central Australia

Angela Wilson [1,*] and Deborah Fearon [2]

[1] BBioMedSci MBBS Hons, Paediatric Senior Registrar, Department of Paediatrics, Alice Springs Hospital, P.O. Box 2234, Alice Springs NT 0871, Australia

[2] FRACP, Head of Department, Department of Paediatrics, Alice Springs Hospital, P.O. Box 2234, Alice Springs NT 0871, Australia; Deborah.fearon@nt.gov.au

* Correspondence: angela.wilson@nt.gov.au; Tel.: +61-(0)-407-882-814

Received: 30 April 2018; Accepted: 6 June 2018; Published: 13 June 2018

Abstract: Few published studies are available describing the prevalence of paediatric strongyloidiasis in endemic areas within Australia. This literature review and exploratory clinical audit presents the first seroprevalence data for paediatric patients in Central Australia. A total of 16.1% (30/186) of paediatric inpatients tested for *Strongyloides stercoralis* in 2016 were seropositive (95% CI: 11.5% to 22.1%). Eosinophilia of unknown aetiology was the most common indication for testing (91.9%). Seropositive patients were significantly more likely to reside in communities outside of Alice Springs ($p = 0.02$). Seropositive patients were noted to have higher mean eosinophil counts with a mean difference of 0.86×10^9/L (95% CI: 0.56 to 1.16, $p < 0.0001$), although the limited utility of eosinophilia as a surrogate marker of strongyloidiasis has been described previously. All seropositive patients were Indigenous. There was no significant difference in ages between groups. There was a male predominance in the seropositive group, although this was not significant ($p = 0.12$). Twelve patients had known human T-lymphotropic virus 1 (HTLV-1) status and all were seronegative. Further research describing the epidemiology of strongyloidiasis in Central Australia is required.

Keywords: strongyloidiasis; *Strongyloides stercoralis*; Indigenous; child health; Aboriginal and Torres Strait Islander; epidemiology; Central Australia

---

1. Introduction

The soil-transmitted helminth *Strongyloides stercoralis* has been described as one of the most neglected of the neglected tropical diseases [1]. Globally, strongyloidiasis is estimated to affect 30 to 370 million people, although data are limited [2,3]. *S. stercoralis* can cause decades-long infection in human hosts [4]. Infection may be clinically silent or cause a range of respiratory, skin, and gastrointestinal symptoms, or fulminant hyperinfection, typically in the setting of immune compromise [5–7].

The *Strongyloides* genus includes over fifty species capable of establishing parasitic infections in a range of animal hosts, and two species are known to infect humans [8]. *Strongyloides fuelleborni* is present in Papua New Guinea and Africa, while *S. stercoralis* is endemic throughout southern Europe, Africa, Asia, the Americas, and the northern two-thirds of Australia [2,9].

Some remote Australian Indigenous communities have *S. stercoralis* seroprevalences approaching 60%, putting them amongst the highest in the world [2,10,11]. Within these communities, Indigenous children have a higher documented prevalence of strongyloidiasis than any other age group [9,12–16].

S. stercoralis disproportionately affects resource-poor populations [17]. Remote Indigenous communities face an inequitable burden of poor health, socioeconomic disadvantage, and barriers to environmental control that impair disease control at a population level [8,18].

Human T-cell lymphotropic virus type 1 (HTLV-1) is an oncogenic virus that infects CD4+ T cells and interferes with Th2 immune responses [19]. HTLV-1 is endemic in Central Australia, and co-infection with *S. stercoralis* is associated with severe strongyloidiasis, *Strongyloides* treatment failure, and increased likelihood of developing T cell lymphoma [5,7,20]. HTLV-1 prevalence in Central Australia is estimated to be approximately from 7.2% to 13.9% among Indigenous adults [20].

Alice Springs Hospital services an extremely remote area of Central Australia that includes the southern half of the Northern Territory and adjacent parts of Western Australia and South Australia. It has a catchment area of approximately 900,000 square km with a population of 48,000 people, of whom 44% are Indigenous Australians (see Figure 1) [21].

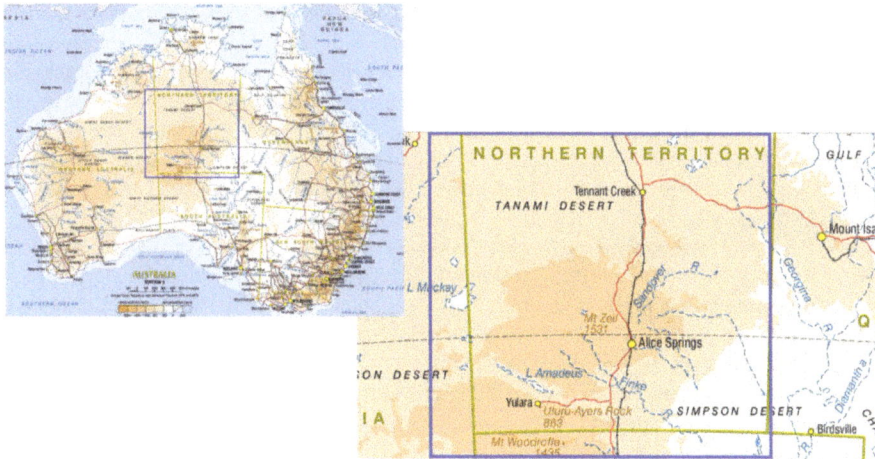

Figure 1. Approximate catchment area of Alice Springs Hospital [21,22].

Over the last three years, the paediatric department has increasingly tested patients with unexplained eosinophilia or other growth, respiratory, or abdominal symptoms for strongyloidiasis, and is in the process of formalising a policy to improve the recognition and management of this condition. HTLV-1 serology is performed on patients with clinical suspicion of immune compromise, particularly in children with chronic suppurative lung disease.

This paper will review of the literature relevant to *S. stercoralis* epidemiology in endemic areas of Australia, and present the results of an audit of *S. stercoralis* testing of paediatric inpatients at Alice Springs Hospital.

2. Review of Endemic Strongyloidiasis Epidemiology in Australia

S. stercoralis has been recognised as a pathogen in Australia for almost a century [23]. Studies examining the prevalence of strongyloidiasis in Australia can be divided into those undertaken in endemic areas and those describing prevalence in groups that have likely acquired it overseas (including migrants and refugee groups and returned military service personnel) [2]. This paper will focus on strongyloidiasis epidemiology in endemic areas within Australia.

The life cycle of *S. stercoralis* is complex and directly relevant to estimates of prevalence [24]. Male and female adults are capable of a single generation of free-living sexual reproduction outside of hosts, and non-infectious rhabditiform larvae moult into parasitic filariform larvae capable of surviving for up to two to three weeks in the environment under optimal conditions [25].

Filariform larvae penetrate host skin and migrate through the lymphatic or venous system to the lungs. They ascend the respiratory tree, are swallowed and migrate to the intestine. Parthenogenic female adults mature and invade the wall of the duodenum and jejunum where they lay up to fifty eggs per day [24]. Eggs hatch into rhabditiform larvae that migrate back into the intestinal lumen.

Larvae may pass into the stool or mature into filariform larvae within the intestine and penetrate back into the host, establishing an auto-infective cycle [24].

A review of existing original research relating to the epidemiology of strongyloidiasis in endemic areas of Australia is presented in Table 1. This table is adapted from [11,18] with additional papers identified from Medline search and reference lists. Articles were located using Medical Subject Headings (MeSH) and text-word terms 'Strongyloides' or 'Strongyloidiasis' and 'Australia'. Papers presenting epidemiological data from *S. stercoralis* endemic areas within Australia were included. Case reports and papers presenting data from other populations were excluded.

Estimates of strongyloidiasis prevalence within endemic areas in Australia vary widely depending on diagnostic method, population surveyed, and season. Community-based studies using faecal larval detection report prevalence rates from <1% to 41%, with substantial increases during the wet season in some locations [10,11,15,26,27]. Agar plate culture for a single stool sample is reported to be less than 60% sensitive [28]. Yield improves with multiple stool examinations and specialised microbiological techniques such as Baermann concentration [28], although this is not available at our health service.

Serology is more sensitive than stool detection of *S. stercoralis* larvae [28]. The sensitivities of various serological assays range from 75.4% to 93.9%, and specificities from 92.2% to 100% [29]. Flannery and White [30] reported the highest seropositivity rate in Australia of 59.6% of individuals tested in one small Northern Territory community. In Central Australia, Einsedel and colleagues reported a seroprevalence of 23.9% among 1126 hospitalised Indigenous adults [20]. No studies examining the seroprevalence of *S. stercoralis* in children in Central Australia were identified.

Children are over-represented in population estimates of strongyloidiasis. A Territory-wide study examining faecal larval detection between 2002 and 2012 found that children under five represented 42.2% of diagnoses, with rates of 3–6% of stool samples examined compared to 1.7% of samples overall [9]. A study of patients diagnosed with strongyloidiasis by faecal microscopy at Royal Darwin Hospital also identified that patients under five years of age were disproportionately represented, with 54% of cases falling in this age group [13].

Growth faltering remains a serious problem in the Northern Territory, affecting about 1 in 7 children under 5 years old in remote communities [31]. Associations between strongyloidiasis and malnutrition are well established but debate remains as to whether strongyloidiasis alone can cause growth faltering or represents an opportunistic infection in a compromised host [1]. The criteria for malnutrition were met by 80% of children diagnosed with strongyloidiasis in one study [13]. In another, Indigenous children with malnutrition were 6.5 times (95% confidence interval [CI]: 1.6 to 26.7) more likely to have *S. stercoralis* than a control group of well-nourished children [14].

Eosinophilia may be the only feature of strongyloidiasis in otherwise asymptomatic hosts, but remains an unreliable marker of strongyloidiasis. Mayer-Cloverdale and colleagues [9] found that just 40.8% of all patients with detectable *S. stercoralis* larvae in their stool had eosinophil counts of 0.5×10^9 cells/L or greater. Eosinophilia was more common in patients under five and was present in 65.5% of positive cases ($p < 0.0001$) [9].

Table 1. Summary of original research describing S. stercoralis epidemiology in endemic areas in Australia.

Author	Location	Sample Size and Demographics	Years Studied	Diagnostic Test	Key Findings
Frith et al., 1974 [26]	NSW: Central Coast	Not stated	1966–1967	Stool examination	4.7% positive on stool microscopy
Jones, 1980 [26]	WA: 20 remote communities	1683 adults and children	1973–1978	Stool microscopy with formol-ether concentration	2% positive on faecal microscopy; Highest infection rate in 15–19 year old age group
Prociv and Luke, 1993 [27]	QLD: 122 remote communities	Children <15 years providing 32,145 faecal samples for diagnosis and disease surveillance	1972–1991	Stool microscopy with formol-ether concentration	Overall infection prevalence of 1.97% positive; Cases found in 52/122 communities; Peak prevalence of 27.5% in one area during wet season vs average prevalence of 12%; Reduction in prevalence from 26.2% to 7% with thiabendazole treatment of infected children
Meloni et al., 1993 [12]	WA: Kimberly region	247 adults and children in five communities	1987–1991	Stool examination	0.25% positive on microscopy; 0.3% in children aged 0 to 13
Gunzburg et al., 1992 [32]	WA: Kimberly region	104 Indigenous children under 5 years old	Not stated	Stool concentration and microscopy	1.2% of samples from children with diarrhoea and 2.1% of samples from well children positive
Fisher et al., 1993 [13]	NT: Darwin	~2000 stool samples from adult and paediatric patients	1991–1992	Stool examination	68 cases of S. stercoralis identified; 54% of diagnoses were in children under 5 years; Eosinophilia noted in 57% of cases
Yiannakou et al., 1992 [33]	QLD: Townsville	14 adult and paediatric cases from 5 year audit	Not stated	Stool examination	9 Indigenous cases, 2 refugees from Vietnam, 1 returned veteran and 2 non-Indigenous patients with no significant travel history
Flannery and White, 1993 [30]	NT: Arnhem Land	29 participants	Not stated	Single stool microscopy; Serology	41% positive on faecal microscopy; 59.6% positive by serological diagnosis
Shield et al., 2015 [15]	NT: Arnhem Land	314 participants including 129 children; 39 underwent serology	1994–1996	Stool microscopy; Serology	19% positive on microscopy; 28% seropositive and 18% equivocal
Aland et al., 1996 [11]	NT: Arnhem Land	300 participants	Not stated	Single stool microscopy	15% positive on faecal microscopy
Page et al., 2006 [34]	NT: Arnhem Land	508 adult and adolescent participants	1996–2002	Serology	35% positive by serological diagnosis at baseline; 78% seroreversion rate of cases with treatment
Kukuruzovic et al., 2002 [14]	NT: Darwin	291 children admitted with diarrhoea and 84 controls	1998–2000	Stool examination	7.2% of stool samples had S. stercoralis detected; 87 children with wasting were 6.5 times (95% CI 1.6 to 26.7) more likely to have S. stercoralis; Hypokalaemia significantly associated with S. stercoralis infection
Einsiedel et al., 2008 [35]	NT: Alice Springs	206 Indigenous adults admitted with blood stream infections	2001–2005	Serology	35.4% were positive by serological diagnosis
Einsiedel and Fernandez, 2008 [5]	NT: Alice Springs	18 Indigenous adults admitted with severe strongyloidiasis	2000–2006	Stool examination; Serology	7/11 patients with severe disease tested for HTLV-1 were positive

Table 1. *Cont.*

Author	Location	Sample Size and Demographics	Years Studied	Diagnostic Test	Key Findings
Einsiedel et al., 2014 [20]	NT: Alice Springs	1126 Indigenous adult inpatients	2000–2010	Serology	23.9% positive by serological diagnosis HTLV-1 positive patients trending towards higher seropositivity rates but not significant (*p* = 0.063)
Mayer-Coverdale et al., 2017 [9]	NT: Territory-wide	22,892 adult and paediatric stool samples provided to NT pathology services	2002–2012	Microscopy with formol-ether concentration	97.7% of cases Indigenous, overall 1.7% positive 42.2% of diagnoses in children under 5 years of age (3–6% positive) Declining rates of diagnosis over time noted
Kearns et al., 2017 [16]	NT: Arnhem Land	859 Indigenous children and adults	2010–2011	Microscopy/culture; Serology	21% seropositive at baseline with 15% equivocal Peak seropositivity in 5–14 year old cohort 89% patients had eosinophilia at baseline 11% had positive faecal microscopy/culture Seroprevalence 2% at 18 months after two mass drug administrations
Hays et al., 2015 [36]	WA: Kimberly region	259 Indigenous adults	2012–2015	Serology	35.3% positive by serological diagnosis (OD > 0.3) Reduction to 5.8% after three years of targeted treatment and follow up of seropositive patients

Abbreviations: NT: Northern Territory; QLD: Queensland; WA: Western Australia; NSW: New South Wales; OD: optic density; HTLV-1: human T-lymphotrophic virus 1.

3. Clinical Audit Methods

Retrospective admission data from Alice Springs Hospital for the 2016 calendar year were obtained. The records of 2071 patients under the age of 16 years old admitted to the paediatric ward were reviewed as part of a departmental audit. Of these, 186 patients who had been tested for *S. stercoralis* were identified. Nonidentifiable coded data relating to patient demographics, clinical presentation, indication for testing, haemoglobin, mean corpuscular volume, eosinophil count, *Strongyloides* serology results, HTLV-1 status (if known), and faecal examination results were collated.

Symptoms at presentation were noted for each patient, with specific reference to growth faltering and gastrointestinal, respiratory, dermatological, and blood stream infections that might be attributable to strongyloidiasis. Growth faltering was defined as weight for age below the 3rd centile, standard weight for height less than two standard deviations below the mean, or crossing of two or more centile lines. Gastrointestinal symptoms included abdominal pain, altered bowel habit, vomiting, and anorexia. Respiratory symptoms included cough, dyspnoea, tachypnoea, chest pain, and pharyngitis. Dermatological manifestations were limited to urticarial rash or larva currens. Pruritus was not included due to the endemic nature of scabies and head lice in this population.

S. stercoralis serology was performed by Western Diagnostic Pathology, using an IgG enzyme-linked immunosorbent assay (ELISA) produced commercially by DRG Instruments. This assay detects IgG directed against the soluble fraction of filariform *S. stercoralis* larvae. The sensitivity of this assay is reported to be 91.2% with a specificity of 93.3% [37]. An optical density of 0.2 or greater is considered positive. In patients from nonendemic areas, a result of 0.2 to 0.4 is considered equivocal.

Statistical analysis was conducted using GraphPad software. Continuous data sets were analysed using unpaired t-tests. Confidence intervals for categorical data were calculated using the modified Wald method, and p values were determined using Chi-square calculations.

This study was conducted in accordance with the Declaration of Helsinki. No identifiable patient data was collected or retained by the investigators.

4. Results

Eosinophilia of unknown aetiology was the indication for testing in 91.9% (171/186) of patients, and seven were tested because of previous eosinophilia. Of the remaining patients, one patient had growth concerns, one was commenced on immunosuppressant medications, and six had gastrointestinal or respiratory presentations suggestive of strongyloidiasis.

Overall, 16.1% (30/186) of patients tested were seropositive for *S. stercoralis* (95% CI: 11.5% to 22.1%). There was no significant age difference between seropositive and seronegative groups ($p = 0.55$) (Table 2, Figures 2 and 3). A male predominance in the seropositive group was observed although the difference was not significant ($p = 0.12$). Seropositive patients were significantly more likely to reside in communities outside of Alice Springs ($p = 0.02$).

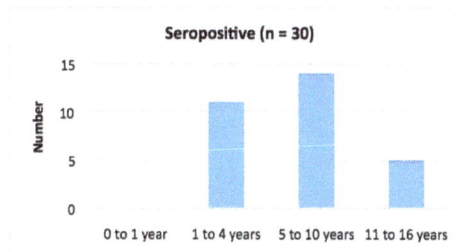

Figure 2. Age distribution in *S. stercoralis* seropositive group.

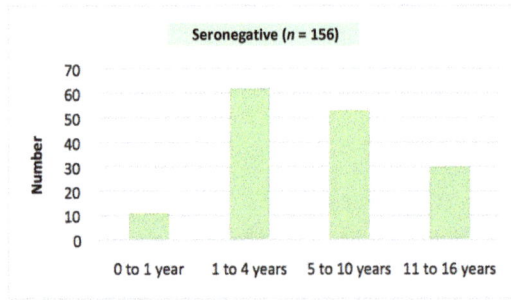

Figure 3. Age distribution in *S. stercoralis* seronegative group.

Table 2. Demographic data, clinical presentation, and investigation results.

Variable	Seronegative (*n* = 156) Number (%)	Seropositive (*n* = 30) Number (%)	*p* Value
Mean Age	6 years 1 month	6 years 7 months	$p = 0.55$
Male Gender	91 (58.3%)	22 (73.3%)	$p = 0.12$
Remote	109 (69.9%)	27 (90.0%)	$p = 0.02$
Indigenous	149 (95.5%)	30 (100%)	$p = 0.24$
Mean serology	N/A	Optic density = 0.84 ± 1.54	
Stool pathogens	17 (36.2%), *n* = 47	5 (62.5%), *n* = 8	$p = 0.16$
Haemoglobin	117.63 ± 25.92 g/L	116.77 ± 27.22 g/L	$p = 0.74$
Mean corpuscular volume	76.578 ± 10.18 fL	76.66 ± 7.72 fL	$p = 0.93$
Mean eosinophil count *	0.96×10^9/L ± 2.13×10^9/L (Range 0.5×10^9/L to 5.3×10^9/L)	1.83×10^9/L ± 1.32×10^9/L (Range 0.6×10^9/L to 4.8×10^9/L)	$p < 0.0001$
Gastrointestinal symptoms	40 (25.6%)	9 (30%)	$p = 0.62$
Respiratory symptoms	42 (26.9%)	7 (23.3%)	$p = 0.68$
Blood stream infection	4 (2.6%)	0 (0%)	$p = 0.37$
Growth faltering	25 (16%)	3 (10%)	$p = 0.4$
HTLV-1 seroprevalence	0/10 (0%)	0/2 (0%)	

* Mean eosinophil count in patients tested for unexplained eosinophilia of $\geq 0.5 \times 10^9$/L (seropositive group *n* = 29, seronegative group *n* = 142).

The data did not support any significant differences in clinical presentation, haemoglobin, or mean corpuscular volume (Figure 4). Four seronegative patients had bloodstream infections, including one patient with cryptococcal disease and three patients with *Staphylococcus aureus* bacteraemia. No patients in either group presented with urticaria or larva currens. No cases of hyperinfection were identified, and none of the 12 patients who had HTLV-1 testing were seropositive.

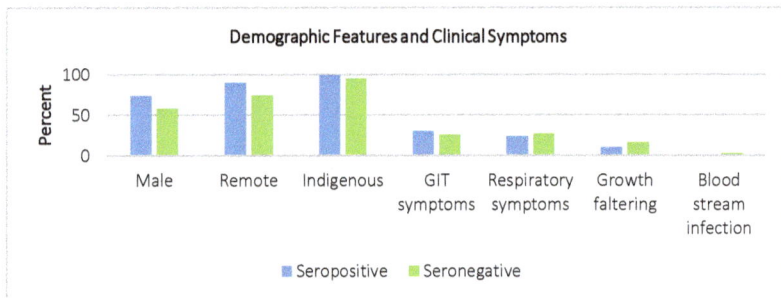

Figure 4. Clinical features during admission. GIT: Gastrointestinal tract.

Within the group of patients tested because of eosinophilia, seropositive patients were noted to have a significantly higher mean eosinophil count with a mean difference of 0.86×10^9/L (95% CI: 0.56 to 1.16, $p < 0.0001$). Of the 55 patients that had a stool sample sent, none had *S. stercoralis* larvae detected (Table 3). There was no significant difference in the rate of other stool pathogens identified between groups ($p = 0.09$).

Table 3. Faecal examination results.

	Seronegative (n = 47/156) Number (%)	Seropositive (n = 8/30) Number (%)
Organism/virus identified	17 (36%)	5 (62.5%)
Strongyloides stercoralis	0	0
Giardia species	5	2
Cryptosporidium parvum	3	2
Blastocystis hominis *	1	0
Trichomonas hominis **	1	0
Entamoeba coli **	1	0
Entamoeba hartmanni **	1	0
Salmonella species	3	0
Campylobacter jejuni	1	0
Norovirus	4	0
Rotavirus	1	0
Adenovirus	1	2
Hymenolepis nana	1	0

* May cause clinically significant infection [38]. ** Not generally considered to cause clinically significant infections [39–41].

The geographical distribution of seropositive and seronegative patients is shown in Figure 5.

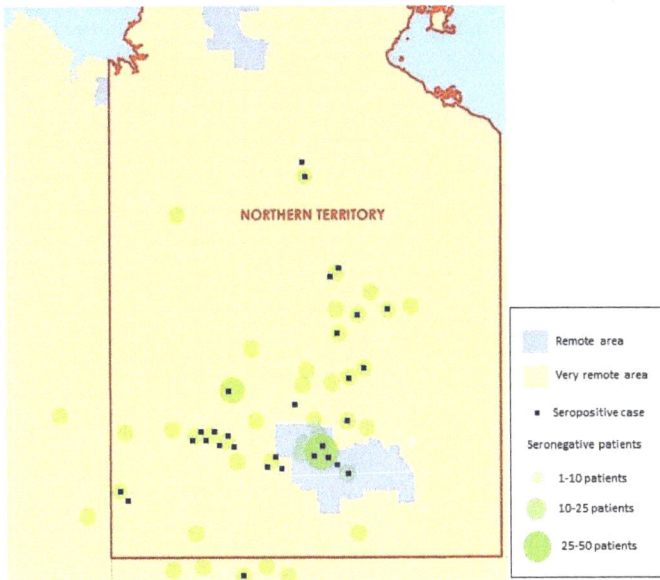

Figure 5. Geographical distribution of seropositive and seronegative cases in Central Australia.

5. Discussion

This exploratory audit highlights many of the universal challenges of understanding and managing *S. stercoralis*. Robust epidemiological data are lacking, clinical features and surrogate markers for infection are poorly sensitive and specific, and microbiological diagnosis is difficult. Although there was a significant difference in mean eosinophil counts, wide ranges and substantial overlap between data sets highlight the limitations of eosinophilia as a clinically useful indicator of possible strongyloidiasis. Further investigation is required to better understand the burden and epidemiology of strongyloidiasis in children in Central Australia.

This audit is limited by small patient numbers, retrospective data collection, and selective population sampling. No reliable conclusions regarding the prevalence of strongyloidiasis among the general paediatric inpatient population or paediatric population in Central Australia can be drawn from this audit. The geographical distribution of cases cannot be used to infer community prevalence but may suggest a clustering of cases in western and northern communities. This is also likely to reflect in part the relative distribution of the remote populations surrounding Alice Springs.

The predominance of remote diagnoses is likely to reflect the ability of *S. stercoralis* to thrive in infrastructure-poor areas, and strongyloidiasis remains a disease predominantly of the poorly resourced in Central Australia [17]. The social determinants of health are starkly relevant in this context, and Einsiedel and Fernandez summarise some of the challenges that remote Indigenous communities face in controlling strongyloidiasis at a population level [5]:

> *Ultimately, strongyloidiasis is a disease of poverty that reflects the appalling socioeconomic situation of Indigenous Australia. In some communities, a median number of 17 persons live in each house, and nearly 50% of dwellings do not have functioning facilities to remove faeces. The endemicity of both S. stercoralis and HTLV-1... renders public education and improvements to housing imperative.*

Socioeconomic disadvantage is associated with higher rates of morbidity and mortality from strongyloidiasis, particularly where this leads to overcrowding, breakdown in sanitation systems, and environmental disease reservoirs from soil contamination [17]. Addressing water, sewerage, and garbage management systems remains fundamental to breaking the cycle of infection and reinfection [8].

Reviews examining other barriers to strongyloidiasis control in Indigenous communities have identified several points for intervention, including the need for improved reporting protocols, increased testing of at-risk individuals, health professional engagement, and community-based monitoring and control programs [8,18,42]. Collaborative community-based initiatives incorporating mass deworming, infrastructure improvements, and culturally safe health education (Figure 6) have demonstrated significant reductions in *Strongyloides* seroprevalences [16,18,42]. One Western Australian study saw the seropositivity in 259 Indigenous adults fall from 35.3% to 5.8% in three years using these strategies [43]. A study in Arnhem Land in the Northern Territory saw seropositivity fall from 21% at baseline to 2% after 18 months of annual mass drug administration [16].

Evidence is emerging that dogs may act as hosts for human strongyloidiasis in some settings [44,45]. Animal services in remote communities are often limited, leading to animal over-population in some areas [46]. Community-based interventions may need to consider incorporating animal management into programs to address this potential reservoir [44].

Within community-based initiatives, further research is needed to inform practices relating to the testing and treatment of Indigenous children. Universal testing of Indigenous people living in endemic areas has been recommended [18,42]. The logistical challenges of implementing universal paediatric testing are substantial in our context. Paediatric blood collection is time-consuming and distressing for patients. Opportunistic blood collection is possible but carries additional costs to health services. Results are rarely available prior to discharge and locating patients for follow-up dosing and serology testing in remote communities is often difficult. Blood spot serology testing is under development and may make this investigation substantially more acceptable to parents and facilitate testing in nurse-led remote clinics where staff may have limited capacity to do paediatric venepuncture [28].

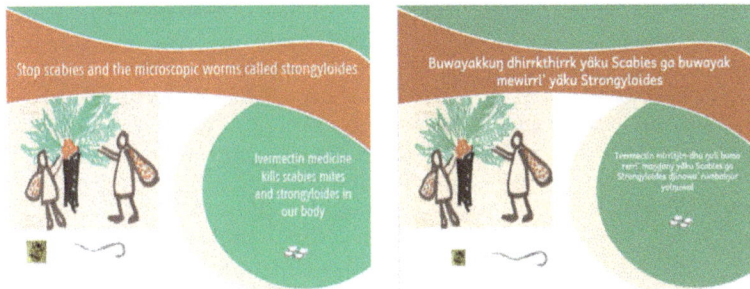

Figure 6. Community education resources produced by Menzies School of Health Research in English and Yolngu.

The safety and tolerability of ivermectin in paediatric patients also requires further investigation. Ivermectin is the mainstay of treatment for strongyloidiasis in adults and older children and has been used in this setting for almost 30 years [47]. The use of ivermectin in children under 15 kilograms or five years of age remains problematic due to a lack of safety data [48], although many health services (including our own) routinely use ivermectin in children under five years old and between ten and fifteen kilograms in weight, at the discretion of the treating specialist.

6. Conclusions

Almost 1 in 6 paediatric patients tested for strongyloidiasis at our health service were found to be seropositive. Remote communities experience an intersection of risk factors that predispose them to a disproportionate burden of disease from *S. stercoralis*. These include poorer sanitation infrastructure, inadequate and overcrowded housing, limited access to health services, very limited access to animal control services, high HTLV-1 prevalence and rates of other chronic comorbidities, and minimal disease surveillance [2,8,17,18,42].

These reflect the global experience of strongyloidiasis as a disease that predominantly affects and exploits the poorly resourced. Management of strongyloidiasis remains inextricably linked to improving the social determinants of health experienced by these communities and controlling environmental reservoirs to reduce the risk of reinfection [17].

Continued advocacy for improvements in basic infrastructure, health service resources and awareness, proactive disease monitoring, and access to effective treatment remains fundamental to the control of strongyloidiasis and other neglected diseases in the most vulnerable communities both within Australia and overseas [3,18].

Author Contributions: Conceptualization, A.W.; methodology, A.W.; formal analysis, A.W.; investigation, A.W.; data curation, A.W.; writing—original draft preparation, A.W.; writing—review & editing, A.W. and D.F.; visualization, A.W.; supervision, D.F.

Conflicts of Interest: The authors declare no conflicts of interest.

References

1. Olsen, A.; van Lieshout, L.; Marti, H.; Polderman, T.; Polman, K.; Steinmann, P.; Stothard, R.; Thybo, R.; Verweij, J.; Magnussen, P. Strongyloidiasis—The most neglected of the neglected tropical diseases? *Trans. R. Soc. Trop. Med. Hyg.* **2009**, *103*, 967–972. [CrossRef] [PubMed]
2. Schar, F.; Trotsdorf, U.; Giardina, F.; Khieu, V.; Muth, S.; Marti, H.; Vounatsou, U.; Odermatt, P. *Strongyloides stercoralis*: Global distribution and risk factors. *PLoS Negl. Trop. Dis.* **2013**, *7*, 1–17. [CrossRef] [PubMed]

3. Bisoffi, Z.; Buonfrate, D.; Montresor, A.; Requena-Mendes, A.; Munoz, J.; Krolewiecki, A.J.; Gotuzzo, E.; Mena, M.A.; Chiodini, P.L.; Anselmi, M.; et al. *Strongyloides stercoralis*: A plea for action. *PLoS Negl. Trop. Dis.* **2013**, *7*, e2214. [CrossRef] [PubMed]
4. Rahmanian, H.; MacFarlane, A.C.; Rowland, K.E.; Einsiedel, L.J.; Neuhaus, S.J. Seroprevalence of *Strongyloides stercoralis* in a South Australian Vietnam veteran cohort. *Aust. N. Z. J. Public Health* **2015**, *39*, 331–335. [CrossRef] [PubMed]
5. Einsiedel, L.; Fernandes, L. *Strongyloides stercoralis*: A cause of morbidity and mortality for indigenous people in Central Australia. *Intern. Med. J.* **2008**, *38*, 697–703. [CrossRef] [PubMed]
6. Page, W.; Speare, R. Chronic strongyloidiasis—Don't look and you won't find. *Aust. Fam. Phys.* **2016**, *45*, 40–44.
7. Buonfrate, D.; Requena-Mendez, A.; Angheben, A.; Munoz, J.; Gobbi, F.; Van Den Ende, J.; Bisoffi, Z. Severe strongyloidiasis: A systematic review of case reports. *BMC Infect. Dis.* **2013**, *13*, 78. [CrossRef] [PubMed]
8. Taylor, M.J.; Garrard, T.A.; O'Donahoo, F.J.; Ross, K.E. Human strongyloidiasis: Identifying knowledge gaps, with emphasis on environmental control. *Res. Rep. Trop. Med.* **2014**, *2014*, 55–63. [CrossRef]
9. Mayer-Coverdale, J.; Crowe, A.; Smith, P.; Baird, R. Trends in *Strongyloides stercoralis* fecal larvae detections in the Northern Territory, Australia: 2002 to 2012. *Trop. Med. Infect. Dis.* **2017**, *2*, 18. [CrossRef]
10. Adams, M.; Page, W.; Speare, R. Strongyloidiasis: An issue in Aboriginal communities. *Rural Remote Health* **2003**, *3*, 152. [PubMed]
11. Johnston, F.H.; Morris, P.S.; Speare, R.; McCarthy, J.; Currie, B.; Ewald, D.; Page, W.; Dempsey, K. Strongyloidiasis: A review of the evidence for Australian practitioners. *Aust. J. Rural Health* **2005**, *13*, 247–254. [CrossRef] [PubMed]
12. Meloni, B.P.; Thompson, R.C.; Hopkins, R.M.; Reynoldson, J.A.; Gracey, M. The prevalence of *Giardia* and other intestinal parasites in children, dogs and cats from aboriginal communities in the Kimberley. *Med. J. Aust.* **1993**, *158*, 157–159. [PubMed]
13. Fisher, D.; McCarry, F.; Currie, B. Strongyloidiasis in the Northern Territory. Under-recognised and under-treated? *Med. J. Aust.* **1993**, *159*, 88–90. [PubMed]
14. Kukuruzovic, R.; Robins-Browne, R.M.; Anstey, N.M.; Brewster, D.R. Enteric pathogens, intestinal permeability and nitric oxide production in acute gastroenteritis. *Pediatr. Infect. Dis. J.* **2002**, *21*, 730–739. [CrossRef] [PubMed]
15. Shield, J.; Aland, K.; Kearns, T.; Gongdjalk, G.; Holt, D.; Currie, B.; Prociv, P. Intestinal parasites of children and adults in a remote Aboriginal community of the Northern Territory, Australia, 1994–1996. *West. Pac. Surveill. Response J.* **2015**, *6*, 44–51. [CrossRef]
16. Kearns, T.M.; Currie, B.J.; Cheng, A.C.; McCarthy, J.; Carapetis, J.C.; Holt, D.C.; Page, W.; Shield, J.; Gundjirryirr, R.; Mulholland, E.; et al. Strongyloides seroprevalence before and after an ivermectin mass drug administration in a remote Australian Aboriginal community. *PLoS Negl. Trop. Dis.* **2017**, *11*, e0005607. [CrossRef] [PubMed]
17. Beknazarova, M.; Whiley, H.; Ross, K. Strongyloidiasis: A disease of socioeconomic disadvantage. *Int. J. Environ. Res. Public Health* **2016**, *13*, 517–532. [CrossRef] [PubMed]
18. Miller, A.; Smith, M.L.; Judd, J.A.; Speare, R. *Strongyloides stercoralis*: Systematic review of barriers to controlling strongyloidiasis for Australian indigenous communities. *PLoS Negl. Trop. Dis.* **2014**, *8*, e3141. [CrossRef] [PubMed]
19. Mirdha, B.R. Human strongyloidiasis: Often brushed under the carpet. *Trop. Gastroenterol.* **2009**, *30*, 1–4. [PubMed]
20. Einsiedel, L.; Spelman, T.; Goeman, E.; Cassar, O.; Arundell, M.; Gessain, A. Clinical associations of humanT-type 1 infection in an indigenous Australian population. *PLoS Negl. Trop. Dis.* **2014**, *8*, e2643. [CrossRef] [PubMed]
21. Northern Territory Government. NT Health Governance: Central Australia Health Service (CAHS). Available online: https://health.nt.gov.au/health-governance/central-australia-health-service (accessed on 5 April 2018).
22. Commonwealth of Australia. 1:20M Australia General Reference Map (A4). Available online: https://ecat.ga.gov.au/geonetwork/srv/eng/search#!a05f7892-cff3-7506-e044-00144fdd4fa6 (accessed on 6 April 2018).
23. Lambert, S.M. Intestinal parasites in north Queensland. *Med. J. Aust.* **1921**, *1921*, 332–336.

24. Jourdan, P.M.; Lamberton, P.H.L.; Fenwick, A.; Addiss, D.G. Soil-transmitted helminth infections. *Lancet* **2017**, *391*, 252–265. [CrossRef]
25. Page, W.; Judd, J.A.; Bradbury, R.D. The unique life cycle of *Strongyloides stercoralis* and implications for public health action. *Trop. Med. Infect. Dis.* **2018**, *3*, 53. [CrossRef]
26. Jones, H.I. Intestinal parasite infections in Western Australian Aborigines. *Med. J. Aust.* **1980**, *2*, 375–380. [PubMed]
27. Prociv, P.; Luke, R. Observations on strongyloidiasis in Queensland aboriginal communities. *Med. J. Aust.* **1993**, *158*, 160–163. [PubMed]
28. Requena-Mendez, A.; Chiodini, P.; Bisoffi, Z.; Buonfrate, D.; Gotuzzo, E.; Munoz, J. The laboratory diagnosis and follow up of strongyloidiasis: A systematic review. *PLoS Negl. Trop. Dis.* **2013**, *7*, e2002. [CrossRef] [PubMed]
29. Bisoffi, Z.; Buonfrate, D.; Sequi, M.; Mejia, R.; Cimino, R.O.; Krolewiecki, A.J.; Albonico, M.; Gobbo, M.; Bonafini, S.; Angheben, A.; et al. Diagnostic accuracy of five serologic tests for *Strongyloides stercoralis* Infection. *PLoS Negl. Trop. Dis.* **2014**, *8*, e2640. [CrossRef] [PubMed]
30. Flannery, G.; White, N. Immunological parameters in northeast Arnhem Land aborigines: Consequences of changing settlement patterns and lifestyles. In *Urban Ecology and Health in the Third World*; Cambridge University Press: Cambridge, UK, 1993; pp. 202–220.
31. McDonald, E.L.; Bailie, R.S.; Rumbold, A.R.; Morris, P.S.; Paterson, B.A. Preventing growth faltering among Australian Indigenous children: Implications for policy and practice. *Med. J. Aust.* **2008**, *188* (Suppl. 8), S84.
32. Gunzburg, S.; Gracey, M.; Burke, V.; Chang, B. Epidemiology and microbiology of diarrhoea in young Aboriginal children in the Kimberley region of Western Australia. *Epidemiol. Infect.* **1992**, *108*, 67–76. [CrossRef] [PubMed]
33. Yiannakou, J.; Croese, J.; Ashdown, L.R.; Prociv, P. Strongyloidiasis in North Queensland: Re-emergence of a forgotten risk group? *Med. J. Aust.* **1992**, *156*, 24–27. [PubMed]
34. Page, W.A.; Dempsey, K.; McCarthy, J.S. Utility of serological follow-up of chronic strongyloidiasis after anthelminthic chemotherapy. *Trans. R. Soc. Trop. Med. Hyg.* **2006**, *100*, 1056–1062. [CrossRef] [PubMed]
35. Einsedel, L.; Fernandez, L.; Woodman, R.J. Racial disparities in infection-related mortality at Alice Springs Hospital, Central Australia, 2000–2005. *Med. J. Aust.* **2008**, *188*, 568–571.
36. Hays, R.; Esterman, A.; Giacomin, P.; Loukas, A.; McDermott, R. Does *Strongyloides stercoralis* infection protect against type 2 diabetes in humans? Evidence from Australian Aboriginal adults. *Diabetes Res. Clin. Pract.* **2015**, *107*, 355–361. [CrossRef] [PubMed]
37. Bon, B.; Houze, S.; Talabani, H.; Magne, D.; Belkadi, G.; Develoux, M.; Senghor, Y.; Chandenier, J.; Ancelle, T.; Hennequin, C. Evaluation of a rapid enzyme-linked immunosorbent assay for diagnosis of strongyloidiasis. *J. Clin. Microbiol.* **2010**, *48*, 1716–1719. [CrossRef] [PubMed]
38. Turkeltaub, J.A.; McCarty, T.R., III; Hotez, P.J. The intestinal protozoa: Emerging impact on global health and development. *Curr. Opin. Gastroenterol.* **2015**, *31*, 38–44. [CrossRef] [PubMed]
39. Meloni, D.; Mantini, C.; Goustille, J.; Desoubeaux, G.; Maakaroun-Vermesse, Z.; Chandenier, J.; Gantois, N.; Duboucher, C.; Fiori, P.L.; Deicas, E.; et al. Molecular identification of *Pentatrichomonas hominis* in two patients with gastrointestinal symptoms. *J. Clin. Pathol.* **2011**, *64*, 933–935. [CrossRef] [PubMed]
40. Calegar, D.A.; Nunes, B.C.; Monteiro, K.J.; Pereira dos Santos, J.; Toma, H.K.; Gomes, T.F.; Lima, M.M.; Boia, M.N.; Carvalho-Costa, F.A. Frequency and molecular characterisation of *Entamoeba histolytica*, *Entamoeba dispar*, *Entamoeba moshkovskii*, and *Entamoeba hartmanni* in the context of water scarcity in northeastern Brazil. *Mem. Inst. Oswaldo Cruz* **2016**, *111*, 114–119. [CrossRef] [PubMed]
41. Zavala, G.A.; Garcia, O.P.; Campos-Ponce, M.; Ronquillo, D.; Caamano, M.C.; Doak, C.M.; Rosado, J.L. Children with moderate-high infection with *Entamoeba coli* have higher percentage of body and abdominal fat than non-infected children. *Pediatr. Obes.* **2016**, *11*, 443–449. [CrossRef] [PubMed]
42. Ross, K.E.; Bradbury, R.S.; Garrard, T.A.; O'Donahoo, F.J.; Shield, J.; Page, W.; Miller, A.; Robertson, G.; Judd, J.A.; Speare, R. The National Strongyloides Working Group in Australia 10 workshops on: Commendations and recommendations. *Aust. N. Z. J. Public Health* **2017**, *41*, 221–223. [CrossRef] [PubMed]
43. Hays, R.; Esterman, A.; McDermott, R. Control of chronic *Strongyloides stercoralis* infection in an endemic community may be possible by pharmacological means alone: Results of a three-year cohort study. *PLoS Negl. Trop. Dis.* **2017**, *11*, e0005825. [CrossRef] [PubMed]

44. Beknazarova, M.; Whiley, H.; Ross, K. Mass drug administration for the prevention of human strongyloidiasis should consider concomitant treatment of dogs. *PLoS Negl. Trop. Dis.* **2017**, *11*, e0005735. [CrossRef] [PubMed]

45. Jaleta, T.G.; Zhou, S.; Bemm, F.M.; Schar, F.; Khieu, V.; Muth, S.; Odermatt, P.; Lok, J.B.; Streit, A. Different but overlapping populations of *Strongyloides stercoralis* in dogs and humans—Dogs as possible source for zoonotic strongyloidiasis. *PLoS Negl. Trop. Dis.* **2017**, *11*, e0005752. [CrossRef] [PubMed]

46. Bradbury, L.; Corlette, S. Dog health program in Numbulwar, a remote aboriginal community in east Arnhem Land. *Aust. Vet. J.* **2006**, *84*, 317–320. [CrossRef] [PubMed]

47. Caumes, E.; Datry, A.; Mayorga, R.; Gaxotte, P.; Danis, M.; Gentilini, M. Efficacy of ivermectin in the therapy of larva currens. *Arch. Dermatol.* **1994**, *130*, 932. [CrossRef] [PubMed]

48. Wilkins, A.L.; Steer, A.C.; Cranswick, N.; Gwee, A. Is it safe to use ivermectin in children less than five years of age and weighing less than 15 kg? *Arch. Dis. Child.* **2018**, *103*, 514–519. [CrossRef] [PubMed]

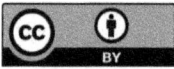

Tropical Medicine and Infectious Disease

MDPI

Article

Application of PCR-Based Tools to Explore *Strongyloides* Infection in People in Parts of Northern Australia

Gemma J. Robertson [1,*], Anson V. Koehler [2], Robin B. Gasser [2], Matthew Watts [3,4], Robert Norton [5] and Richard S. Bradbury [6]

1   Public and Environmental Health, Forensic and Scientific Services, Health Support Queensland, Brisbane, QLD 4108, Australia
2   Department of Veterinary Biosciences, The University of Melbourne, Melbourne, VIC 3053, Australia; anson.koehler@unimelb.edu.au (A.V.K.); robinbg@unimelb.edu.au (R.B.G.)
3   Centre for Infectious Diseases and Microbiology, Institute for Clinical Pathology and Medical Research NSW Health Pathology, Westmead Hospital, Westmead, NSW 2145, Australia; matthew.watts@health.nsw.gov.au
4   Marie Bashir Institute for Infectious Diseases and Biosecurity, University of Sydney, Westmead, NSW 2145, Australia
5   Pathology Queensland, The Townsville Hospital, Townsville, QLD 4814, Australia; Robert.Norton@health.qld.gov.au
6   School of Health, Medical and Applied Sciences, Central Queensland University, North Rockhampton, QLD 4700, Australia; r.bradbury@cqu.edu.au
*   Correspondence: Gemma.Robertson@health.qld.gov.au; Tel.: +61-1800-000-777

Received: 12 October 2017; Accepted: 1 December 2017; Published: 8 December 2017

Abstract: Strongyloidiasis, which is caused by infection with the nematode *Strongyloides stercoralis*, is endemic to areas of northern Australia. Diagnosis in this region remains difficult due to the distances between endemic communities and diagnostic laboratories, leading to lengthy delays in stool processing for microscopy and culture. PCR represents a viable solution to this difficulty, having potential for high sensitivity detection of *S. stercoralis*, even in older, unpreserved faecal samples. We prospectively collected 695 faecal specimens that were submitted to The Townsville Hospital Microbiology Laboratory from the North Queensland region for routine parasitological examination, and subjected them to a *Strongyloides* sp. real-time (q)PCR. Results were confirmed with a novel nested conventional PCR assay targeting the 18S rRNA gene, followed by single-strand conformation polymorphism analysis (SSCP). Of the 695 specimens tested, *S. stercoralis* was detected in three specimens (0.4%) by classical parasitological methods (direct microscopy and formyl-ether acetate concentration), whereas 42 positives were detected by qPCR (6.0%). Conventional PCR confirmed the real-time PCR results in 24 of the samples (3.5%). Several apparent false-positive results occurred at higher cycle times (C_t) in the qPCR. Use of real-time PCR in these populations is promising for the enhanced detection of disease and to support eradication efforts.

Keywords: strongyloidiasis; *Strongyloides stercoralis*; Australia; PCR; SSCP

1. Introduction

Strongyloidiasis is an intestinal helminthic disease of humans with protean clinical presentations, including acute enteritis, chronic asymptomatic infection, or a potentially fatal hyperinfection syndrome [1]. The causative agent, *Strongyloides stercoralis*, is a nematode that is endemic to tropical and sub-tropical regions of the world. The parasitic life cycle includes an auto-infective component, and, therefore, without the appropriate treatment, infection with this nematode can persist for decades [1].

Estimates indicate that 30–370 million people are infected with this parasite worldwide [2]. This variation in estimated burden of infection is attributable to a number of factors, the most important being the difficulty in achieving an accurate diagnosis of infection, particularly in people with low-burden, chronic strongyloidiasis [3,4].

There is a paucity of detailed information regarding the prevalence and distribution of autochthonous strongyloidiasis in Australia, and methodologies vary considerably among studies. Prevalences of 0.26% and 1.9% were recorded from surveys in north Western Australia in 1993 and 1997, using low-sensitivity diagnostic techniques (direct microscopy, $ZnSO_4$ flotation, and Kato-Katz) [4,5]. In the Northern Territory, prevalences that were reported ranged from 7.2 to 59.6% (direct microscopy, concentration techniques, serology) [6–9]. This wide range in prevalence is reflective of the difficulties in diagnosis of this disease, with many traditional faecal microscopy methods having poor sensitivity for the detection of strongyloidiasis. The most comprehensive investigation published to date on strongyloidiasis in Australia was from Queensland [10], a state that includes the Tropical North. This study was conducted via the Aboriginal Health Program (AHP), which was established by the State Health Department in 1972. Single formalin-fixed stool samples that were collected from children in Aboriginal and Torres Strait Islander (ATSI) communities were sent to a central laboratory, where they underwent formol-ether concentration (FEC) and were examined by trained microscopists [10]. The overall annual prevalence ranged from 0 to 4.7% between 1972 and 1991, based on annual reports, with an average overall prevalence of 1.97% [10]. Two communities within the north-west region, Doomadgee and Mornington Island (Gununa), had a remarkably high prevalence (up to 26.0% and 27.5%, respectively). Based on results from the AHP data, strongyloidiasis was most prevalent in northern coastal areas of the state and was associated with areas of high rainfall, humidity, and temperature [10]. These data have not been updated for over 25 years, and the current prevalence of strongyloidiasis in Queensland is unknown. In each of these studies [4–10], the prevalence of infection is likely to be underestimated because of the low sensitivity of the diagnostic methods that were used [11–13]. Although comparisons of prevalence among geographic locations are unreliable due to the distinct methods that are employed among studies, strongyloidiasis is known to be common in residents of remote ATSI communities, north of the Tropic of Capricorn [14].

The Townsville Hospital Microbiology Laboratory (TTHML) services a large geographical area that is home to a diverse sociodemographic population, including a large ATSI population that lives in several small communities (including Doomadgee and Mornington Island) remote to the laboratory location. The majority of the population is concentrated within the major centre of Townsville, a regional city with a historically low prevalence of strongyloidiasis [10]. Despite the rate of detection of strongyloidiasis decreasing by ~40% since 2003 statewide (unpublished data), the methodologies that were utilised to detect these infections at TTHML do not offer confidence that the number of infections has reduced in real terms. Techniques such as agar plate culture and the Baermann sedimentation method [15], are the gold standard for the detection of infection with *S. stercoralis*. However, several factors been persistent barriers to their implementation in the Australian diagnostic laboratory setting. These factors include: long specimen transport times after collection in remote communities, potential exposure to extremes of temperature during transit, variable sensitivities of different diagnostic methodologies [15–18], intermittent shedding and uneven distribution of larvae in faeces [19], limited viability of larvae [20], subjectivity in the interpretation of morphological characteristics of larvae for differentiation from hookworms [1], limited resources and technical complexity of the assay, and the risk of infection to laboratory staff [21–23]. Modified concentration techniques (e.g., FLOTAC) [24] have emerged as alternatives to the gold standard (i.e., agar plate and Baermann methods), but the sensitivity and specificity of these methods vary considerably in the published literature [25–28]. The introduction of formalin-ether-acetate concentration (FEAC; Mini-Parasep kit, Apacor, Berkshire, UK) at TTHML in 2012 may have led to a reduction in the detection of infected patients; product information for this kit, as provided by the manufacturer, indicates that this system should not be used for the detection of *Strongyloides* larvae [29]. It is likely that this methodology concentrates out helminth larvae from the sediment, leading to false negatives. For these reasons, serological methods have been heavily relied upon for diagnosis and management of strongyloidiasis in Queensland, due to analyte stability [30], favourable sensitivity and specificity profiles [31], and their utility for monitoring the antibody response following treatment [32]. Nonetheless, the variations in sensitivity and specificity [33], and interassay variability [34], present limitations for serological techniques, particularly when they are used as the sole diagnostic tool.

Molecular diagnostic methods offer an attractive solution to many of the problems that are inherent to the diagnosis of *Strongyloides* infection using faecal samples in northern Australian diagnostic laboratories. The most commonly used and widely validated molecular diagnostic test for the detection of strongyloidiasis worldwide is the real-time PCR that was developed by Jaco Verweij and co-workers [35], which uses a DNA region in the small subunit of the nuclear rRNA (18S) gene as a marker. A loop-mediated isothermal amplification method has also been developed, which shows major potential for implementation in areas with minimal laboratory infrastructure [36]. In the present study, we used the real-time method [35] in a diagnostic service laboratory in Queensland for the diagnosis of *Strongyloides* sp. infection in communities with a low apparent prevalence of strongyloidiasis, and then employed PCR-based mutation scanning [37] to assess levels of genetic variation within *Strongyloides* sp. from these communities.

2. Materials and Methods

2.1. Ethics

Approval for specimen collection and analysis was given by The Townsville Hospital and Health Service Human Research Ethics Committee, reference number HREC/14/QTHS/4.

2.2. Specimen Collection and Study Site

Stool specimens that were sent to TTHML for investigation of parasitic infections were collected over a one-year period (January–December 2014). Faecal specimens for parasitological examination are sent to TTHML from a large geographic area (478,446 km^2), comprising the North West, Northern, and Mackay regions of Queensland (Figure 1). Across this area, the average daily temperature ranges from 17.3 °C to 30.2 °C, with an average rainfall of 702 mm per year [38]. The total human population of these regions is 431,300, with 224,700 (52.1%), 171,600 (39.8%), and 35,000 (8.1%) people residing in the Northern, Mackay, and North West regions, respectively. In the North West region, the proportion of the population that identify as ATSI is 21.7%, more than three times the proportion in the Northern and Mackay regions (7.1% and 4.1%, respectively). However, all of the regions have a higher proportion of ATSI residents as compared to the state as a whole, with Indigenous residents comprising 3.6% of the entire Queensland population [38].

Both fresh and formalin fixed faecal samples are received from the North West and Northern regions, while only fixed specimens (that are unsuitable for PCR testing) are received from the Mackay region. Specimens from the North West region are refrigerated during transport. A distinction was not made between inpatients and outpatients, due to the chronicity of *Strongyloides* infection. Specimens were aliquoted into 100% ethanol at a 1:5 dilution using approximately 1 g of stool and were stored at 4 °C.

2.3. Microscopy

All of the specimens with a request for ova, cysts, and parasites (OCP) underwent direct microscopy and FEAC using the Mini-Parasep Faecal Parasite Concentrator (Apacor, Wokingham, UK). Briefly, 0.4 g of faeces was introduced to the Mini-Parasep mixing chamber, along with 3.3 mL of SAF and one drop of Triton-X-100. The tube was sealed with the filtration unit and thoroughly vortexed to emulsify the specimen. Tubes were left to stand for 30 min to complete the fixation process. The tube was then inverted and centrifuged at 500 *g* for 5 min, and the supernatant was discarded. A wet preparation of the sediment in both saline and Lugol's iodine was examined for ova, cysts, and helminths at ×100 and ×400 under a light microscope, followed by the preparation of permanent smears using a modified iron-haematoxylin stain for examination at ×1000. Requests specifically asking for detection of a hookworm or *Strongyloides* infection were also processed using the Harada-Mori technique, as previously described [39]. The sediment was examined at ×400 under a light microscope for larvae.

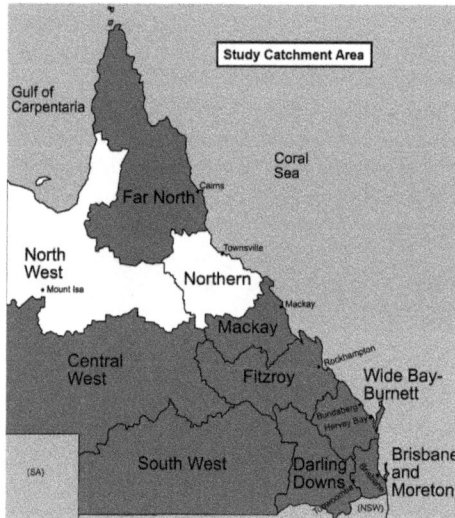

Figure 1. Fresh faecal specimens sampled for *Strongyloides* PCR were submitted from laboratories in the regions indicated. 90.7% of specimens received came from patients residing in these areas, and 95% of specimens positive by qPCR came from patients residing in these areas. Two positive specimens came from the Far North and Central West regions, and one specimen came from a small community (not shown) just over the western border of the North West region.

2.4. DNA Extraction

Ethanol-preserved faecal specimens were centrifuged at 10,000× *g* for 10 min and the supernatant discarded. Specimens were then resuspended in 1 mL of sterile saline and were left overnight at 4 °C. Following centrifugation at 10,000× *g* for 10 min, the supernatant was discarded, and DNA was extracted from the pellet using the PowerSoil DNA Isolation Kit (Mo Bio Laboratories, Carlsbad, CA, USA), according to the manufacturer's instructions, and was stored at −80 °C.

2.5. Real-Time PCR

This PCR assay was performed using primers (forward 5′-GAA TTC CAA GTA AAC GTA AGT CAT TAG C-3′, reverse 5′-TGC CTC TGG ATA TTG CTC AGT TC-3′) and probe (FAM-5′-ACA CAC CGG CCG TCG CTG C-3′-BHQ1) targeting a 101 bp region of the 18S rRNA gene (cf. GenBank accession number AF279916), as described by Verweij et al. [35], using a reaction volume of 25 µL [40]. The PCR mixture comprised 0.3 µM of each primer, 0.1 µM of probe, 5 mM $MgCl_2$, 0.1 mg/mL bovine serum albumin (BSA) (Fisher Biotec, Australia), and 5 µL of DNA template in a final volume of 25 µL of PCR buffer (HotStarTaq Master Mix, QIAGEN, Hilden, Germany). PCR was performed on a Corbett Rotor-Gene 6000 (QIAGEN) under the following conditions: 15 min at 95 °C, followed by 45 cycles of 15 s at 95 °C, and 30 s at 60 °C. Detection and analysis of products was performed using Corbett Rotor Gene 6000 Series Software (QIAGEN, Hilden, Germany). Thresholds were determined at each run visually, with a cut-off cycle time (C_t) of 40.

Specimens with amplification detected up to a C_t value of 40 had a repeat amplification that was performed to confirm the result. Duplicate results of $C_t < 40$ were considered as PCR positive, while those that failed to produce a product on repeat amplification were considered PCR equivocal. Real-time PCR results were compared to the results of microscopic testing (direct microscopy and FEAC) to determine sensitivity and specificity.

2.6. PCR-Based Single-Strand Conformation (SSCP) Analysis and Sequencing

All of the genomic DNA samples that were shown to be test-positive by real-time PCR were subjected to nested PCR utilising new pairs of primers designed to the 18S rRNA gene using Geneious [41] and Primer3 software [42]. The primer pair Strong155F (5′-TAA AGG AAT TGA CGG AAG GGC A-3′) and Strong578R (5′-TCC CAG TTA CGT AAT GTT TTC AAT GTT-3′) was used in the primary PCR to amplify a 423 bp region, and secondary primer pairs Strong198F (5′-GCT AAA TTT GAC TCA ACA CGG GAA-3′) and Strong492R (5′-CCC GGA CAT CTA AGG GCA TC-3′) were used to amplify a 294 bp region of the gene.

Nested PCR was carried out in 50 μL containing 10 mM Tris-HCl (pH 8.4), 50 mM KCl (Promega, Madison, WI, USA), 3.0 mM of $MgCl_2$, 200 μM of each deoxynucleotide triphosphate, 50 pmol of each primer, and 1 U of GoTaq (Promega) DNA polymerase. PCR reactions were performed on a Veriti thermal cycler (Applied Biosystems, Foster City, CA, USA) under the following conditions: initial denaturation at 94 °C/5 min, denaturation, annealing, and extension cycles of 30 s at 94 °C, 30 s at 64 °C, and 30 s at 72 °C for 35 cycles, followed by a final extension of 72 °C for 5 min. The quality, size, and intensity of individual PCR amplicons were assessed by electrophoresis (7 V/cm) in 1.5% agarose gels using TBE (65 mM Tris-HCl, 27 mM boric acid, 1 mM EDTA, pH 9; Bio-Rad, Hercules, CA, USA) as the buffer. Following electrophoresis, gels were stained with ethidium bromide and their size was estimated by comparison to PhiX174-*Hae*III (Promega, Madison, WI, USA) markers (Figure 2).

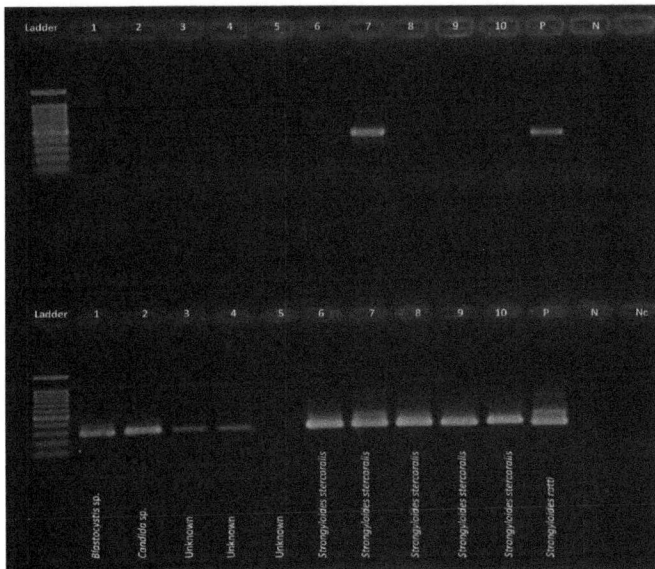

Figure 2. Conventional nested PCR testing a subset of samples, with primary PCR on the top row and secondary PCR on the bottom row. A 100 bp ladder (Promega) is used as a marker in the first lane. *Strongyloides ratti* was used as the positive control along with negative controls. The primers are non-specific therefore the single strand conformational polymorphism (SSCP) method was employed (see Figure 3).

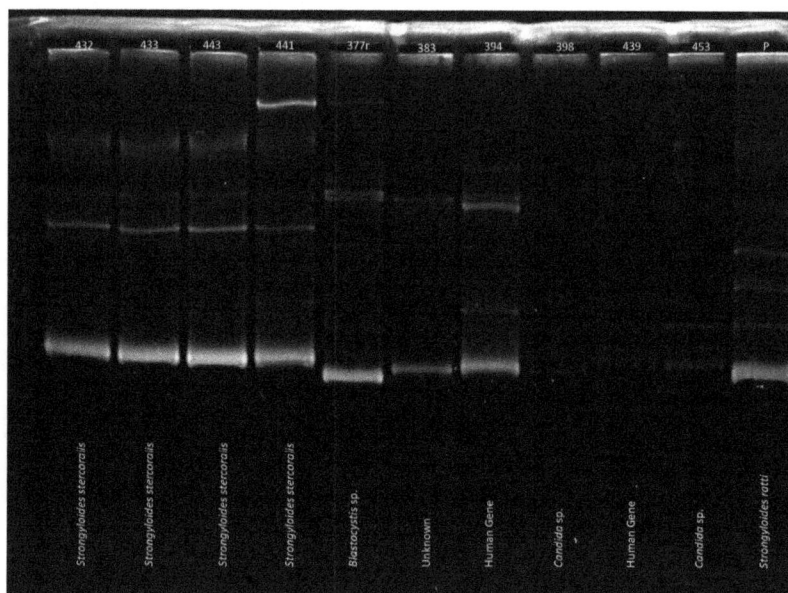

Figure 3. Sample single-strand conformational polymorphism (SSCP) gel, with text denoting results of sequencing. The banding profile for *Strongyloides stercoralis* is easily distinguishable from the other profiles which included *Blastocystis* sp., *Candida* sp. and human genes. Note prominent extra band in lane 441, which is most likely the result of conformers linked to sequence variability or background amplification.

SSCP analysis [37] was used to scan for sequence variation within and among 18S amplicons. In brief, 1 μL of each secondary amplicon was mixed with 5 μL of DNA sequencing-stop solution (Promega) and 5 μL of H$_2$O, heat-denatured at 94 °C/30 min, snap-cooled on a freeze-block (−20 °C), and then subjected to electrophoresis at 74 V at 7.4 °C (constant) for 16 h in a GMA Wide Mini S-2 × 25 gel in a SEA 2000 rig (Elchrom Scientific AG, Cham, Switzerland) using TAE buffer (40 mM Tris base, 20 mM acetic acid, 1.0 mM EDTA, Bio-Rad, USA). A control sample (extracted DNA of *S. ratti*) was included on each gel to ensure the reproducibility of profiles representing this sample among gels. Subsequently, 5 μL aliquots of individual amplicons representing all distinct electrophoretic profiles were treated with ExoSAP-IT® (Affymetrix, Santa Clara, CA, USA), according to the manufacturer's instructions, and then subjected to direct, automated sequencing (BigDye Terminator v.3.1 chemistry, Applied Biosystems, Foster City, CA, USA).

2.7. Eosinophil Counts and Strongyloides Serology

The most recent eosinophil counts (within three months) and *Strongyloides* serology (Bordier IVD EIA, Crissier, Switzerland; somatic antigens from larvae of *Strongyloides ratti*) results for each patient were extracted from the laboratory information system, where available. The reference ranges for *Strongyloides* serology are as follows: signal-to-cut off (S/CO) > 1.1 is considered positive; S/CO between 0.9–1.1 is considered equivocal, and S/CO < 0.9 is negative. The reference range for eosinophil count is dependent upon age and is reported using standard cut-offs that are produced by Pathology Queensland.

2.8. Statistical Analysis

The Student's *t*-test (in Microsoft Excel version 15.0.1911.1000) was used to assess the statistical difference between C_t values; a *p*-value of < 0.05 was considered to be significant.

3. Results

3.1. Patient Demographics and Specimen Selection

Over the period January to December 2014, 1912 faecal specimens were submitted to TTHML for diagnosis of parasitic infection: 1080 (56.5%) originated from the Northern region laboratory, 463 (24.2%) from the Mackay region laboratory, and 369 (19.3%) from the North West region laboratory. Fresh faecal specimens accounted for 1449 of the total, and, of these, 706 (48.7%) were sampled for real-time PCR. Specimens were selected based on volume available for sampling, demographic spread, and resource constraints. Eleven specimens were misplaced; the final number of specimens that were able to undergo DNA extraction and PCR was 695 (48.0%). The average age of participants was 43.3 years (median 53 years, range one month to 97 years; 48.8% male, 51.2% female). A relative majority of samples came from patients aged more than 60 years (34.9%) (Figure 4). Thirty (4.2%) specimens were from patients residing in the Mackay region, 499 (70.6%) from patients residing in the Northern region, 141 (20.0%) from patients residing in the North West region, and 36 (5.1%) from patients residing in other areas (predominantly the Far North region) (Figure 1).

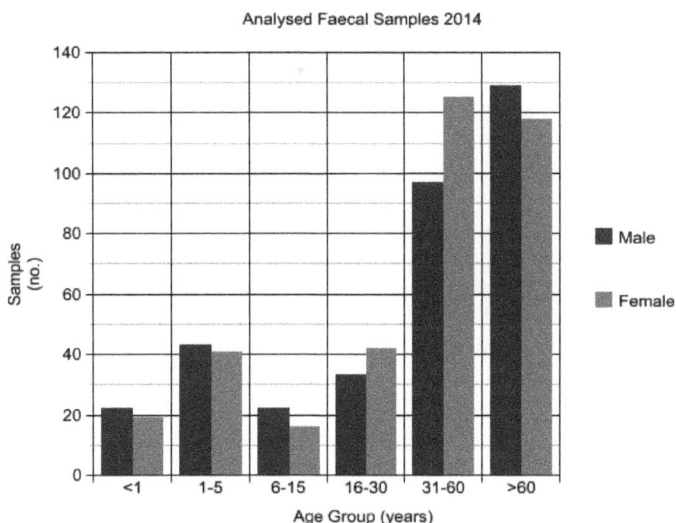

Figure 4. Demographics of patient faecal samples received at Townsville Hospital Microbiology Laboratory (TTHML) in 2014 and assessed by *Strongyloides* sp. qPCR.

3.2. Microscopy, Harada-Mori Culture and Real-Time PCR Results

Of the 695 faecal samples, five samples from three people were test-positive for larvae of *S. stercoralis* by microscopy, but no larvae were detected in any samples by Harada-Mori culture. By contrast, 42 samples were test-positive by real-time PCR, with a mean C_t value of 34.44 (median 36.34, geometric mean 33.97, range 18.77 to 39.33) (Table 1), and 12 samples were equivocal, with a mean C_t value of the initial positive result being 38.46 (median 38.37, geometric mean 38.44, range 36.32 to 39.96). By comparison to microscopy on FEAC samples, the sensitivity of the PCR was 100% (95% CI 47.82–100.00%), while specificity was 94.91% (95% CI 93.05–96.39%). It should be noted that calculations of sensitivity and specificity are not in comparison to a gold standard test, and will therefore overestimate sensitivity and underestimate specificity. Six samples were deemed low-level positives, with C_t values ranging from 40.28 to 42.13 on duplicate runs, and were included for further analysis. Twenty-two (36.7%) of the test-positive, equivocal, and low-level samples were from the North West region, and 35 (58.3%) were from the Northern region (Figure 1). One test-positive sample was from the Central West region, one equivocal specimen was from the Far North, and another equivocal specimen a short distance across the border into the Northern Territory. All five samples that were shown to contain *S. stercoralis* larvae by microscopy were test-positive by real-time PCR, with a mean C_t value of 25.61 (median 23.72, geometric mean 24.79, range 18.77 to 35.25). Numbers positive by microscopy were too few to allow for the statistical comparison of C_t values by the Student's *t*-test.

3.3. PCR-SSCP Analysis and Sequencing

PCR-based mutation scanning was conducted on 60 samples that were test positive (*n* = 42), equivocal (*n* = 12), or low-level positive (*n* = 6) (Table 1). Twenty-five of the 42 positive samples (59.5%) and five of the 12 equivocal samples (41.7%) contained DNA sequences that were consistent with *S. stercoralis* by sequencing and SSCP. Ten of the positive samples, five of the equivocal samples, and one of the low-level positive samples demonstrated non-specific amplification by nested PCR. These were further characterised by sequencing as human gene (*n* = 5), *Blastocystis hominis* (*n* = 4), *Candida* sp. (*n* = 3), *Saccharomyces* sp. (*n* = 2), *Hymenolepis nana* (*n* = 1), or *Entamoeba coli* (*n* = 1).

The *S. stercoralis* sequences that were generated showed no sequence variability; however, two samples were found to have an extra band by SSCP analysis, which could represent conformers that are linked to sequence variability or background amplification (Figure 3). One sample came from a patient in the regional city of Townsville, while the other sample came from a patient in Charters Towers, approximately 150 km south-west. Further characterisation of the hypervariable region IV is required to determine the significance of these results.

3.4. Comparison of Serology and Eosinophilia with qPCR Results

Twelve PCR test-positive and equivocal samples (20.0%), for which no *S. stercoralis* larvae were detected by microscopy, were from people who had eosinophilia and/or antibodies against *Strongyloides* (Table 1). These 12 samples had a mean C_t value of 34.17 (median 35.96, geometric mean 33.85, range 25.66 to 38.84). When the 11 PCR test-positive and equivocal samples for which no eosinophil count was available were excluded from the analysis, C_t values were significantly higher for those with eosinophilia than for those without by a Student's *t*-test (*p* = 0.0135).

Sixteen patients that were included in this study had *Strongyloides* serology testing within the previous two years, 11 of which yielded positive titres. Only six of these serology-positive patients showed positive (*n* = 5) or equivocal (*n* = 1) results in the real-time PCR. All of these six had serology collected within three months of faecal specimen collection (range two days–three months). By nested PCR, four yielded *Strongyloides* sequences, whilst one yielded a sequence from *B. hominis*. One patient with positive serology and with equivocal real-time PCR yielded sequences for *Entamoeba coli* by nested PCR. Five of the 16 patients tested had returned positive serology in the previous two years, two on the same day as faecal specimen collection (range, one day–one year, nine months), but tested negative by real-time PCR. The treatment history of these patients is unknown.

Thirteen of those positive by real-time PCR also showed eosinophilia; nine of these yielded *Strongyloides* sequences by nested PCR, with the remaining four amplifying sequences of *B. hominis*, *H. nana*, human gene, and *Saccharomyces* sp. Only one sample with an elevated eosinophil count was equivocal by real-time PCR, which yielded a *Candida* sp. sequence on nested PCR. A single sample with equivocal results, but no eosinophilia, had a reactive *Strongyloides* serology titre.

Table 1. Characteristics of patients with faecal samples submitted for diagnostic testing that yielded positive, equivocal or low level amplification *Strongyloides* sp. 18S rRNA real-time PCR compared to confirmatory testing using a second nested *Strongyloides* sp. 18S rRNA PCR with SSCP and sequencing. Values in bold are positive/above the normal range; * same patient; ^ another specimen on the same patient was PCR negative; Eos: eosinophil; nd: not done; SSCP: single strand conformation polymorphism; NW: North West; NTH: North; CW: Central West.

Age (Years)	Gender	Place of Residence	Region	Real-time PCR	Mean C_t Value	Nested PCR	Sequence Identity/SSCP Homology	*Strongyloides* Serology	Eosinophil Count ($\times 10^9$/L)	Parasites Detected by FEAC Microscopy
2	F	Doomadgee *	NW	Positive	18.77	Detected	*S. stercoralis*	nd	nd	*S. stercoralis*
2	F	Doomadgee *	NW	Positive	19.16	Detected	*S. stercoralis*	nd	0.57	*S. stercoralis*
51	F	Doomadgee	NW	Positive	23.72	Detected	*S. stercoralis*	Reactive (3.1)	0.43	*S. stercoralis*
41	F	Doomadgee	NW	Positive	25.66	Detected	*S. stercoralis*	Reactive (1.6)	0.93	
2	F	Doomadgee *	NW	Positive	31.13	Detected	*S. stercoralis*	nd	3.69	*S. stercoralis*
9	M	Doomadgee	NW	Positive	35.25	Detected	*H. nana*	nd	2.84	*S. stercoralis, H. nana, B. hominis, E. nana*
70	M	Aurukun *	NW	Positive	27.44	Detected	*S. stercoralis*	nd	0.89	*B. hominis*
70	M	Aurukun *	NW	Positive	28.00	Detected	*S. stercoralis*	nd	0.72	*B. hominis*
28	M	Mount Isa	NW	Positive	28.10	Detected	*S. stercoralis*	nd	nd	*B. hominis*
66	M	Mount Isa	NW	Positive	36.27	Detected	*B. hominis*	nd	0.02	
30	M	Mount Isa	NW	Positive	36.41	Detected	*S. stercoralis*	nd	0.41	
61	M	Magnetic Island	NTH	Positive	31.15	Detected	*S. stercoralis*	nd	nd	
28	M	Magnetic Island	NTH	Positive	35.69	Detected	*S. stercoralis*	nd	0.30	
64	F	Magnetic Island	NTH	Positive	35.93	Detected	Human gene	nd	0.60	
51	F	Magnetic Island	NTH	Positive	36.12	Detected	*S. stercoralis*	nd	nd	
36	M	Townsville	NTH	Positive	31.86	Detected	*S. stercoralis*	Reactive (4.0)	1.27	*B. hominis*
70	M	Townsville	NTH	Positive	34.12	Detected	*S. stercoralis*	nd	0.13	*B. hominis*
40	M	Townsville	NTH	Positive	36.10	Detected	*S. stercoralis*	Reactive (3.1)	1.48	*H. nana, B. hominis, Entamoeba coli*
<1	F	Townsville	NTH	Positive	36.13	Detected	*S. stercoralis*	nd	0.00	
58	M	Townsville	NTH	Positive	36.57	Detected	*S. stercoralis*	nd	0.10	
<1	M	Townsville	NTH	Positive	37.08	Detected	*S. stercoralis*	nd	nd	
14	F	Townsville	NTH	Positive	37.31	Detected	*S. stercoralis*	nd	nd	
39	F	Townsville	NTH	Positive	38.51	Not Detected	Candida sp.	nd	0.08	
69	F	Townsville	NTH	Positive	38.97	Detected	Candida sp.	nd	0.46	
51	F	Townsville	NTH	Positive	39.33	Not Detected		nd	0.20	
43	F	Jundah	CW	Positive	34.32	Detected	*B. hominis*	nd	0.04	*B. hominis*
67	F	Mornington Island	NW	Positive	35.08	Detected	*B. hominis*	Reactive (4.1)	2.14	
1	M	Mornington Island	NW	Positive	36.96	Detected	Human gene	nd	8.04	*G. intestinalis*
35	M	Normanton	NW	Positive	35.81	Detected	*S. stercoralis*	nd	1.90	
36	M	Palm Island	NTH	Positive	36.53	Detected	*S. stercoralis*	nd	0.25	

Table 1. *Cont.*

Age (Years)	Gender	Place of Residence	Region	Real-time PCR	Mean C$_t$ Value	Nested PCR	Sequence Identity/SSCP Homology	Strongyloides Serology	Eosinophil Count (×10⁹/L)	Parasites Detected by FEAC Microscopy
<1 y	M	Palm Island	NTH	Positive	38.37	Not Detected		nd	nd	
1	M	Palm Island	NTH	Positive	38.48	Detected	Human gene	nd	nd	
20	F	Palm Island	NTH	Positive	38.84	Detected	*S. stercoralis*	nd	0.62	
78	M	Ayr	NTH	Positive	36.63	Detected	*S. stercoralis*	nd	0.14	
1	M	Cloncurry	NW	Positive	36.81	Not Detected		nd	nd	*B. hominis; E. nana*
94	F	Home Hill	NTH	Positive	36.95	Not Detected		nd	0.12	*B. hominis*
80	F	Greenvale	NTH	Positive	37.01	Detected	*S. stercoralis*	nd	0.09	
11	F	Charters Towers	NTH	Positive	37.15	Detected	*S. stercoralis*	nd	nd	
79	M	Hughenden	NW	Positive	37.66	Detected	*Saccharomyces* sp.	nd	1.05	
27	M	Camooweal	NW	Positive	38.12	Detected	*Saccharomyces* sp.	nd	0.25	*G. intestinalis*
84	M	Ingham	NTH	Positive	38.40	Not Detected		nd	0.09	*B. hominis*
63	F	Ingham	NTH	Positive	38.53	Not Detected		nd	0.09	

4. Discussion

This study provides clear evidence of strongyloidiasis in North Queensland. The majority of PCR positive specimens (36.0%) came from the north-west region of Queensland, out of proportion to the number of samples that were submitted from that area (142, or 20.1%). This is consistent with the known epidemiology of the region and the very remote nature of the North West, with consequent difficulties in the delivery of health services, sanitation, and effective health education to the many of the small communities scattered throughout that region.

The primary difficulty in determining positive and negative predictive values for *Strongyloides* PCR in this low prevalence population was the absence of a sensitive gold standard comparator. In an attempt to overcome this limitation, a sensitive, but not specific, nested PCR with subsequent SSCP and sequencing was performed. Previous studies of the efficacy of real-time PCR for the diagnosis of strongyloidiasis have either been performed in endemic, high-prevalence settings, or in patients with a high pre-test probability as a result of travel to an endemic region [34,35,43]. Such patient cohorts provide a high likelihood of true positive results, and thus a high positive predictive value for the test performed. The setting of a regional diagnostic laboratory in North Queensland offered a unique opportunity to determine the efficacy of this methodology in an endemic, but low-prevalence, environment on a large sample cohort. *Strongyloides* sp. real-time PCR was positive in 37 more specimens than were detected by microscopy, supporting previous studies demonstrating the low sensitivity of FEAC for *Strongyloides* detection [11,13,43,44]. All *Strongyloides* cultures were negative in this study; however, this may have been due to delays during transport, the chilling of faecal samples during shipment, and the low larval load in most samples [20], as demonstrated by the large number of microscopy negative results.

In the absence of a gold standard, it is not clear if all the positive real-time PCR results are true positives. Positive results were obtained from patient samples where the residence was not in an area of known transmission, or without supporting laboratory markers, such as eosinophilia, though the limited value of eosinophilia as a predictor for strongyloidiasis has been discussed in previous studies [45]. Based upon the limited clinical information that is available, it was not possible to determine if these patients were exposed in the past. The reported specificity of the primers employed, based upon sequence analysis of amplicons, has approached 100% in almost all of the previously published papers [46–49]. However, in a recent *Strongyloides* PCR-based survey of samples from Cambodia and Timor Leste, primer-dimers led to false-positive results [50]. Altering the forward primer sequence slightly led to an improvement in the performance of the PCR, based upon the assessments made on specimens from the Northern Territory of Australia (Holt D, personal communication). It is possible that a similar phenomenon affected the results from this study, and further investigation is warranted.

Thirteen samples showing C_t values of less than 40 on initial PCR were negative or had a C_t >40 upon repeat testing; at least one of these were found to be true *S. stercoralis* infections by nested PCR and sequencing. Using sequencing and SSCP of the nested PCR products as a confirmatory test substantiated that at least 31 of the samples that were tested contained *S. stercoralis*. While the nested PCR primers also led to non-specific amplification, this does not exclude lower concentrations of *Strongyloides* DNA in the affected samples, with preferential non-specific amplification. Investigations into PCR efficiency have demonstrated preferential amplification for G-C-rich templates over those with a significant A-T composition [51]. In the case of *Strongyloides stercoralis*, the whole genome sequence has an A-T content of 78% [52].

In terms of the most appropriate C_t cut-off value for the RT-PCR, some studies have utilised a C_t cut-off of 35 cycles [50,53]. However, some specimens in this study with *Strongyloides* sp. detected by microscopy, and others with eosinophilia and/or reactive serology, had C_t values of over 35. Similarly, Sultana et al. found that the sensitivity of the same RT-PCR that was employed in this study was low in samples with a low larval load, with only 5/32 samples delivering positive results and all with C_t

values between 36–38 [40]. While a C_t cut-off value of 35 may be too low to detect low larval burden, a higher C_t cut-off may include false-positive reactions [54].

The ability to speciate *Strongyloides* by nested PCR was limited as the primers targeted the hypervariable region IV of the 18S rRNA gene, a section of genome containing only four single nucleotide polymorphisms (SNP) [55]. The low specificity of these primers in a mixed specimen, such as faeces, limits its application in diagnostics, and may make it for suitable for use on cultured larvae. When sequenced, the products that confirmed the presence of the amplified DNA as *Strongyloides stercoralis* were identical, without the presence of SNPs. Interestingly, this was the case despite two extracts identified as *S. stercoralis* by sequencing demonstrating an extra band on SSCP analysis. Whether this reflects an increased resolution of SSCP for detection of *S. stercoralis* genotypes or the paucity of available genomic data for *Strongyloides* species, has not been determined and warrants further investigation.

This study indicated that the currently employed methods for the detection of *S. stercoralis* in north Queensland (direct microscopy, FEAC, and Harada-Mori) were not able to detect the majority of cases of strongyloidiasis. Transport time and refrigeration, as lower temperatures kill larvae, limits the applicability of conventional culture techniques for the routine diagnosis of strongyloidiasis in this setting [56]. The use of the qPCR for the detection of *Strongyloides* DNA in stool samples increased the diagnostic sensitivity, and would assist with individual diagnoses, screening, and public health interventions to eradicate this neglected disease.

Acknowledgments: This study was funded through the generous support of the Pathology Queensland Study, Education, and Research Fund. We are grateful to Professor Adrian Miller for reviewing the draft manuscript. Molecular work at the University was supported by a grant from the Australian Research Council (ARC LP160101299; RBG and AVK). This paper is dedicated to the memory of our friend and colleague, Emeritus Professor Rick Speare. Rick's incredible work in strongyloidiasis, Indigenous health, and public health more broadly, were an inspiration to all of us, and his kindness, mentoring spirit, and generosity are missed by us all.

Author Contributions: G.J.R. and R.V.B. conceived and designed the experiments, with assistance from R.N.; G.J.R. and A.V.K. performed the experiments; G.J.R., A.V.K., R.B.G., M.W. and R.V.B. analysed the data; G.J.R. prepared the original manuscript, with editing and analysis from A.V.K., R.B.G., M.W., R.N. and R.V.B.

Conflicts of Interest: The authors declare no conflict of interest. Richard Bradbury is co-authoring this paper in his personal capacity and in his capacity as an adjunct academic at Central Queensland University.

References

1. Cook, G.C. *Strongyloidiasis: A Major Roundworm Infection of Man*; Grove, D.I., Ed.; Taylor & Francis: London, UK, 1989; ISBN 978-0-85066-732-5.
2. Bisoffi, Z.; Buonfrate, D.; Montresor, A.; Requena-Méndez, A.; Muñoz, J.; Krolewiecki, A.J.; Gotuzzo, E.; Mena, M.A.; Chiodini, P.L.; Anselmi, M.; et al. *Strongyloides stercoralis*: A plea for action. *PLoS Negl. Trop. Dis.* **2013**, *7*, e2214. [CrossRef] [PubMed]
3. Nielsen, P.B.; Mojon, M. Improved diagnosis of *Strongyloides stercoralis* by seven consecutive stool specimens. *Zent. Bakteriol. Mikrobiol. Hyg. A* **1987**, *263*, 616–618. [CrossRef]
4. Meloni, B.P.; Thompson, R.C.; Hopkins, R.M.; Reynoldson, J.A.; Gracey, M. The prevalence of *Giardia* and other intestinal parasites in children, dogs and cats from aboriginal communities in the Kimberley. *Med. J. Aust.* **1993**, *158*, 157–159. [PubMed]
5. Reynoldson, J.A.; Behnke, J.M.; Pallant, L.J.; Macnish, M.G.; Gilbert, F.; Giles, S.; Spargo, R.J.; Thompson, R.C. Failure of pyrantel in treatment of human hookworm infections (*Ancylostoma duodenale*) in the Kimberley region of north west Australia. *Acta Trop.* **1997**, *68*, 301–312. [CrossRef]
6. Fisher, D.; McCarry, F.; Currie, B. Strongyloidiasis in the Northern Territory. Under-recognised and under-treated? *Med. J. Aust.* **1993**, *159*, 88–90. [PubMed]
7. Einsiedel, L.J.; Woodman, R.J. Two nations: Racial disparities in bloodstream infections recorded at Alice Springs Hospital, central Australia, 2001–2005. *Med. J. Aust.* **2010**, *192*, 567–571. [PubMed]
8. Kukuruzovic, R.; Robins-Browne, R.M.; Anstey, N.M.; Brewster, D.R. Enteric pathogens, intestinal permeability and nitric oxide production in acute gastroenteritis. *Pediatr. Infect. Dis. J.* **2002**, *21*, 730–739. [CrossRef] [PubMed]

9.   Johnston, F.H.; Morris, P.S.; Speare, R.; McCarthy, J.; Currie, B.; Ewald, D.; Page, W.; Dempsey, K. Strongyloidiasis: A review of the evidence for Australian practitioners. *Aust. J. Rural Health* **2005**, *13*, 247–254. [CrossRef] [PubMed]

10.   Prociv, P.; Luke, R. Observations on strongyloidiasis in Queensland aboriginal communities. *Med. J. Aust.* **1993**, *158*, 160–163. [PubMed]

11.   Anamnart, W.; Pattanawongsa, A.; Intapan, P.M.; Maleewong, W. Albendazole stimulates the excretion of *Strongyloides stercoralis* larvae in stool specimens and enhances sensitivity for diagnosis of strongyloidiasis. *J. Clin. Microbiol.* **2010**, *48*, 4216–4220. [CrossRef] [PubMed]

12.   Bartlett, M.S.; Harper, K.; Smith, N.; Verbanac, P.; Smith, J.W. Comparative evaluation of a modified zinc sulfate flotation technique. *J. Clin. Microbiol.* **1978**, *7*, 524–528. [PubMed]

13.   Steinmann, P.; Zhou, X.-N.; Du, Z.-W.; Jiang, J.-Y.; Wang, L.-B.; Wang, X.-Z.; Li, L.-H.; Marti, H.; Utzinger, J. Occurrence of *Strongyloides stercoralis* in Yunnan Province, China, and comparison of diagnostic methods. *PLoS Negl. Trop. Dis.* **2007**, *1*, e75. [CrossRef] [PubMed]

14.   Loukas, A. *Neglected Tropical Diseases—Oceania*; Springer International Publishing: Cham, Switzerland, 2016; ISBN 978-3-319-43148-2.

15.   Koga, K.; Kasuya, S.; Khamboonruang, C.; Sukavat, K.; Nakamura, Y.; Tani, S.; Ieda, M.; Tomita, K.; Tomita, S.; Hattan, N. An evaluation of the agar plate method for the detection of *Strongyloides stercoralis* in northern Thailand. *J. Trop. Med. Hyg.* **1990**, *93*, 183–188. [PubMed]

16.   Panosian, K.J.; Marone, P.; Edberg, S.C. Elucidation of *Strongyloides stercoralis* by bacterial-colony displacement. *J. Clin. Microbiol.* **1986**, *24*, 86–88. [PubMed]

17.   Arakaki, T.; Iwanaga, M.; Kinjo, F.; Saito, A.; Asato, R.; Ikeshiro, T. Efficacy of agar-plate culture in detection of *Strongyloides stercoralis* infection. *J. Parasitol.* **1990**, *76*, 425–428. [CrossRef] [PubMed]

18.   Koga, K.; Kasuya, S.; Ohtomo, H. How effective is the agar plate method for *Strongyloides stercoralis*? *J. Parasitol.* **1992**, *78*, 155–156. [CrossRef] [PubMed]

19.   Dreyer, G.; Fernandes-Silva, E.; Alves, S.; Rocha, A.; Albuquerque, R.; Addiss, D. Patterns of detection of *Strongyloides stercoralis* in stool specimens: Implications for diagnosis and clinical trials. *J. Clin. Microbiol.* **1996**, *34*, 2569–2571. [PubMed]

20.   De J. Inês, E.; Souza, J.N.; Santos, R.C.; Souza, E.S.; Santos, F.L.; Silva, M.L.S.; Silva, M.P.; Teixeira, M.C.A.; Soares, N.M. Efficacy of parasitological methods for the diagnosis of *Strongyloides stercoralis* and hookworm in faecal specimens. *Acta Trop.* **2011**, *120*, 206–210. [CrossRef] [PubMed]

21.   Herwaldt, B.L. Laboratory-acquired parasitic infections from accidental exposures. *Clin. Microbiol. Rev.* **2001**, *14*, 659–688. [CrossRef] [PubMed]

22.   De Kaminsky, R.G. Evaluation of three methods for laboratory diagnosis of *Strongyloides stercoralis* infection. *J. Parasitol.* **1993**, *79*, 277–280. [CrossRef] [PubMed]

23.   Soulsby, H.M.; Hewagama, S.; Brady, S. Case series of four patients with strongyloides after occupational exposure. *Med. J. Aust.* **2012**, *196*, 444. [CrossRef] [PubMed]

24.   Cringoli, G. FLOTAC, a novel apparatus for a multivalent faecal egg count technique. *Parassitologia* **2006**, *48*, 381–384. [PubMed]

25.   Intapan, P.M.; Maleewong, W.; Wongsaroj, T.; Singthong, S.; Morakote, N. Comparison of the quantitative formalin ethyl acetate concentration technique and agar plate culture for diagnosis of human strongyloidiasis. *J. Clin. Microbiol.* **2005**, *43*, 1932–1933. [CrossRef] [PubMed]

26.   Glinz, D.; Silué, K.D.; Knopp, S.; Lohourignon, L.K.; Yao, K.P.; Steinmann, P.; Rinaldi, L.; Cringoli, G.; N'Goran, E.K.; Utzinger, J. Comparing diagnostic accuracy of Kato-Katz, Koga agar plate, ether-concentration, and FLOTAC for *Schistosoma mansoni* and soil-transmitted helminths. *PLoS Negl. Trop. Dis.* **2010**, *4*, e754. [CrossRef] [PubMed]

27.   Knopp, S.; Mgeni, A.F.; Khamis, I.S.; Steinmann, P.; Stothard, J.R.; Rollinson, D.; Marti, H.; Utzinger, J. Diagnosis of soil-transmitted helminths in the era of preventive chemotherapy: Effect of multiple stool sampling and use of different diagnostic techniques. *PLoS Negl. Trop. Dis.* **2008**, *2*, e331. [CrossRef] [PubMed]

28.   Marchi Blatt, J.; Cantos, G.A. Evaluation of techniques for the diagnosis of *Strongyloides stercoralis* in human immunodeficiency virus (HIV) positive and HIV negative individuals in the city of Itajaí, Brazil. *Braz. J. Infect. Dis.* **2003**, *7*, 402–408. [PubMed]

29.   Moody, A.; Rao, S.; Subirats, M. *Evaluation of Parasep SF, Ether and Ethyl Acetate Free Faecal Concentrators*; Apacaor: Berkshire, UK, 2013.

30. Mounsey, K.; Kearns, T.; Rampton, M.; Llewellyn, S.; King, M.; Holt, D.; Currie, B.J.; Andrews, R.; Nutman, T.; McCarthy, J. Use of dried blood spots to define antibody response to the *Strongyloides stercoralis* recombinant antigen NIE. *Acta Trop.* **2014**, *138*, 78–82. [CrossRef] [PubMed]
31. Requena-Méndez, A.; Chiodini, P.; Bisoffi, Z.; Buonfrate, D.; Gotuzzo, E.; Muñoz, J. The laboratory diagnosis and follow up of strongyloidiasis: A systematic review. *PLoS Negl. Trop. Dis.* **2013**, *7*, e2002. [CrossRef] [PubMed]
32. Page, W.A.; Dempsey, K.; McCarthy, J.S. Utility of serological follow-up of chronic strongyloidiasis after anthelminthic chemotherapy. *Trans. R. Soc. Trop. Med. Hyg.* **2006**, *100*, 1056–1062. [CrossRef] [PubMed]
33. Schaffel, R.; Nucci, M.; Carvalho, E.; Braga, M.; Almeida, L.; Portugal, R.; Pulcheri, W. The value of an immunoenzymatic test (enzyme-linked immunosorbent assay) for the diagnosis of strongyloidiasis in patients immunosuppressed by hematologic malignancies. *Am. J. Trop. Med. Hyg.* **2001**, *65*, 346–350. [CrossRef] [PubMed]
34. Sudarshi, S.; Stümpfle, R.; Armstrong, M.; Ellman, T.; Parton, S.; Krishnan, P.; Chiodini, P.L.; Whitty, C.J.M. Clinical presentation and diagnostic sensitivity of laboratory tests for *Strongyloides stercoralis* in travellers compared with immigrants in a non-endemic country. *Trop. Med. Int. Health* **2003**, *8*, 728–732. [CrossRef] [PubMed]
35. Verweij, J.J.; Canales, M.; Polman, K.; Ziem, J.; Brienen, E.A.T.; Polderman, A.M.; van Lieshout, L. Molecular diagnosis of *Strongyloides stercoralis* in faecal samples using real-time PCR. *Trans. R. Soc. Trop. Med. Hyg.* **2009**, *103*, 342–346. [CrossRef] [PubMed]
36. Watts, M.R.; James, G.; Sultana, Y.; Ginn, A.N.; Outhred, A.C.; Kong, F.; Verweij, J.J.; Iredell, J.R.; Chen, S.C.-A.; Lee, R. A loop-mediated isothermal amplification (LAMP) assay for *Strongyloides stercoralis* in stool that uses a visual detection method with SYTO-82 fluorescent dye. *Am. J. Trop. Med. Hyg.* **2014**, *90*, 306–311. [CrossRef] [PubMed]
37. Gasser, R.B.; Hu, M.; Chilton, N.B.; Campbell, B.E.; Jex, A.J.; Otranto, D.; Cafarchia, C.; Beveridge, I.; Zhu, X. Single-strand conformation polymorphism (SSCP) for the analysis of genetic variation. *Nat. Protoc.* **2006**, *1*, 3121–3128. [CrossRef] [PubMed]
38. Queensland Government. Queensland Regional Profiles. Queensland Government Statistician's Office. 2016. Available online: http://statistics.qgso.qld.gov.au/qld-regional-profiles (accessed on 4 January 2016).
39. World Health Organization. *CCTA/WHO African Conference on Ancylostomiasis*; World Health Organization Technical Report Series No. 255; World Health Organization: Geneva, Switzerland, 1963.
40. Sultana, Y.; Jeoffreys, N.; Watts, M.R.; Gilbert, G.L.; Lee, R. Real-time polymerase chain reaction for detection of *Strongyloides stercoralis* in stool. *Am. J. Trop. Med. Hyg.* **2013**, *88*, 1048–1051. [CrossRef] [PubMed]
41. Kearse, M.; Moir, R.; Wilson, A.; Stones-Havas, S.; Cheung, M.; Sturrock, S.; Buxton, S.; Cooper, A.; Markowitz, S.; Duran, C.; et al. Geneious Basic: An integrated and extendable desktop software platform for the organization and analysis of sequence data. *Bioinformatics* **2012**, *28*, 1647–1649. [CrossRef] [PubMed]
42. Untergasser, A.; Cutcutache, I.; Koressaar, T.; Ye, J.; Faircloth, B.C.; Remm, M.; Rozen, S.G. Primer3—New capabilities and interfaces. *Nucleic Acids Res.* **2012**, *40*, e115. [CrossRef] [PubMed]
43. Ten Hove, R.J.; van Esbroeck, M.; Vervoort, T.; van den Ende, J.; van Lieshout, L.; Verweij, J.J. Molecular diagnostics of intestinal parasites in returning travellers. *Eur. J. Clin. Microbiol. Infect. Dis.* **2009**, *28*, 1045–1053. [CrossRef] [PubMed]
44. Sithithaworn, P.; Srisawangwong, T.; Tesana, S.; Daenseekaew, W.; Sithithaworn, J.; Fujimaki, Y.; Ando, K. Epidemiology of *Strongyloides stercoralis* in north-east Thailand: Application of the agar plate culture technique compared with the enzyme-linked immunosorbent assay. *Trans. R. Soc. Trop. Med. Hyg.* **2003**, *97*, 398–402. [CrossRef]
45. Naidu, P.; Yanow, S.K.; Kowalewska-Grochowska, K.T. Eosinophilia: A poor predictor of *Strongyloides* infection in refugees. *Can. J. Infect. Dis. Med. Microbiol.* **2013**, *24*, 93–96. [PubMed]
46. Schär, F.; Odermatt, P.; Khieu, V.; Panning, M.; Duong, S.; Muth, S.; Marti, H.; Kramme, S. Evaluation of real-time PCR for *Strongyloides stercoralis* and hookworm as diagnostic tool in asymptomatic schoolchildren in Cambodia. *Acta Trop.* **2013**, *126*, 89–92. [CrossRef] [PubMed]
47. Sitta, R.B.; Malta, F.M.; Pinho, J.R.; Chieffi, P.P.; Gryschek, R.C.B.; Paula, F.M. Conventional PCR for molecular diagnosis of human strongyloidiasis. *Parasitology* **2014**, *141*, 716–721. [CrossRef] [PubMed]

48. Sharifdini, M.; Mirhendi, H.; Ashrafi, K.; Hosseini, M.; Mohebali, M.; Khodadadi, H.; Kia, E.B. Comparison of nested polymerase chain reaction and real-time polymerase chain reaction with parasitological methods for detection of *Strongyloides stercoralis* in human fecal samples. *Am. J. Trop. Med. Hyg.* **2015**, *93*, 1285–1291. [CrossRef] [PubMed]

49. Saugar, J.M.; Merino, F.J.; Martín-Rabadán, P.; Fernández-Soto, P.; Ortega, S.; Gárate, T.; Rodríguez, E. Application of real-time PCR for the detection of *Strongyloides* spp. in clinical samples in a reference center in Spain. *Acta Trop.* **2015**, *142*, 20–25. [CrossRef] [PubMed]

50. Llewellyn, S.; Inpankaew, T.; Nery, S.V.; Gray, D.J.; Verweij, J.J.; Clements, A.C.A.; Gomes, S.J.; Traub, R.; McCarthy, J.S. Application of a multiplex quantitative PCR to assess prevalence and intensity of intestinal parasite infections in a controlled clinical trial. *PLoS Negl. Trop. Dis.* **2016**, *10*, e0004380. [CrossRef] [PubMed]

51. Polz, M.F.; Cavanaugh, C.M. Bias in template-to-product ratios in multitemplate PCR. *Appl. Environ. Microbiol.* **1998**, *64*, 3724–3730. [PubMed]

52. Hunt, V.L.; Tsai, I.J.; Coghlan, A.; Reid, A.J.; Holroyd, N.; Foth, B.J.; Tracey, A.; Cotton, J.A.; Stanley, E.J.; Beasley, H.; et al. The genomic basis of parasitism in the *Strongyloides* clade of nematodes. *Nat. Genet.* **2016**, *48*, 299–307. [CrossRef] [PubMed]

53. Janwan, P.; Intapan, P.M.; Thanchomnang, T.; Lulitanond, V.; Anamnart, W.; Maleewong, W. Rapid detection of *Opisthorchis viverrini* and *Strongyloides stercoralis* in human fecal samples using a duplex real-time PCR and melting curve analysis. *Parasitol. Res.* **2011**, *109*, 1593–1601. [CrossRef] [PubMed]

54. Caraguel, C.G.B.; Stryhn, H.; Gagné, N.; Dohoo, I.R.; Hammell, K.L. Selection of a cutoff value for real-time polymerase chain reaction results to fit a diagnostic purpose: Analytical and epidemiologic approaches. *J. Vet. Diagn. Investig.* **2011**, *23*, 2–15. [CrossRef] [PubMed]

55. Hasegawa, H.; Sato, H.; Fujita, S.; Nguema, P.P.M.; Nobusue, K.; Miyagi, K.; Kooriyama, T.; Takenoshita, Y.; Noda, S.; Sato, A.; et al. Molecular identification of the causative agent of human strongyloidiasis acquired in Tanzania: Dispersal and diversity of *Strongyloides* spp. and their hosts. *Parasitol. Int.* **2010**, *59*, 407–413. [CrossRef] [PubMed]

56. Shiwaku, K.; Chigusa, Y.; Kadosaka, T.; Kaneko, K. Factors influencing development of free-living generations of *Strongyloides stercoralis*. *Parasitology* **1988**, *97 Pt 1*, 129–138. [CrossRef] [PubMed]

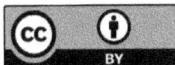

Tropical Medicine and Infectious Disease

MDPI

Review

The Health Effects of Strongyloidiasis on Pregnant Women and Children: A Systematic Literature Review

Matthew Paltridge * and Aileen Traves

College of Medicine and Dentistry, James Cook University, Smithfield QLD 4878, Australia;
Aileen.Traves@jcu.edu.au
* Correspondence: matthew.paltridge@my.jcu.edu.au; Tel.: +61-400-872-750

Received: 28 April 2018; Accepted: 15 May 2018; Published: 18 May 2018

Abstract: Strongyloidiasis is a helminth infection that remains under-researched despite its ability to cause significant illness. Women and children may be at particular risk of health consequences from this parasite. This systematic literature review aims to examine research on the long-term health effects that strongyloidiasis has in pregnant women and children. We conducted a structured search using multiple databases to collect all primary studies discussing health effects of strongyloidiasis in the aforementioned groups. The review included 20 results: 16 primary studies and four case reports. The methodological quality of studies was substandard, and there was substantial heterogeneity to the statistical analysis and outcomes assessed in the literature. Statistically significant associations were found between strongyloidiasis and low birth weight, as well as wasting. No links were found between strongyloidiasis and anaemia. Due to testing methods used in the studies, the prevalence of *Strongyloides stercoralis* in these studies was probably under-estimated. Current research is suggestive that strongyloidiasis has long-term adverse health effects on the offspring of infected mothers and in chronically-infected children. Data analysis was hindered by both methodological and statistical flaws, and as such, reliable conclusions regarding the health impacts could not be formed.

Keywords: Strongyloidiasis; low birth weight; wasting

---

1. Introduction

Strongyloidiasis is a Neglected Tropical Disease (NTD) caused by the infection of a host with the soil-transmitted nematode of the *Strongyloides* genus. Humans are most commonly infected by *S. stercoralis*. However, *S. fuelleborni* has also been observed to infect humans in Papua New Guinea (PNG). *S. stercoralis* is believed to infect over 370 million people worldwide [1].

Strongyloidiasis was originally identified as a disease to look for primarily in returned travellers, refugees, or war veterans [2,3]. The life cycle of *S. stercoralis* grants it the ability to autoinfect hosts, thereby allowing the parasites to persist chronically in individuals. The parasite was believed to exist in the small intestines of hosts in a predominantly asymptomatic state, but it occasionally caused low-grade epigastric pain and diarrhoea. Studies have instead shown that intermittently symptomatic strongyloidiasis is more common than asymptomatic infection [4]. As more precise serological tests are being developed, recent data is showing that the prevalence of *Strongyloides* infections remains consistently underestimated [2,5].

There are a variety of testing methods currently utilised to detect *S. stercoralis* infection. However, they differ greatly in their accuracy [6]. The current gold standard as recognised by the Centers for Disease Control and Prevention (CDC) is seven stool samples using specialised testing techniques such as the Baermann concentration or nutrient agar plate cultures [7]. While studies typically relied on stool samples, modern serological techniques have been proven to be more accurate and practical for use in research [8].

Strongyloidiasis has also been associated with life-threatening illness. Immunosuppression allows the parasite to multiply rapidly in the small intestine and migrate through the gut to the bloodstream and other organs. This is called disseminated strongyloidiasis (DS) or hyperinfection syndrome (HS), which has a mortality rate of 85–100% from overwhelming sepsis [9]. Common conditions that cause adequate immunosuppression include HTLV-1 infection, malignancy, and exogenous corticosteroid administration [10].

While researchers have been able to shed light on the acute health effects of strongyloidiasis, the long-term consequences of this infection have not yet been fully identified. One of the main hypothesised chronic effects of strongyloidiasis is malnutrition; however, there is insufficient evidence to be certain. Milner et al. have postulated a model by which malabsorption occurs in *S. stercoralis*-infected patients, where the infection causes oedema and inflammation of the small intestine walls and prevents nutrient uptake [11]. While this is an old study that has struggled to be replicated in similar projects, a theoretical mechanism of malabsorption exists for *S. strongyloides*, suggesting that the parasite may well lead to malnutrition [12]. If this is the case, chronic strongyloidiasis has a direct clinical relevance to particular sub-groups of society that are most susceptible to harm from malnutrition, such as pregnant women, infants, and children.

Pregnant women are most likely to be affected by strongyloidiasis through two mechanisms: acute severe infection due to immunosuppression, or chronic nutritional deficiencies. Physiological changes during pregnancy cause a level of immunosuppression in the mother, placing her at an increased risk of HS or DS [13,14]. While pregnancy alone has not been observed to cause severe strongyloidiasis, corticosteroids are often administered to women when clinicians suspect a preterm delivery, and this combined effect may immunosuppress the mothers sufficiently to cause severe infection [15]. Some parasitic infections have also been known to cause anaemia during pregnancy, and theoretically *S. stercoralis* may do the same [16,17].

When looking at the risks to pregnant women, the risks to their unborn fetuses must also be considered. The offspring of infected mothers may be placed at an increased risk of harm from the effects of maternal malnutrition. Multiple studies have researched whether maternal helminth infections are a risk factor for poor pregnancy outcomes, such as intra-uterine growth restriction (IUGR) or low birth weight (LBW). While there is evidence to suggest that this may be the case, it remains unsubstantiated [18–21]. Helminth genera such as *Ascaris* or *Ancylostoma* tend to be the focus of such studies; thus there is insufficient literature to demonstrate whether strongyloides does or does not contribute to LBW as well. This is an important gap in knowledge, because if strongyloidiasis does in fact lead to LBW, this means that clinicians are not appropriately screening and treating populations in endemic areas.

Children more generally may also be affected if they become chronically infected during their childhood. Chronic diseases in childhood that produce poor growth are a particular public health concern due to the long term multifactorial consequences they have on individuals and society [22,23]. If strongyloides does cause malabsorption, this will affect the growth and development of children and leave them at an increased risk of poor health outcomes later in life. Insufficient literature is available to determine whether this is the case.

As an NTD, there is a lack of adequate research analysing the effects of strongyloides. Very few studies mention the specific consequences for pregnant women and children, and no systematic reviews have been performed studying the chronic health effects of strongyloidiasis. Those studies that do discuss chronic harm present enough theoretical and observational evidence to hypothesise that there are major health impacts on these sub-groups of the population, justifying the need for a more expansive review of the literature. This review aims to systematically summarise current evidence on the long-term effects that chronic strongyloidiasis has on pregnant women, their offspring, and infected children in general. By doing so, we hope to determine whether these sub-groups are at a potentially higher risk of harm than the rest of the population and highlight current gaps in research.

2. Materials and Methods

This systematic literature review was conducted and reported according to the Preferred Reporting Items for Systematic Reviews and Meta-Analyses (PRISMA) guidelines (Appendix A) [24]. The review focuses on primary studies that measured the health outcomes of strongyloides infections in pregnant women, the offspring of infected women, and children who were chronically infected during their childhood. The review has been structured according to the 'Narrative Synthesis' format described by Mays et al., for ease of reading and in order to easily draw conclusions between studies with different objectives and designs [25]. The review was registered with the PROSPERO International Prospective Register of Systematic Reviews (ID: CRD42017069403). Specific questions this review attempts to answer include: what are the current acute and chronic health effects that strongyloidiasis poses to these cohorts, and, what gaps remain in the literature studying chronic strongyloidiasis?

2.1. Search Strategy

The search strategy was based on the database sources of Medline, PubMed, CINAHL, Web of Science, Informit, The Cochrane Collaboration, Scopus, and Google Scholar. A subsequent snowball search of the reference lists of included full text articles was conducted to find further relevant sources. References were stored using EndNote X8™.

The search strategy was centred around six key concepts highlighted in Table 1: 'strongyloidiasis', 'severe disease', 'pregnancy', 'infant', 'immune status', and 'eosinophilia'. 'Severe disease' was defined as any disease classified in the article as disseminated strongyloidiasis (DS) or hyperinfection syndrome (HS). Pregnancy included the presence of a live fetus at any week of gestation. 'Immune status' was used to find references to immunosuppressed populations in which strongyloidiasis may occur, such as HIV or HTLV1-infected cohorts.

Table 1. Concepts and synonyms used in search strategy.

#	Concept	Key Words
1	Strongyloidiasis	Strongyl * OR Anguillulose
2	Severity of disease	Disseminat * OR Hyperinfect * OR Severe OR Fatal OR Mortality OR Morbidity OR Death *
3	Pregnancy	Pregnan * OR Mother * OR Matern * OR Antenat * OR Natal OR Perinat *
4	Infant	Neonat * OR Newborn OR Infant * OR Baby * OR Fetus * OR Foetus * OR Fetal OR Preterm OR Child OR Prematur * OR Low Birth Weight OR LBW OR Birth Weight OR Intrauterine Growth Restriction OR IUGR OR FGR OR SGA
5	Immune status	Immunocompromised OR Tumour OR Cancer OR Haematolog * OR Lymphom * OR Leukaem * OR Neoplas * OR Malignan * OR HIV OR HTLV1 OR Rheumat * OR Diabet * OR Transplant * OR Steroid * OR Corticosteroid * OR Immunosuppress * OR Glucocorticoid * OR Sepsis
6	Eosinophilia	Eosin *

* keywords were truncated with asterisks added, to locate all forms of the word during the literature search.

Synonyms were drafted with the help of other strongyloidiasis-related literature reviews [6,26,27]. Search terms were modified to fit with the search requirements of each database used, including the use of MeSH terms for PubMed. Literature searching commenced on 26 July 2017 and was completed on 9 August 2017. The full search strategy outlining the combinations of terms used is depicted in Table 2.

Table 2. Combinations of key words used in search strategy.

Number Search	Combination
1.	1 + 3
2.	1 + 6
3.	1 + 2 + 3
4.	1 + 2 + 6
5.	1 + 3 + 4
6.	1 + 3 + 5
7.	1 + 3 + 6
8.	1 + 4 + 6
9.	1 + 5 + 6

2.2. Data Collection and Analysis

Titles and then abstracts were screened for potential inclusion. The full texts were then read to determine their eligibility according to the search criteria. If the full text could not be found, attempts were made to contact the authors or other institutions to access a full text. Articles that met the criteria were included for analysis.

A standardised spreadsheet was used to extract data from the full text articles. Data items obtained included study date, sample size, country, funding sources, ethics approval, characteristics of participants, outcomes measured, method of testing for *S. stercoralis*, statistical analysis performed, prevalence of strongyloidiasis, eosinophilia, limitations or confounding factors, and results of outcomes measured. Thematic analysis involving the simple pooling of data items was performed. Included studies and their data points were presented in both individual and aggregated tables. Due to the articles being primarily observational studies with a heterogeneous range of outcomes studied, meta-analysis was not performed.

2.3. Inclusion Criteria

We included all quantitative studies that tested for *Strongyloides* infections in cohorts of pregnant women, newborns, or children aged 0 to 18 years of age. If the study cohort focused on children, articles were only included if they measured the long-term effects on participants. Articles were included regardless of what outcomes they measured, such as haemoglobin (Hb) levels, neurocognitive function, or anthropometry. Types of research that were included in this review consisted of randomised control trials, observational studies, and individual case reports. Case reports were included due to the limited results that we found in our scoping searches prior to the formal literature search. By including case reports on top of the more rigorous primary literature, we can present a full landscape of current studies of strongyloidiasis in pregnant women and children.

2.4. Exclusion Criteria

Epidemiological studies that only commented on risk factors for infection (rather than outcomes) were excluded. Animal studies were excluded as no studies specifically looking at strongyloidiasis in pregnant animals were identified. Conference proceedings, poster presentations, and abstracts without a full text were also excluded. No language restrictions or date ranges were placed on included texts.

We hypothesised that there would be very little literature discussing srongyloidiasis in pregnant women and their children, and that many of the studies may have suboptimal methodological quality. As such, we did not exclude studies based on their methodology or statistical analysis used, as if they were found to be of generally poor quality, this would be an important limitation of current research to discuss.

2.5. Methodological Quality

A quality assessment of the observational studies was conducted according to a scale specifically generated for this review (Table 3). The scale is a modification of previously validated tools and used criteria from the Quality Appraisal for Cadaveric Studies (QUACS) scale first used by Smith et al., the Newcastle-Ottawa Scale (NOS), and an independent scale used in a similar systematic literature review [28–30]. QUACS and NOS have been validated as accurate tools to use in observational studies; however, specific items were added to the scale to make it more applicable for assessing the studies included in this review [31]. Due to the heterogeneous nature of methodologies and results used, we refrained from providing a score to assess and compare quality.

Table 3. Quality assessment tool used for observational studies.

	Low Risk	Medium Risk	High Risk
Objective stated	Aims and objectives fully described with reasons for why they are important	Aims and objectives described, no reasons given for having these aims	Aims and objectives not fully described
Ethics and funding	Mentioned, no conflicts	Mentioned, potential conflicts of interest	Not mentioned or conflicts of interest
Methods described	Methods discussed and are reliable	Methods discussed, but may not be reliable	Methods not fully discussed
Details context of group	Participant characteristics outlined with discussion of how an accurate sample was ensured	Participant characteristics outlined	Participant characteristics not fully outlined
Inclusion criteria, exclusion criteria, sample size	Fully described with reasons given	Fully described	Not adequately described
Education of researchers	Education given, researchers have appropriate experience or qualifications	Education given, experience or qualifications not mentioned	Education and experience is not discussed
Methodological bias discussed and addressed	Efforts made to identify and solve potential bias	Mention of potential bias in methodology	No mention of bias in methodology
More than one researcher	More than one researcher	N/A	Only one researcher
Statistical analysis appropriate	Multivariate logistic regression is used	Chi square analysis is used	Any other form of analysis is used
Results presented thoroughly	Results fully and accurately described	Only partial results given	Important results omitted or not thoroughly described
Study discussed in context	Results analysed according to other studies	Results are analysed, some mention of current context	Results analysed with no mention to other research
Clinical implications of results	Direct clinical application of results is discussed	Mention of clinical relevance is made	No mention of clinical implications of results
Limitations and confounding factors	Study discussed limitations and confounding factors comprehensively	Some discussion of limitations and confounding factors	No discussion of limitations or confounding factors

N/A: not applicable.

Case series were assessed for quality according to the Joanna Briggs Institute Critical Appraisal Tool: Checklist for Case Reports [32]. The risk of bias evaluations was not used to exclude studies from data synthesis but rather would be utilised to comment on the current gaps in literature and accuracy of results.

3. Results

Database and reference list searching returned 1666 unique results, of which 94 were considered eligible for full-text review. The full texts of 29 sources could not be found, even after attempts were made to contact authors, libraries, and institutions to access a copy. These studies were decades old, focused on other parasites, and from the citation information available did not indicate that they would add further use to this review or significantly change the conclusions. This left 65 full-text articles that were read in full. Based on our inclusion and exclusion criteria, 45 articles were then excluded. Thirty-nine full texts were excluded as they were either found to be irrelevant or were solely epidemiological studies and did not measure health outcomes of their participants. Six studies were found to be review articles and were subsequently excluded. This left a total of 20 studies for inclusion.

Sixteen articles were sourced from electronic library databases, while the remaining four studies were individually added from the Google Scholar search; no further articles were added after reviewing the reference lists of included full-texts. Sixteen studies were original research papers while four articles were individual case reports that discussed *Strongyloides* in pregnant women. Countries in which studies were performed included Australia (1), France (1), Ghana (2), Guatemala (1), India (1), Kenya (1), Nigeria (1), Papua New Guinea (3), Peru (2), Tanzania (1), Thailand (2), Uganda (2), Unites States of America (USA, 2) and Venezuela (1). Publication dates of the articles ranged from 1989 until 2015. The outcomes of the search strategy are summarised in Appendix B. For the purpose of clarity, the research papers will be discussed separately to the case studies.

3.1. Study Characteristics

Participant demographics included pregnant women (3), pregnant women and their newborn children (5), or only infected children (8). Participants were mostly from low socio-economic environments, and hygiene was typically stated as poor in the studies. Only one study focused specifically on *S. stercoralis* infections, and two studies focused on *S. fuelleborni*. The majority of studies either surveyed all helminth infections in their cohorts, or their main focus was on other helminths, malaria, or HIV, and happened to include data on strongyloidiasis. The study settings included in-hospital environments (3), community settings (10), or antenatal and postnatal clinics (3) (Table 4).

3.2. Quality Assessment

Overall, the methodological rigour of the literature was of a low quality. With regard to the prospective studies, 16 were cohort studies while only one was a case-control study; there were no randomised controlled trials included. The studies were found to vary widely in their study designs, attempts to control bias, and outcomes measured (Appendix C, Figure A3).

Nine studies used logistic regression, while five studies use chi-square analysis. The majority of studies did not consider or report potential bias being present in their studies and took limited steps to prevent this from affecting their results. Many studies did not adequately discuss their inclusion and exclusion criteria, sample sizes, or the involvement of researchers in data collection. The cohorts were often arbitrarily chosen and not adequately matched. Many of the studies were quoted to be using data from other larger trials without discussing any potential bias in these results. The majority of studies only reported data selectively and did not specify the non-significant results.

Case reports were overall of a high quality and comprehensively discussed the clinical relevance of their patients (Appendix C, Figure A4).

3.3. Risk of Bias of Included Studies

Generally, the literature did not appropriately comment on potential limitations or confounding factors to their research. Some commonly mentioned limitations amongst studies included small sample sizes, small prevalence data of *S. stercoralis*, inappropriate testing methods, and inability to follow-up with included participants.

Table 4. Study Characteristics.

Author, Year, Country	Study Design	Participant Characteristics	Sample Size	Length of Review	Setting	Prevalence
Baidoo et al., (2010), Ghana [33]	Prospective observational cohort study	Pregnant women	108	12 months	Community	2%
Barnish et al., (1989), Papua New Guinea [34]	Prospective observational cohort study	Children <5 years	12	NR	Community	63%
Cabada et al., (2014), Peru [35]	Prospective observational cohort study	Amazonian clan members, all ages	215	NR	Community	6%
Mangklabruks et al., (2012), Thailand [36]	Prospective observational cohort study	Newborns followed from antenatal clinic visits	2184	1 year 9 months	Antenatal and postnatal clinics	0.8%
Dada-Adegbola et al., (2004), Nigeria [37]	Prospective observational cohort study	Children <5 years with diarrhoea	227	NR	Hospital	5.3%
Dreyfuss et al., (2001), Tanzania [38]	Prospective observational cohort study	HIV-infected pregnant women and their newborns	822	NR	Antenatal and postnatal clinics	1.78%
Egger et al., (1990), Thailand [39]	Prospective observational cohort study	Children 3–8 years	343	NR	Community	25.4%
Herrera et al., (2006), Peru [40]	Prospective observational case-control study	Community members <20 years	100	1 month	Community	27%
King et al., (2004), Papua New Guinea [41]	Prospective observational cohort study	Children <5 years	179	4 months	Community	27%
LaBeaud et al., (2015), Kenya [42]	Prospective observational cohort study	Mothers and their infants <3 years	545	3 years	Community	NR
Muhangi et al., (2007), Uganda [43]	Prospective observational cohort study	Pregnant women	2507	1 year 7 months	Hospital	12.3%
Nampijja et al., (2012), Uganda [44]	Prospective observational cohort study	Mothers and their infants <15 months	983	2 years	Antenatal and postnatal clinics	13%
Phuanukoonnon et al., (2013), Papua New Guinea [45]	Prospective observational cohort study	Pregnant women	201	1 year 5 months	Community	3%
Verhagen et al., (2013), Venezuela [46]	Prospective observational cohort study	Children 4–17 years	390	1 year 6 months	Community	7.9%
Villar et al., (1989), Guatemala [47]	Prospective observational cohort study	Mothers and their newborns	14,914	1 year 9 months	Community	0.4%
Yatich et al., (2010), Ghana [48]	Prospective observational cohort study	Mothers and their newborns	746	2 months	Hospital	3.9%

NR: not reported.

3.4. Prevalence

The prevalence of *S. stercoralis* in the studies was typically low, with a mean prevalence of 12.3% and the median prevalence being 6%. Studies with mixed urban and rural cohorts found that the prevalence of strongyloidiasis was higher in participants from rural areas. A few studies noted that their prevalence data was unreliable due to using suboptimal testing methods that have been proven to be inaccurate for detecting *S. stercoralis* [6].

3.5. Method of Testing

All the studies included in this review used various methods of stool-sample analysis to determine the rates of *S. stercoralis* infections in their cohorts. Methods included the Baermann (3 studies), Kato-Katz (4), Ritchie (1), formol-ether concentration (2), simple smear technique (1), volume dilution method (1), or were unspecified (4). No studies utilised serological testing. Single samples with limited follow-up were used, rather than the serial testing of multiple specimens.

3.6. Effects on LBW

Four studies measured the effect that *S. stercoralis* infection in pregnant women had on the birth weight of their offspring [36,38,47,48]. Two studies, one in Thailand and one in Tanzanian HIV-infected mothers, found odds ratios of 4.93 (95% CI 1.47, 16.50) and 4.23 (95% CI 1.24, 14.41), respectively, that LBW was caused by strongyloidiasis (Table 5) [36,38]. One study in Ghana found an odds ratio of 2.1 (95% CI 0.97, 4.49) for LBW, small for gestational age (SGA), or preterm delivery [48]. The fourth study found a non-significant increased risk of IUGR; the study attributed a low prevalence of strongyloidiasis to the failure to achieve a statistically significant result [47]. IUGR was predominantly seen in malnourished women who had strongyloidiasis, and the study authors hypothesised this as a possible cause rather than the helminth itself. None of the studies measured the length of duration of *S. stercoralis* infection in the pregnant mother, or the intensity of larval output as an indicator of the severity of the infection.

3.7. Anthropometry

Five studies analysed whether there were long term effects of *Strongyloides* infections on the nutrition and growth of infected children (Table 6) [39–42,46]. Three studies found that strongyloidiasis was associated with decreased weight-for-height or weight-for-age z-scores. However, not all of these were statistically significant [39,40,46]. These measurements are more typically used to determine wasting, which is an acute indicator of malnutrition, rather than the more chronic indicator of stunting. One study found a statistically significant relationship between strongyloidiasis and decreased height-for-age z-score ($p < 0.01$), which is used to measure stunting [39]. One study found that at 30 months of age, children with strongyloidiasis had a decreased head circumference ($p = 0.002$); this same study did not find any significant link to other anthropometric measures. One study found no statistically significant relationships between stunting, wasting, and *S. stercoralis* infections, but did note that the intensity of infection was associated with decreased weight-for-age and weight-for-height z-scores, within the *Strongyloides*-infected population ($p = 0.02$, 0.016 respectively) [41]. Another article found that children infected with strongyloidiasis were substantially more likely to suffer from marasmus or kwashiorkor when compared to non-infected children ($p = 0.001$) [40]. The majority of studies also found that polyparasitism was more strongly associated with lower z-scores of all the anthropometric measures when compared to solely *S. stercoralis* infection.

Table 5. Methodology and outcomes of *Strongyloides* infections.

Study	Only *S. stercoralis* Is Assessed	Results Are Aggregated	Testing Method for *S. stercoralis*	Statistical Analysis	Results
33	No	Yes	Stool; formol-ether concentration method	Chi-square test	Helminth infections are a predictor of iron-deficiency anaemia in pregnant women
34	No	No	Stool; not specified	Correlation coefficient	Heavy infection predisposes to poor growth
35	No	No	Stool; Kato-Katz method	Chi-square test	High rates of anaemia and malnutrition in children. Helminth infections not associated with these outcomes. *Strongyloides* was not managed by treatment
36	No	Yes	Not specified	Multivariate logistic regression	Odds ratio of 4.93 of *Strongyloides*/hookworm infection in pregnancy causing LBW (95% CI 1.47, 16.50)
37	Yes	N/A	Stool; formol-ether concentration methods	Logistic regression	Higher rates of malnutrition in *Strongyloides*-infected children. Malnutrition may increase the risk of contracting *Strongyloides*
38	No	No	Stool; Kato-Katz method	Multivariate logistic regression	Odds ratio of 4.23 for *Strongyloides* causing LBW (95% CI 1.24, 14.41)
39	No	No	Stool; simple smear technique	Chi-square test	Lower mean height-for-age z-score ($p < 0.01$)
40	No	No	Stool; Baermann method	Multivariate logistic regression	Malnutrition more common in *Strongyloides* infections. No relationship between *Strongyloides* and anthropometry
41	No	No	Stool; volume dilution method	Logistic regression	*Strongyloides* associated with decreased weight-for-age z-score ($p < 0.05$). Not associated with weight-for-height z-score ($p < 0.05$)
42	No	No	Stool; Ritchie method	Logistic regression	*Strongyloides* at 30 months is associated with decreased head circumference ($p = 0.002$)
43	No	No	Stool; Kato-Katz method	Logistic regression	No relationship between *Strongyloides* and anaemia
44	No	No	Stool; Kato-Katz method	Logistic regression	Negative impact on language function of infants ($p < 0.05$). Non-significant impact on gross motor, sociocognition, and self-care
45	No	Yes	Stool; not specified	Chi-square test	No relationship to anaemia
46	No	No	Stool; Baermann and Kato-Katz methods	Multivariate logistic regression	No relationship to anaemia. Non-significant relationship between weight-for-age and BMI-for-age
47	No	No	Not specified	Multivariate logistic regression	Increased risk of IUGR. Malnourished women with *Strongyloides* most at risk
48	No	No	Stool; Baermann method	Chi-square and *t*-test	Malaria co-infection had higher rates of pre-term delivery, small-for-gestational-age, and LBW ($p < 0.05$)

N/A: not applicable.

Table 6. Anthropometric changes associated with *S. stercoralis* infections.

Study	Weight-for-Age z-Score	Weight-for-Height z-Score	Height-for-Age z-Score	Head Circumference z-Score
39	NR	-1.01 (p = NS)	-2.03 ($p < 0.01$)	NR
40	Positive association (p = 0.045)	NR	No association (p = 0.24)	NR
41	No association	No association	No association	NR
42	No association	No association	No association	-1.69 (p = 0.002) at 30 months
43	NR	-0.24 (p = NS)	NR	NR

NR: not reported.

Generally, consensus from the studies was that malnutrition either predisposes participants to *S. stercoralis* infections or chronic strongyloidiasis may cause malnutrition. Due to their study designs, firm conclusions could not be made to determine whether strongyloidiasis is a risk factor or consequence of malnutrition. This issue becomes further complicated when considering that strongyloidiasis was seen more commonly in populations of lower socio-economic status, as malnutrition is also more commonly observed in these groups.

3.8. Strongyloidiasis and Anaemia

Five studies measured whether *S. stercoralis* contributed to maternal anaemia [33,35,43,45,46]. One study found that helminth infections were a predictor of iron-deficiency anaemia. However, the helminths were not differentiated in the results so conclusions cannot be made about the effects of *S. stercoralis* [33]. The other four studies found no relationship between strongyloidiasis and anaemia.

3.9. Case Reports

Four case reports were found as part of the literature search that fulfilled our inclusion criteria (Table 7) [49–52]. All four cases describe women who presented at varying stages of gestation with predominantly gastrointestinal or respiratory symptoms. Two cases were classified as HS, one as DS, and one was symptomatic but non-disseminated. Corticosteroids preceded two of the cases, and in both of these cases the patients were found to have either HS or DS. Two women had HTLV-1 co-infections, which has been previously noted as a common occurrence. Two women required ICU admissions, and one patient died from cardiorespiratory arrest secondary to septic shock. Fetal demise also occurred in the patient who passed away [48].

All patients were treated with ivermectin. Of the three women who survived, all underwent spontaneous vaginal births to healthy babies, with no complications. They made a full recovery from the infection, although one mother re-presented a year later, again pregnant and suffering from gastrointestinal symptoms [50]. She was found to have been re-infected with *S. stercoralis*.

Table 7. Summary of case reports.

Author, Year, Country	Country of Origin, Gestation	Presenting Complaint	HS or DS?	Corticosteroids Administered	Treatment	Outcome
Buresch et al., 2015, USA [49]	Haiti, 25 weeks	Chest pain, dyspnoea, copious bilious vomiting	HS	Betamethasone 12 mg, 2 doses 24 h apart	Ivermectin	Septic shock, SIRS, cardiopulmonary arrest, fetal demise
Heaton et al., 2002, USA [52]	Ethiopia, 9 weeks	Diarrhoea, epigastric pain, vomiting	None	None	Ivermectin 200 μg/kg	SVB at term, cleared of infection
Malézieux-Picard et al., 2016, France [50]	Burkina Faso, 32 weeks	Abdominal pain, anorexia, constipation, weight loss	HS	Betamethasone 12 mg stat	Ivermectin 200 μg/kg/day for 3 days	SVB, recovered from infection
Prasad et al., 2016, India [51]	India, 39 weeks	Cough, watery diarrhoea	DS	None	Ivermectin 12 mg	SVB, cleared of infection

SVB: spontaneous vaginal birth.

4. Discussion

This review aimed to summarise current literature that analysed the long-term health outcomes of strongyloidiasis on pregnant women, their offspring, and children. Our findings suggest that there are enduring consequences for children that are either born to infected mothers, or who are chronically infected early in their development. To our knowledge, this is the first systematic literature review that attempts to determine the possibility of chronic health effects caused by strongyloidiasis in these subgroups.

The small number of studies that investigated the birth outcomes of newborns with infected mothers found that there is an association between strongyloidiasis and LBW. The 95% confidence intervals of these studies were large, despite always showing positive associations with LBW. Research has consistently recognised LBW to have lasting impacts on the morbidity and mortality of these newborns, as per the Barker and Brenner hypotheses [53]. The reliability of strongyloidiasis causing LBW is still questionable, as studies were conducted in developing countries with participants that had a range of other comorbidities (such as HIV). Therefore, further research and analysis of this potential risk factor is required. If strongyloidiasis is confirmed to cause LBW, the infection should be treated like other known risk factors for LBW, and women should receive appropriate prenatal screening and treatment [54].

Studies that measured the anthropometry of infected infants and children generally agreed that strongyloidiasis did result in a negative impact on their growth. Wasting and stunting are long-term detriments to the wellbeing of children, and research has established that they lead to increased medical comorbidities, reduced schooling, and reduced economic productivity [55,56]. The main effects of strongyloidiasis were only seen in the more acute measurement of wasting, rather than the more chronic indicator of stunting, thus the clinical implications of this finding are less certain. However, a study conducted by Richard et al. found that wasting was associated with stunting and the long-term effects that go with this [57]. Therefore, strongyloidiasis is likely to have clinically significant impacts on the health of people infected during childhood. Ivermectin should be used as part of existing community and school-based deworming initiatives in endemic areas, to prevent the enduring consequences of wasting.

The assessment of strongyloidiasis affecting the growth of children is affected by the small number of included articles that commented on these measurements. Studies also did not publish their full results lists, and the differences in cohort characteristics were large. Epidemiologically, the studies were unable to determine if strongyloidiasis was more common in malnourished children or if the disease process itself caused malnutrition. As the studies were cross-sectional, no studies looked at whether children had been chronically infected with strongyloidiasis. In order to confidently conclude that *S. stercoralis* does in fact cause deficiencies in growth and therefore have direct clinical consequences, longitudinal studies of affected participants with larger sample sizes need to be performed.

Several studies noted a range of common epidemiological risk factors which may lead to a greater risk of infants and pregnant women contracting this infection. Absence of footwear, other household members already being infected, and poor sanitation facilities, were all emphasised in the studies as potential risk factors. This poses another challenge to public health strategies, as newborns can quickly become chronically infested from their mothers or family members. Even if strongyloidiasis does not cause LBW, maternal infection can still cause chronic health effects due to the high likelihood of passing on their infection early in childhood and causing malnutrition, wasting or stunting. Interventions targeting water, sanitation, and hygiene (WASH) may provide a solution to reducing these epidemiological risk factors and therefore the long-term consequences of strongyloidiasis [58].

Based on the review findings, anaemia should not be considered a potential complication of *S. stercoralis* infections. This is in contrast to other helminths such as hookworm, which have been more strongly linked with anaemia [59]. Studies that have observed the clinical manifestations of strongyloidiasis in different cohorts have produced conflicting results regarding anaemia [60,61]. The primary reason why we are still not sure whether *S. stercoralis* causes anaemia is because both are typically common in under-nourished, socio-economically poorer populations with increased health comorbidities. This makes the task of attributing anaemia to the helminth difficult.

There is a paucity in literature looking at the effects of *S. stercoralis* infection on pregnant women, their offspring, and infected children. The only literature that could be found that mentions pregnant women with severe infection were case studies; no prospective studies could be found in which pregnancy was researched as a potential risk factor of HS or DS. Likewise, very little information currently exists to determine whether *S. stercoralis* infection in the mother is an independent risk factor for LBW, SGA, IUGR, or preterm delivery. As there were so few studies found analysing these variables, this may suggest a publication bias is present which has inflated the health effects strongyloidiasis has on these populations.

Although only a few case reports exist that discuss strongyloidiasis in pregnancy, the ones found in this review showed that this infection can cause severe or ultimately fatal complications. Pregnant women are already immunosuppressed and thus may be at a higher risk of hyperinfection syndrome. Clinicians must currently rely on individual cases for information on the possible disease course of strongyloidiasis or look elsewhere to different population groups. Corticosteroids preceded 50% of the onset of HS, although the sample was small. In areas endemic to *S. stercoralis*, women giving preterm birth or who are immunosuppressed are at risk of these severe complications and should be screened accordingly.

There is reason to believe that the prevalence and therefore the health effects of strongyloidiasis is underestimated in the current literature. The majority of studies only included *S. stercoralis* as one of many parasites tested. As the researchers were not directly focusing on strongyloidiasis they accordingly did not use accurate diagnostic tests and therefore are likely to have missed a significant amount of *S. stercoralis* infections in their participants. Even amongst stool samples, the gold standard of seven serial samples was not performed [1]. This may have had the potential to understate the longitudinal consequences strongyloidiasis had on children and thereby prevented studies from achieving statistical significance. This failure to achieve significance and the substantially low prevalence data compared to other helminths may have resulted in unpublished data, creating a relative publication bias in the literature reviewed. Healthcare providers would benefit from more accurate prevalence data in order to appropriately manage these subgroups. Therefore, the convenient and reliable serological tests should be used in further studies on strongyloidiasis.

If strongyloidiasis does indeed lead to adverse health effects in infants, this has direct clinical implications for endemic areas. This review strengthens arguments for increased screening and treatment of pregnant women to confer the best possible outcome for their children. Ivermectin has been proven to be safe in pregnancy, despite not currently being used due to its assigned pregnancy category of B3 [62]. The clinicians in all four case reports used ivermectin and no complications were observed. It is the opinion of the authors that there is enough favourable evidence to support the use of ivermectin in pregnancy, particularly given the significance of the consequences to mothers and children. Health practitioners in endemic areas would benefit from further clarification of whether this drug is appropriate for use in pregnant women.

The findings outlined in this review need to be considered with caution, as only a small number of studies have currently looked at these effects and their methodological quality may be considered suboptimal. While some studies did achieve statistical significance in their findings, they often occurred in small samples, in participants with comorbidities such as HIV or malnutrition, and in countries in developing nations; thus, their findings cannot be generalised.

Limitations

A number of limitations to this review have been identified and must be taken into consideration when analysing the findings. Studies reviewed used varying methods of statistical analysis, which were presented and compared despite some results not being statistically significant or insufficiently powered. Many studies were conducted decades ago in vastly different contexts, using less accurate testing methods. It was unfortunate that some studies aggregated the results of *S. stercoralis* with other helminths such as hookworm; these were still included in the review. A significant proportion of our included full-texts also could not be found. Meta-analysis could not be performed and thus only simple pooling of results was possible. Due to the marked variation in the outcomes assessed by different studies, the findings were compared between cohorts that varied dramatically in their characteristics. Because of these limitations, a level of bias in the findings was unavoidable, despite taking steps to ensure transparency and academic rigour.

5. Conclusions

In conclusion, current research is suggestive that maternal strongyloidiasis is a risk factor for LBW. However, a lack of literature and sub-optimal study designs prevents this from being a certainty. Chronic infection in childhood is most strongly associated with wasting and may potentially lead to stunting. Due to similar issues, current research is unable to ascertain whether strongyloidiasis leads to malnutrition or is just more commonly found in the malnourished. The strongest conclusion gleaned from this literature review was that the prevalence of strongyloidiasis was very likely underestimated, due to the methods of testing and lack of focus on this specific helminth in the study designs. In order to truly determine whether pregnant women, their offspring, and infected children are in fact susceptible sub-groups of the population, further longitudinal research utilising modern serological techniques and control groups is required.

Funding: This research received no external funding.

Acknowledgments: We are grateful to Caroline de Costa and Robyn McDermott for their support in producing this review. This paper is dedicated to the memory of Emeritus Professor Rick Speare. His contributions to the field of parasitology are an inspiration that will continue to guide future researchers for years to come.

Conflicts of Interest: The authors declare no conflict of interest.

Appendix A

Section/topic	#	Checklist item	Reported on page #
TITLE			
Title	1	Identify the report as a systematic review, meta-analysis, or both.	1
ABSTRACT			
Structured summary	2	Provide a structured summary including, as applicable: background; objectives; data sources; study eligibility criteria, participants, and interventions; study appraisal and synthesis methods; results; limitations, conclusions and implications of key findings; systematic review registration number.	1
INTRODUCTION			
Rationale	3	Describe the rationale for the review in the context of what is already known.	2
Objectives	4	Provide an explicit statement of questions being addressed with reference to participants, interventions, comparisons, outcomes, and study design (PICOS).	3
METHODS			
Protocol and registration	5	Indicate if a review protocol exists, if and where it can be accessed (e.g., Web address), and, if available, provide registration information including registration number.	3
Eligibility criteria	6	Specify study characteristics (e.g., PICOS, length of follow-up) and report characteristics (e.g., years considered, language, publication status) used as criteria for eligibility, giving rationale	3
Information sources	7	Describe all information sources (e.g., databases with dates of coverage, contact with study authors to identify additional studies) in the search and date last searched	3
Search	8	Present full electronic search strategy for at least one database, including any limits used, such that it could be repeated.	4
Study selection	9	State the process for selecting studies (i.e., screening, eligibility, included in systematic review, and, if applicable, included in the meta-analysis).	4
Data collection process	10	Describe method of data extraction from reports (e.g., piloted forms, independently, in duplicate) and any processes for obtaining and confirming data from investigators.	4
Data items	11	List and define all variables for which data were sought (e.g., PICOS, funding sources) and any assumptions and simplifications made.	4
Risk of bias in individual studies	12	Describe methods used for assessing risk of bias of individual studies (including specification of whether this was done at the study or outcome level), and how this information is to be used in any data synthesis.	5
Summary measures	13	State the principal summary measures (e.g., risk ratio, difference in means).	4
Synthesis of results	14	Describe the methods of handling data and combining results of studies, if done, including measures of consistency (e.g., I², I³) for each meta-analysis.	4

Figure A1. *Cont.*

Section/topic	#	Checklist item	Reported on page #
Risk of bias across studies	15	Specify any assessment of risk of bias that may affect the cumulative evidence (e.g., publication bias, selective reporting within studies).	5
Additional analyses	16	Describe methods of additional analyses (e.g., sensitivity or subgroup analyses, meta-regression), if done, indicating which were pre-specified.	N/A
RESULTS			
Study selection	17	Give numbers of studies screened, assessed for eligibility, and included in the review, with reasons for exclusions at each stage, ideally with a flow diagram.	6
Study characteristics	18	For each study, present characteristics for which data were extracted (e.g., study size, PICOS, follow-up period) and provide the citations.	9
Risk of bias within studies	19	Present data on risk of bias of each study and, if available, any outcome level assessment (see item 12).	8
Results of individual studies	20	For all outcomes considered (benefits or harms), present, for each study: (a) simple summary data for each intervention group (b) effect estimates and confidence intervals, ideally with a forest plot.	6
Synthesis of results	21	Present results of each meta-analysis done, including confidence intervals and measures of consistency.	N/A
Risk of bias across studies	22	Present results of any assessment of risk of bias across studies (see Item 15).	8
Additional analysis	23	Give results of additional analyses, if done (e.g., sensitivity or subgroup analyses, meta-regression [see Item 16]).	N/A
DISCUSSION			
Summary of evidence	24	Summarize the main findings including the strength of evidence for each main outcome; consider their relevance to key groups (e.g., healthcare providers, users, and policy makers).	11
Limitations	25	Discuss limitations at study and outcome level (e.g., risk of bias), and at review-level (e.g., incomplete retrieval of identified research, reporting bias).	13
Conclusions	26	Provide a general interpretation of the results in the context of other evidence, and implications for future research.	14
FUNDING			
Funding	27	Describe sources of funding for the systematic review and other support (e.g., supply of data); role of funders for the systematic review.	14

Figure A1. Preferred Reporting Items for Systematic Reviews and Meta-Analyses (PRISMA) checklist.

Appendix B

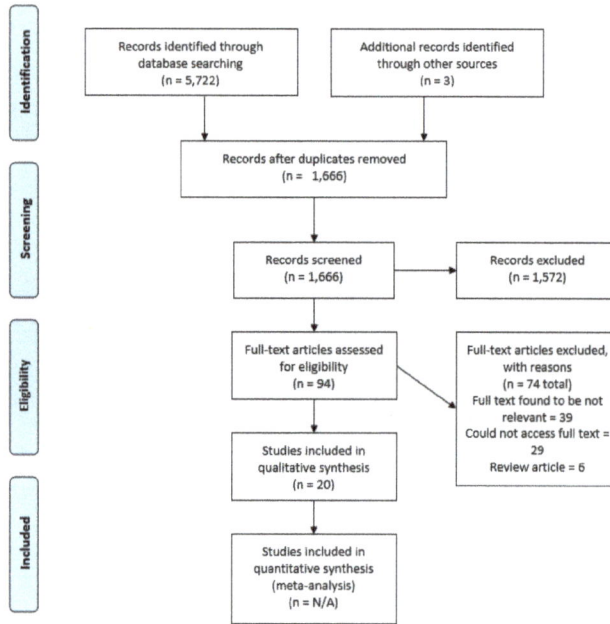

Figure A2. PRISMA flow diagram.

Appendix C

		Objective stated	Ethics and funding	Methods described	Details context of group	Inclusion, exclusion, sample size	Education of researchers	Methodological bias discussed and addressed	More than one researcher	Statistical analysis appropriate	Results presented thoroughly	Study discussed in context	Clinical implications of results	Limitations and confounding factors
33		M	H	M	H	H	M	H	H	M	L	L	M	H
34		H	H	M	H	H	M	H	H	H	M	H	H	M
35		L	L	M	L	H	M	H	H	M	L	M	L	H
36		L	L	H	L	M	H	H	L	L	L	L	L	L
37		L	H	M	M	H	M	H	H	M	M	M	M	H
38		L	L	M	L	M	M	H	L	L	L	L	L	H
39		M	H	M	M	H	M	H	H	M	M	L	M	H
40		L	H	L	H	M	M	H	L	L	H	H	H	H
41		H	H	M	H	H	M	H	H	L	M	M	H	H
42		M	L	M	L	M	M	M	L	L	M	L	L	L
43		M	L	M	M	M	M	M	H	L	L	M	M	M
44		M	L	M	M	M	M	M	L	L	L	L	M	M
45		H	L	H	H	H	M	H	H	M	L	M	H	H
46		M	L	L	L	M	M	M	L	L	L	M	M	M
47		M	H	H	M	H	M	M	L	L	L	M	L	M
48		M	L	L	M	H	M	H	H	M	L	M	L	M

Legend:
- L — Low Risk
- M — Medium Risk
- H — High

Figure A3. Quality assessment scale.

	Y	Yes
	NA	Not Applicable
	N	No

	Demographics described	History	Current clinical condition	Diagnostic tests appropriate	Treatment clearly described	Post-intervention condition	Adverse events identified	Takeaway lessons
49	Y	Y	Y	Y	Y	Y	Y	Y
50	Y	Y	Y	Y	Y	N	NA	Y
50	Y	Y	Y	Y	Y	Y	Y	Y
51	Y	Y	Y	Y	Y	N	NA	Y

Figure A4. Quality assessment according to JBI Critical Appraisal Tool: Checklist for Case Reports.

References

1. Bisoffi, Z.; Buonfrate, D.; Montresor, A.; Requena-Méndez, A.; Muñoz, J.; Krolewiecki, A.J.; Gotuzzo, E.; Mena, M.A.; Chiodini, P.L.; Anselmi, M.; et al. *Strongyloides stercoralis*: A plea for action. *PLoS Negl. Trop. Dis.* **2013**, *7*, e2214. [CrossRef] [PubMed]

2. Puthiyakunnon, S.; Boddu, S.; Li, Y.; Zhou, X.; Wang, C.; Li, J.; Chen, X. Strongyloidiasis—An insight into its global prevalence and management. *PLoS Negl. Trop. Dis.* **2014**, *8*, e3018. [CrossRef] [PubMed]

3. Caumes, E.; Keystone, J.S. Acute strongyloidiasis: A rarity. Chronic strongyloidiasis: A time bomb! *J. Travel Med.* **2011**, *18*, 71–72. [CrossRef] [PubMed]

4. Grove, D.I. Human strongyloidiasis. *Adv. Parasitol.* **1996**, *38*, 251–309. [PubMed]

5. Siddiqui, A.A.; Berk, S.L. Diagnosis of *Strongyloides stercoralis* infection. *Clin. Infect. Dis.* **2001**, *33*, 1040–1047. [CrossRef] [PubMed]

6. Requena-Méndez, A.; Chiodini, P.; Bisoffi, Z.; Buonfrate, D.; Gotuzzo, E.; Muñoz, J. The laboratory diagnosis and follow up of strongyloidiasis: A systematic review. *PLoS Negl. Trop. Dis.* **2013**, *7*, e2002. [CrossRef] [PubMed]

7. Centers for Disease Control. Resources for Health Professionals. Strongyloidiasis Website. Published 2016. Updated 19 August 2017. Available online: https://www.cdc.gov/parasites/strongyloides/health_professionals/index.html (accessed on 27 August 2017).

8. Shield, J.M.; Page, W. Effective diagnostic tests and anthelmintic treatment for *Strongyloides stercoralis* make community control feasible. *P. N. G. Med. J.* **2008**, *51*, 105–119. [PubMed]

9. Mejia, R.; Nutman, T.B. Screening, prevention, and treatment for hyperinfection syndrome and disseminated infections caused by *Strongyloides stercoralis*. *Curr. Opin. Infect. Dis.* **2012**, *25*, 458–463. [CrossRef] [PubMed]

10. Kassalik, M.; Mönkemüller, K. *Strongyloides stercoralis* Hyperinfection syndrome and disseminated disease. *Gastroenterol. Hepatol.* **2011**, *7*, 766–768.

11. Milner, P.; Irvine, R.; Barton, C.; Bras, G.; Richards, R. Intestinal malabsorption in *Strongyloides stercoralis* infestation. *Gut* **1965**, *6*, 574. [CrossRef] [PubMed]

12. Kotcher, E.; Miranda, M.; Esquivel, R.; Peña-Chavarría, A.; Donohugh, D.L.; Baldizón, C.; Acosta, A.; Apuy, J.L. Intestinal malabsorption and helminthic and protozoan infections of the small intestine. *Gastroenterology* **1966**, *50*, 366–371. [PubMed]

13. Robinson, D.P.; Klein, S.L. Pregnancy and pregnancy-associated hormones alter immune responses and disease pathogenesis. *Horm. Behav.* **2012**, *62*, 263–271. [CrossRef] [PubMed]

14. Mor, G.; Cardenas, I. The immune system in pregnancy: A unique complexity. *Am. J. Reprod. Immunol.* **2010**, *63*, 425–433. [CrossRef] [PubMed]

15. Roberts, D.; Dalziel, S. Antenatal corticosteroids for accelerating fetal lung maturation for women at risk of preterm birth. *Cochrane Database Syst. Rev.* **2006**. [CrossRef]

16. McClure, E.M.; Meshnick, S.R.; Mungai, P.; Malhotra, I.; King, C.L.; Goldenberg, R.L.; Hudgens, M.G.; Siega-Riz, A.M.; Dent, A.E. The association of parasitic infections in pregnancy and maternal and fetal anemia: A cohort study in coastal Kenya. *PLoS Negl. Trop. Dis.* **2014**, *8*, e2724. [CrossRef] [PubMed]

17. Tay, S.C.K.; Nani, E.A.; Walana, W. Parasitic infections and maternal anaemia among expectant mothers in the Dangme East District of Ghana. *BMC Res. Notes* **2017**, *10*, 3. [CrossRef] [PubMed]

18. Aderoba, A.K.; Iribhogbe, O.I.; Olagbuji, B.N.; Olokor, O.E.; Ojide, C.K.; Ande, A.B. Prevalence of helminth infestation during pregnancy and its association with maternal anemia and low birth weight. *Int. J. Gynaecol. Obstet.* **2015**, *129*, 199–202. [CrossRef] [PubMed]

19. Salam, R.A.; Haider, B.A.; Humayun, Q.; Bhutta, Z.A. Effect of administration of antihelminthics for soil-transmitted helminths during pregnancy. *Cochrane Database Syst. Rev.* **2015**. [CrossRef] [PubMed]

20. Imhoff-Kunsch, B.; Briggs, V. Antihelminthics in pregnancy and maternal, newborn and child health. *Paediatr. Perinat. Epidemiol.* **2012**, *26* (Suppl. S1), 223–238. [CrossRef] [PubMed]

21. Fairley, J.K.; Bisanzio, D.; King, C.H.; Kitron, U.; Mungai, P.; Muchiri, E.; King, C.L.; Malhotra, I. Birthweight in offspring of mothers with high prevalence of helminth and malaria infection in coastal Kenya. *Am. J. Trop. Med. Hyg.* **2013**, *88*, 48–53. [CrossRef] [PubMed]

22. Prendergast, A.J.; Humphrey, J.H. The stunting syndrome in developing countries. *Paediatr. Int. Child Health* **2014**, *34*, 250–265. [CrossRef] [PubMed]

23. Martins, V.J.B.; Toledo Florêncio, T.M.M.; Grillo, L.P.; do Carmo P Franco, M.; Martins, P.A.; Clemente, A.P.; Santos, C.D.; de Fatima A Vieira, M.; Sawaya, A.L. Long-lasting effects of undernutrition. *Int. J. Environ. Res. Public Health* **2011**, *8*, 1817–1846. [CrossRef] [PubMed]

24. Moher, D.; Liberati, A.; Tetzlaff, J.; Altman, D.G.; The PRISMA Group. Preferred Reporting Items for Systematic Reviews and Meta-Analyses: The PRISMA Statement. *PLoS Med.* **2009**, *6*, e1000097. [CrossRef] [PubMed]

25. Mays, N.; Pope, C.; Popay, J. Systematically reviewing qualitative and quantitative evidence to inform management and policy-making in the health field. *J. Health Serv. Res. Policy* **2005**, *10* (Suppl. S1), 6–20. [CrossRef] [PubMed]

26. Buonfrate, D.; Requena-Mendez, A.; Angheben, A.; Muñoz, J.; Gobbi, F.; Van Den Ende, J.; Bisoffi, Z. Severe strongyloidiasis: A systematic review of case reports. *BMC Infect. Dis.* **2013**, *13*, 78. [CrossRef] [PubMed]

27. Miller, A.; Smith, M.L.; Judd, J.A.; Speare, R. *Strongyloides stercoralis*: Systematic review of barriers to controlling strongyloidiasis for Australian Indigenous communities. *PLoS Negl. Trop. Dis.* **2014**, *8*, e3141. [CrossRef] [PubMed]

28. Smith, T.O.; Nichols, R.; Gilding, E.; Donell, S.T. Are location, proportion and length of VM patellar attachment aetiological factors in patellofemoral dysfunction? A systematic review. *Eur. J. Orthop. Surg. Traumatol.* **2009**, *19*, 63–73. [CrossRef]

29. Hu, A.S.Y.; Menon, R.; Gunnarsson, R.; de Costa, A. Risk factors for conversion of laparoscopic cholecystectomy to open surgery—A systematic literature review of 30 studies. *Am. J. Surg.*. [CrossRef] [PubMed]

30. Lo, C.K.-L.; Mertz, D.; Loeb, M. Newcastle-Ottawa Scale: Comparing reviewers' to authors' assessments. *BMC Med. Res. Methodol.* **2014**, *14*, 45. [CrossRef] [PubMed]

31. Wilke, J.; Krause, F.; Niederer, D.; Engeroff, T.; Nürnberger, F.; Vogt, L.; Banzer, W. Appraising the methodological quality of cadaveric studies: Validation of the QUACS scale. *J. Anat.* **2015**, *226*, 440–446. [CrossRef] [PubMed]

32. The Joanna Briggs Institute. Checklist for Case Reports. Critical Appraisal Tools Website. Published 2017. Available online: http://joannabriggs.org/research/critical-appraisal-tools.html (accessed on 27 August 2017).

33. Baidoo, S.; Tay, S.; Obiri-Danso, K.; Abruquah, H. Intestinal helminth infection and anaemia during pregnancy: A community based study in Ghana. *Afr. J. Bacteriol. Res.* **2010**, *2*, 9–13.

34. Barnish, G.; Harari, M. Possible effects of *Strongyloides fuelleborni*-like infections on children in the Karimui area of Simbu Province. *P. N. G. Med. J.* **1989**, *32*, 51–54. [PubMed]

35. Cabada, M.M.; Lopez, M.; Arque, E.; White, A.C. Prevalence of soil-transmitted helminths after mass albendazole administration in an indigenous community of the Manu jungle in Peru. *Pathog. Glob. Health* **2014**, *108*, 200–205. [CrossRef] [PubMed]

36. Chiang Mai Low Birth Weight Study Group; Mangklabruks, A.; Rerkasem, A.; Wongthanee, A.; Rerkasem, K.; Chiowanich, P.; Sritara, P.; Pruenglampoo, S.; Yipintsoi, T.; Tongsong, T.; et al. The risk factors of low birth weight infants in the northern part of Thailand. *J. Med. Assoc. Thail.* **2012**, *95*, 358–365. [PubMed]

37. Dada-Adegbola, H.O.; Bakare, R.A. Strongyloidiasis in children five years and below. *West Afr. J. Med.* **2004**, *23*, 194–197. [CrossRef] [PubMed]

38. Dreyfuss, M.L.; Msamanga, G.I.; Spiegelman, D.; Hunter, D.J.; Urassa, E.J.; Hertzmark, E.; Fawzi, W.W. Determinants of low birth weight among HIV-infected pregnant women in Tanzania. *Am. J. Clin. Nutr.* **2001**, *74*, 814–826. [CrossRef] [PubMed]

39. Egger, R.J.; Hofhuis, E.H.; Bloem, M.W.; Chusilp, K.; Wedel, M.; Intarakhao, C.; Saowakontha, S.; Schreurs, W.H. Association between intestinal parasitoses and nutritional status in 3-8-year-old children in northeast Thailand. *Trop. Geogr. Med.* **1990**, *42*, 312–323. [PubMed]

40. Herrera, J.; Marcos, L.; Terashima, A.; Alvarez, H.; Samalvides, F.; Gotuzzo, E. Factors associated with *Strongyloides stercoralis* infection in an endemic area in Peru. *Rev. Gastroenterol. Peru* **2006**, *26*, 357–362. [PubMed]

41. King, S.E.; Mascie-Taylor, C. '*Strongyloides fuelleborni kellyi*' and other intestinal helminths in children from Papua New Guinea: Associations with nutritional status and socioeconomic factors. *P. N. G. Med. J.* **2004**, *47*, 181–191. [PubMed]

42. LaBeaud, A.D.; Nayakwadi Singer, M.; McKibben, M.; Mungai, P.; Muchiri, E.M.; McKibben, E.; Gildengorin, G.; Sutherland, L.J.; King, C.H.; King, C.L.; et al. Parasitism in children aged three years and under: Relationship between infection and growth in rural coastal Kenya. *PLoS Negl. Trop. Dis.* **2015**, *9*, e0003721. [CrossRef] [PubMed]

43. Muhangi, L.; Woodburn, P.; Omara, M.; Omoding, N.; Kizito, D.; Mpairwe, H.; Nabulime, J.; Ameke, C.; Morison, L.A.; Elliott, A.M. Associations between mild-to-moderate anaemia in pregnancy and helminth, malaria and HIV infection in Entebbe, Uganda. *Trans. R. Soc. Trop. Med. Hyg.* **2007**, *101*, 899–907. [CrossRef] [PubMed]

44. Nampijja, M.; Apule, B.; Lule, S.; Akurut, H.; Muhangi, L.; Webb, E.L.; Lewis, C.; Elliott, A.M.; Alcock, K.J. Effects of maternal worm infections and anthelminthic treatment during pregnancy on infant motor and neurocognitive functioning. *J. Int. Neuropsychol. Soc.* **2012**, *18*, 1019–1030. [CrossRef] [PubMed]

45. Phuanukoonnon, S.; Michael, A.; Kirarock, W.S.; Pomat, W.S.; van den Biggelaar, A.H. Intestinal parasitic infections and anaemia among pregnant women in the highlands of Papua New Guinea. *P. N. G. Med. J.* **2013**, *56*, 119–125. [PubMed]

46. Verhagen, L.M.; Incani, R.N.; Franco, C.R.; Ugarte, A.; Cadenas, Y.; Sierra Ruiz, C.I.; Hermans, P.W.; Hoek, D.; Campos Ponce, M.; de Waard, J.H.; et al. High malnutrition rate in Venezuelan Yanomami compared to Warao Amerindians and Creoles: Significant associations with intestinal parasites and anemia. *PLoS ONE* **2013**, *8*, e77581. [CrossRef] [PubMed]

47. Villar, J.; Klebanoff, M.; Kestler, E. The effect on fetal growth of protozoan and helminthic infection during pregnancy. *Obstet. Gynecol.* **1989**, *74*, 915–920. [PubMed]

48. Yatich, N.J.; Jolly, P.E.; Funkhouser, E.; Agbenyega, T.; Rayner, J.C.; Ehiri, J.E.; Turpin, A.; Stiles, J.K.; Ellis, W.O.; Jiang, Y.; et al. The effect of malaria and intestinal helminth coinfection on birth outcomes in Kumasi, Ghana. *Am. J. Trop. Med. Hyg.* **2010**, *82*, 28–34. [CrossRef] [PubMed]

49. Buresch, A.M.; Judge, N.E.; Dayal, A.K.; Garry, D.J. A fatal case of strongyloidiasis in pregnancy. *Obstet. Gynecol.* **2015**, *126*, 87–89. [CrossRef] [PubMed]

50. Malezieux-Picard, A.; Saint-Paul, M.C.; Dellamonica, J.; Courjon, J.; Tieulié, N.; Marty, P.; Fuzibet, J.G.; Collomp, R.; Marinho, J.A.; Queyrel, V. Severe intestinal obstruction due to *Strongyloides stercoralis* in a pregnant woman. *Med. Mal. Infect.* **2017**, *47*, 429–431. [CrossRef] [PubMed]

51. Prasad, M.; Chauhan, A.; Chamariya, S.; Kuyare, S.; Koticha, A. A case of strongyloidiasis in pregnancy. **2017**, *6*, 1130–1131. [CrossRef]

52. Heaton, J.; Shippey, S.; Macri, C.; Macedonia, C. Intestinal helminthes infestation in pregnancy: A case report and literature review. *Mil. Med.* **2002**, *167*, 954–955. [PubMed]

53. Reyes, L.; Manalich, R. Long-term consequences of low birth weight. *Kidney Int.* **2005**, *68*, S107–S111. [CrossRef] [PubMed]

54. Herceg, A. *Improving Health in Aboriginal and Torres Strait Islander Mothers, Babies and Young Children: A Literature Review*; Commonwealth Department of Health and Ageing: Canberra, Australia, 2005.

55. Huynh, D.T.T.; Estorninos, E.; Capeding, R.Z.; Oliver, J.S.; Low, Y.L.; Rosales, F.J. Longitudinal growth and health outcomes in nutritionally at-risk children who received long-term nutritional intervention. *J. Hum. Nutr. Diet.* **2015**, *28*, 623–635. [CrossRef] [PubMed]

56. Olofin, I.; McDonald, C.M.; Ezzati, M.; Flaxman, S.; Black, R.E.; Fawzi, W.W.; Caulfield, L.E.; Danaei, G.; Nutrition Impact Model Study (anthropometry cohort pooling). Associations of suboptimal growth with all-cause and cause-specific mortality in children under five years: A pooled analysis of ten prospective studies. *PLoS ONE* **2013**, *8*, e64636. [CrossRef] [PubMed]

57. Richard, S.A.; Black, R.E.; Gilman, R.H.; Guerrant, R.L.; Kang, G.; Lanata, C.F.; Mølbak, K.; Rasmussen, Z.A.; Sack, R.B.; Valentiner-Branth, F.; et al. Wasting is associated with stunting in early childhood. *J. Nutr.* **2012**, *142*, 1291–1296. [CrossRef] [PubMed]

58. Strunz, E.C.; Addiss, D.G.; Stocks, M.E.; Ogden, S.; Utzinger, J.; Freeman, M.C. Water, sanitation, hygiene, and soil-transmitted helminth infection: A systematic review and meta-analysis. *PLoS Med.* **2014**, *11*, e1001620. [CrossRef] [PubMed]

59. Bethony, J.; Brooker, S.; Albonico, M.; Geiger, S.M.; Loukas, A.; Diemert, D.; Hotez, P.J. Soil-transmitted helminth infections: Ascariasis, trichuriasis, and hookworm. *Lancet* **2006**, *367*, 1521–1532. [CrossRef]

60. Carrilho, G.F.; Da Costa, G.M.; Olivi, M.J.; Vicentini, V.; Anibal, F.D.F. Anemia in patients with intestinal parasitic infection. *Rev. Ibero-Latinoam. Parasitol.* **2011**, *70*, 206–211.

61. Kightlinger, L.K.; Seed, J.R.; Kightlinger, M.B. The epidemiology of *Ascaris lumbricoides*, *Trichuris trichiura*, and hookworm in children in the Ranomafana rainforest, Madagascar. *J. Parasitol.* **1995**, *81*, 159–169. [CrossRef] [PubMed]

62. Ndyomugyenyi, R.; Kabatereine, N.; Olsen, A.; Magnussen, P. Efficacy of ivermectin and albendazole alone and in combination for treatment of soil-transmitted helminths in pregnancy and adverse events: A randomized open label controlled intervention trial in Masindi district, western Uganda. *Am. J. Trop. Med. Hyg.* **2008**, *79*, 856–863. [PubMed]

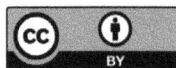

Tropical Medicine and
Infectious Disease

MDPI

Review

The Unique Life Cycle of *Strongyloides stercoralis* and Implications for Public Health Action

Wendy Page [1,2,*], Jenni A. Judd [3] and Richard S. Bradbury [4]

1 Miwatj Health Aboriginal Corporation, Nhulunbuy, NT 0881, Australia
2 Public Health and Tropical Medicine, James Cook University, Cairns, QLD 4870, Australia
3 Centre for Indigenous Health Equity Research, School of Health, Medical and Applied Sciences,
   Central Queensland University, Bundaberg, QLD 4670, Australia; j.judd@cqu.edu.au
4 School of Health, Medical and Applied Sciences, Central Queensland University,
   Rockhampton, QLD 4700, Australia; r.bradbury@cqu.edu.au
* Correspondence: wendy.page@my.jcu.edu.au; Tel.: +61-407-601-449

Received: 27 April 2018; Accepted: 21 May 2018; Published: 25 May 2018

Abstract: *Strongyloides stercoralis* has one of the most complex life cycles of the human-infecting nematodes. A common misconception in medical and public health professions is that *S. stercoralis* in its biology is akin to other intestinal nematodes, such as the hookworms. Despite original evidence provided by medical and veterinary research about this unique helminth, many assumptions have entered the scientific literature. This helminth is set apart from others that commonly affect humans by (a) the internal autoinfective cycle with autoinfective larvae randomly migrating through tissue, parthenogenesis, and the potential for lifelong infection in the host, the profound pathology occurring in hyperinfection and systemic manifestations of strongyloidiasis, and (b) a limited external cycle with a single generation of free-living adults. This paper aims to review and discuss original research on the unique life cycle of *S. stercoralis* that distinguishes it from other helminths and highlight areas where increased understanding of the parasite's biology might lead to improved public health prevention and control strategies.

Keywords: *Strongyloides stercoralis*; strongyloidiasis; life cycle; public health; control; biology

1. Introduction

Strongyloides stercoralis is distinguished amongst intestinal helminths by several factors of its biology, most impressively by its autoinfective life cycle (Figure 1), leading to potential lifelong infection and capacity to kill its human host, decades after initial infection. Strongyloidiasis affects an estimated 370 million people worldwide, based on data from 2013 [1]. Previously quoted estimates of 30 to 100 million people date back to 1989 [2]. The disease remains endemic in all tropical and sub-tropical countries worldwide, particularly in countries with developing infrastructure but also in developed nations such as the United States of America, Australia, Spain, and Italy [3]. Seroprevalence in some Latin American and African countries reaches in excess of 20% [4,5], and seroprevalence in excess of 40% has been reported in parts of South East Asia [6]. Rates of infection are concerningly high amongst refugees arriving from these countries when sensitive serological tests are employed, reaching 46% amongst Sudanese and 23% amongst Somalian refugees entering the USA in 2007 [7].

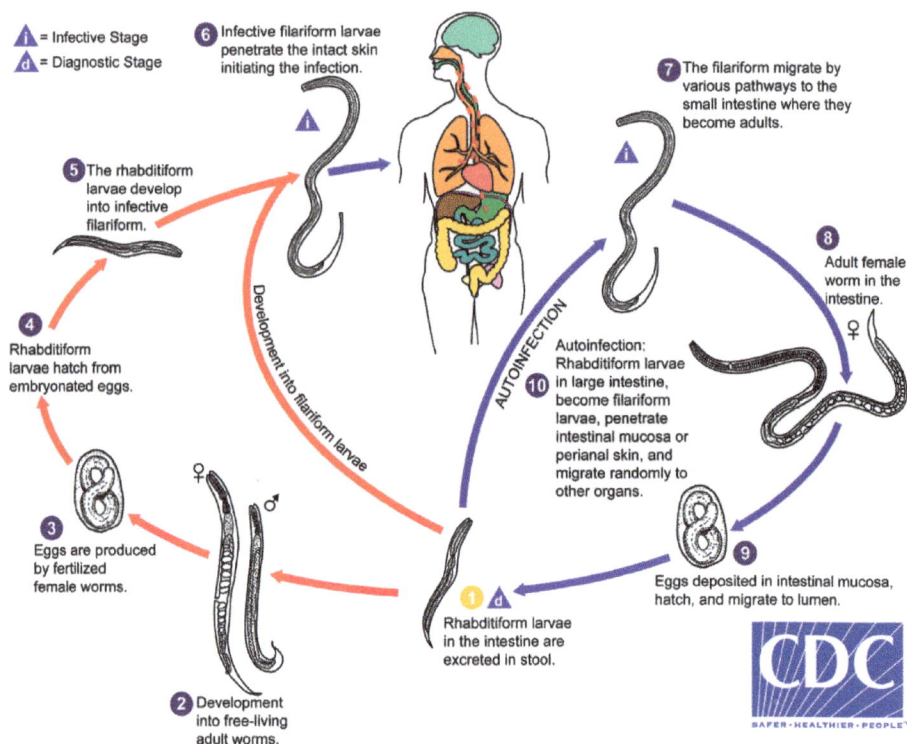

Figure 1. The life cycle of *Strongyloides stercoralis*. Distinctive features include (**a**) random migration of autoinfective larvae, (**b**) embryonated egg rapidly hatches to rhabditiform larvae, and (**c**) single generation of free-living male and female adults. Source: CDC DPDx: (https://www.cdc.gov/dpdx/), with permission.

The reported prevalence in immigrants and refugees may, in fact, be an underestimate due to a reliance on insensitive microscopic methods for diagnosis. Single-dose albendazole is now a standard treatment for helminthic infection amongst refugees entering the United States. This treatment did reduce rates of strongyloidiasis in incoming refugees when tested by insensitive microscopic methods [8], although such methods do not detect very low–intensity infections. Albendazole treatment has a reported cure rate of 62–69%, depending on dosage regimen, as compared to 88–96% for ivermectin [9]. However, in many cases, these data were also based on insensitive faecal microscopic methods prior to the availability or routine application of faecal PCR and agar plate culture for the detection of larvae. Incomplete eradication of residual larvae after anthelmintic treatment resulting in recrudescence due to parthenogenesis and the autoinfective cycle needs more attention from researchers at this time.

Some developed countries retain limited, focal, endemic transmission of strongyloidiasis. Such environmental transmission often occurs in geographically limited foci or 'hot spots'. Examples are remote Indigenous communities in Australia, where up to 59.6% of people tested seropositive for disease, with Indigenous and non-Indigenous residents being affected [10,11]. Studies of residents of rural East Tennessee in the late 1980s found a prevalence of 6.1% amongst hospitalized patients, almost certainly an underestimate given the insensitive microscopic method used for diagnosis [12].

Also, of particular concern to these developed countries is the prevalence of infection in travellers returned from highly endemic nations, with one study finding that *S. stercoralis* was the fifth most common clinical pathogen identified in returned international travellers presenting with infectious gastrointestinal disease [13]. Veterans of overseas conflicts are another important group in these countries at risk of long-term strongyloidiasis. A recent study of Australian Vietnam veterans found a *S. stercoralis* seropositivity rate of 11.6%, 40 years after the end of Australian involvement in that conflict [14]. The burden of disease in veterans of more recent conflicts and peacekeeping operations remains largely unexplored. These infections may present a hidden burden to the local health system many decades later if infected immigrants and returned travellers are immunosuppressed and develop severe systemic disease.

Developing strategies to reduce morbidity and mortality from strongyloidiasis in endemic areas requires a clear understanding of the idiosyncratic life cycle of *S. stercoralis*. Perhaps due to development of superficially similar rhabditiform into filariform stages of larvae at one point in its lifecycle, the overall biology of *S. stercoralis* is often confused with that of the hookworms, despite being very disparate. This paper highlights misunderstandings and errors in the interpretation of the parasite's biology that may be hampering effective prevention, control, and eradication efforts worldwide.

2. Modes of Transmission to Human Host

Transmission of infective larvae to the human host is almost exclusively depicted in scientific literature as being transdermal. Looss first demonstrated this process in 1904 by self-inoculating and infecting himself with *S. stercoralis* via exposing his skin to several hundred filariform larvae and subsequently finding larvae in his faeces 64 days after exposure [15]. Although not usually indicated in life cycle charts, and not the usual mode of transmission, experimentation by Wilms demonstrated oral ingestion of larvae by a human volunteer resulted in a shorter duration of 17 days before larvae were identified in faeces [16]. Transmission from human donor to human recipient can occur with organ transplantation [17].

3. The Internal Autoinfective Cycle—Ordered Pathway and Random Migration

S. stercoralis demonstrates remarkable persistence within the host due to its autoinfective cycle. The traditional pathway of infection is via infective filariform larvae entering the skin (transdermal) and being carried through the circulation to the right side of the heart and from there to the lungs. At this point, the larvae migrate through the alveoli, ascend the trachea and are coughed up and swallowed into the oesophagus. From there, larvae travel to the small intestine where they mature into parasitic female adults (Figure 2a). The parasitic females burrow into the lining of the gut and produce eggs that do not require fertilization from a parasitic male (parthenogenesis) and hatch in the mucosa. This blood-pulmonary pathway was described by Fülleborn in 1914, who examined the tracheae and oesophagi of transdermally-infected dogs [18]: 'The first major studies were done in 1914 in tracheotomized dogs by Fülleborn (1914), who concluded that the majority of larvae passed via the bloodstream to the lungs, ascended the respiratory tree, were swallowed, then arrived in the small bowel where they completed their development' [18,19].

Importantly, the blood-pulmonary pathway is not the only route by which *S. stercoralis* larvae may reach the human gut. Schad and his colleagues observed a lower number of larvae than would be expected in the lungs of dogs with massive hyperinfection, thus questioning the assumption that autoinfective larvae only followed the ordered traditional pulmonary-tracheal pathway [20]. Further studies monitored the pathways of migration of radiolabeled *S. stercoralis* larvae in 10-day-old pups [21]. This work demonstrated that larvae not only enter the gastrointestinal tract via traversing the trachea but also randomly migrate through the viscera and other tissue directly to the duodenum. In the findings of these studies, the authors considered random migration to be a significant part of the infective life cycle of *S. stercoralis* in dogs and likely to occur in other hosts, such as humans [21–23]. This work, whilst convincing and exquisitely performed, had not entered the medical literature [24], possibly due to the veterinary nature of the original study. The majority of current texts still only refer to a cardiopulmonary-tracheal migration phase for infective larvae.

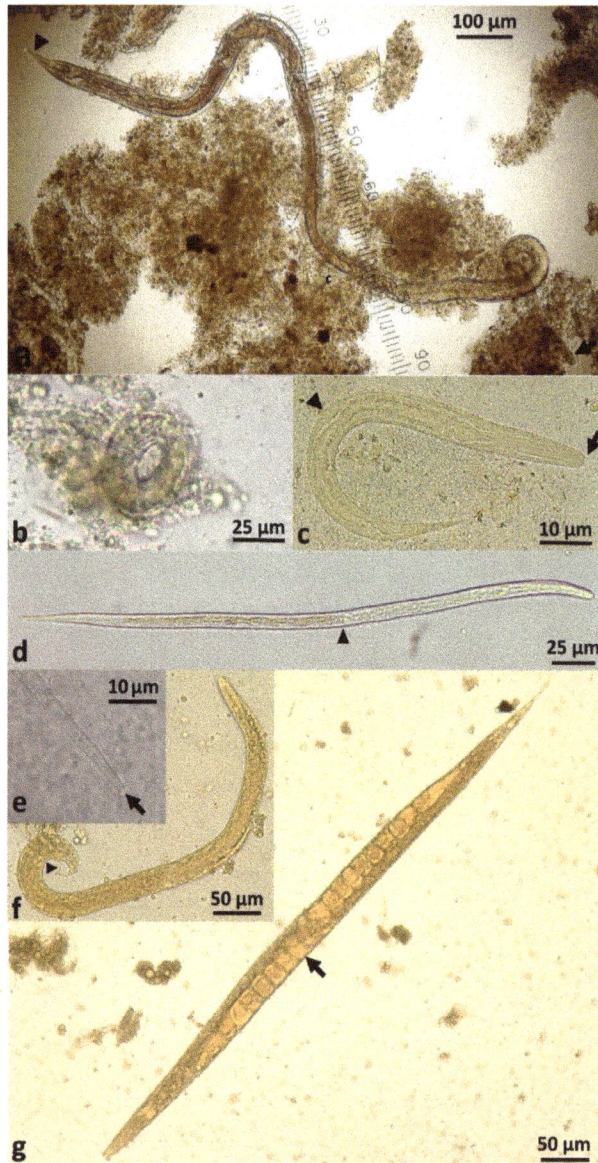

Figure 2. The life stages of *Strongyloides stercoralis*; (**a**) parasitic female with tapering anterior (arrow) and pointed caudal extremity (dart); (**b**) embryonated egg; (**c**) rhabditiform larva in faeces with short buccal cavity (arrow) and rhomboid genital primordium (dart); (**d**) filariform larva with oesophago-intestinal junction at mid-body (dart); (**e**) notched tail of the filariform larva (arrow); (**f**) free-living male with prominent spicule (dart); and (**g**) gravid free-living female with eggs in uterus (arrow). Note: Figure 2a,b are from faeces of a patient with hyperinfection; these life stages are not seen in patient faeces in the absence of severe hyperinfection. Figure attributions: (**a,b,e**): Dr Richard Bradbury, Central Queensland University; (**d**): Emeritus Professor John Goldsmid, University of Tasmania; (**c,f,g**): CDC DPDx web site (https://www.cdc.gov/dpdx/). Reproduced with permission.

Based on the migration of infective filariform larvae after cutaneous inoculation into dogs, it seems unlikely that the autoinfective larvae only follow an ordered route during chronic infection. The currently accepted assumption, that autoinfective larvae invading the tissues take the ordered pulmonary-tracheal pathway back to the small intestine and that random migration only occurs during disseminated infection, is unsupported by scientific studies. An exponential increase in numbers of *S. stercoralis* with dysregulation of the autoinfective cycle [24] resulting in multiple end-organ failure, are more likely to be the reason, rather than a change in migratory pathway.

Potential misunderstandings of larval migration have also led to the clinical manifestations of chronic strongyloidiasis being limited only to the skin, lungs and gastrointestinal tract, with extension to other organs then categorised under disseminated and hyperinfection. Biopsies and clinical specimens from the former three sites are generally easier to obtain. However, random migration throughout the organs may be occurring in limited numbers without disseminated disease or hyperinfection. This hypothesis explains the finding of *S. stercoralis* in 'ectopic sites' such as the parotid gland [25] and pericardial fluid [26] in cases of chronic strongyloidiasis, without apparent systemic disease. Recurrent meningitis without fatal dissemination [27–29] suggests the autoinfective larvae are transporting enteric bacteria on its random migratory pathway during chronic infection. Although categorised as a soil-transmitted helminth, the perception that *S. stercoralis* may benefit from broadening its category to a 'tissue parasite' [30] is supported by the apparent random migration of autoinfective larvae in the tissues, the burrowing of the parasitic female into the intestinal mucosa, and the common need for serologic evaluation for diagnosis. The more recent category of strongyloidiasis as a neglected tropical disease is warranted.

Corticosteroids, Hyperinfection and Dissemination

Disseminated strongyloidiasis in humans has a very high case fatality rate, with 68.5% of 244 cases analysed in a recent systematic review having a fatal outcome [17]. If the increasing rate of prescriptions for corticosteroids and the relative lack of awareness of strongyloidiasis within the medical profession in first-world countries continues, *S. stercoralis* will likely become a growing clinical challenge, particularly in the context of increased immigration from and travel to highly endemic countries. Buonfrate and colleagues' systematic review of 244 case reports (171 having at least hyperinfection and 73 with confirmed systemic disease) [17], found corticosteroid use was associated in 67% of all cases. Many of these patients had other sources of immunosuppression, such as leukaemia, organ transplantation, multiple myeloma, and cancer, but corticosteroids remain an outstanding common factor. Solid organ transplant recipients made up 11.5% of cases (10% having concomitant corticosteroid use) [17]. The fatality rate was 68% in this group. Ten percent of all studied cases carried human T-cell leukaemia virus type 1 (HTLV-1), a viral blood disease endemic in several areas of the world with high rates of strongyloidiasis, including Okinawa and Australian Indigenous communities [31,32], and associated with disseminated strongyloidiasis. Patients with HIV made up 13% of cases, with only 3% of those HIV-positive individuals also taking corticosteroids [17]. A handful of patients had alcoholism or severe malnutrition as underlying pathologies. An apparently healthy patient developed hyperinfection and died despite being given thiabendazole [17].

The close association of corticosteroids with hyperinfection, sometimes leading to systemic disease, may be due to more than just host immunosuppression. Observational studies noted a strong association between corticosteroids and disseminated strongyloidiasis and suggested that immunosuppression alone did not precipitate dissemination. Genta observed that, in many cases, patients developed massive disseminated disease within 10 days of receipt of corticosteroids, where no larvae were detectable in their faeces prior to beginning immunosuppressive therapy [24]. In one case report, a single sub-conjunctival injection of dexamethasone triggered severe disseminated disease [33]. Ectopic production of adrenocorticotropic hormone (ACTH), which stimulates secretion of glucocorticoids, and ACTH treatment in two patients, also led to disseminated disease [34,35]. Genta also noted that in many cases, patients do not present with other diseases aligned with immunosuppression, such as candidiasis, reactivation of cytomegalovirus or toxoplasmosis (Genta, 1992). He surmised that corticosteroid treatment promoted ecdysis (moulting) of rhabditiform larvae in the gut and transformation to autoinfective larvae, thereby rapidly increased helminth load via autoinfection and caused systemic disease [24].

More recent work has explored this hypothesis in the laboratory. The steroid/thyroid hormone receptor from filariform larvae of *S. stercoralis* [36] and the steroid hormone dafachronic acids (DAs), which regulate the growth of *Caenorhabditis elegans* nematodes, also determines dauer arrest or reproduction growth in *S. stercoralis* [37]. Treatment with glucocorticoids was found to be necessary to induce hyperinfection in mice even when they were already severely immunocompromised [38].

4. The Eggs of *Strongyloides stercoralis*—Rarely Seen

In contrast to other intestinal nematodes, *S. stercoralis* larvae, rather than eggs, are passed in faeces. The parasitic female produces thin-shelled, ellipsoid eggs at early cleavage stage, which rapidly embryonate (Figure 2b) and then hatch in the crypts of Lieberkühn in the intestinal mucosa [39]. Eggs are only passed in faeces in cases of severe hyperinfection.

Embryonated eggs of *S. stercoralis* have occasionally been found in bronchoalveolar aspirates of patients with systemic strongyloidiasis [1]. The presence of eggs from parasitic adults [40] in respiratory specimens is a poor prognostic sign, as eggs are rarely seen, and is indicative of severe, life-threatening infection.

5. Developmental Pathways after Hatching

The eggs of the parasitic female rapidly develop and emerge as first-stage rhabditiform larvae. These rhabditiform larvae (L1) migrate to the intestinal lumen, where they feed on their passage along the intestinal tract. There are three separate developmental pathways that the larvae may undergo.

1. Internal autoinfective cycle: first-stage rhabditiform larvae moult to second-stage rhabditiform and further moult to become autoinfective filariform (L3) larvae that do not leave the human host. These autoinfective larvae migrate through the host to become parasitic adult females living in the small intestine and producing further offspring by parthenogenesis. In this way, *S. stercoralis* remains in intimate contact with its host. This autoinfective cycle, a distinguishing feature of *S. stercoralis*, allows the worms to maintain infection for many decades in the human host, in one case lasting for up to 65 years [41]. As described above, this internal autoinfective cycle ensures long-term survival of this species independent of the external environment.

2. External direct or homogonic cycle: Larvae leave the human host via faeces to the external environment. First-stage rhabditiform larvae moult to second-stage rhabditiform larvae and moult a second time to become infective filariform third-stage larvae (L3i) (Supplementary Video S1). These active, non-feeding filariform larvae may survive in a suitable environment for up to two weeks [19,20] until finding a new host. This cycle is referred to as the direct external cycle or the homogonic cycle.

3. External indirect or heterogonic cycle: Larvae leave the human host via faeces. First-stage rhabditiform larvae undergo four moults to become (i) rhabditiform free-living adult females (Supplementary Video S2) or alternatively, (ii) rhabditiform free-living adult males [20].

These free-living adults are further part of the indirect external or heterogonic development cycle. They mate, and the females produce eggs that are passed and rapidly hatch to become rhabditiform larvae (Figure 2c). In senile older females, eggs will develop to larvae within the uterus and escape from the decaying mother's body [42]. These rhabditiform larvae feed on bacteria from the faecally-contaminated soil and then moult as in the homogonic cycle to become infective, non-feeding filariform larvae (L3i) (Figure 2d). *S. stercoralis* larvae typically live for less than three weeks, even in soil under optimal conditions with a temperature of 20–28 °C and high moisture. Larvae die rapidly in unfavourable conditions, impeding faecal diagnostic tests in remote laboratories that rely on viable larvae [43]. This generation of filariform larvae are definitively unable to develop into free-living adults [44] (Figure 2f,g) and have only one goal—to find a human host, failing which they will die within two weeks or less in the environment [20]. The male and female free-living adult worms only live for 2–4 days [44–46]. This single free-living generation amplifies the number of infective filariform larvae in the environment seeking a human host [20,47]. The duration of time in the environment of the external cycle is limited to three weeks maximum in an optimum environment [20,30,46].

6. The Single Generation of the Free-Living Cycle

The false perception that *S. stercoralis* may survive in the environment in a cycle of unlimited generations of free-living adults may have been perpetuated by observations of morphologically-similar free-living rhabditoid nematodes from soil in culture. Speare noted in 1989 that 'It is important to be able to differentiate rhabditoids from *Strongyloides*. Failure to do so has led to a number of authors presenting rhabditoids as evidence of recurrent free-living generations of *S. stercoralis*' [48]. Faecal cultures can be easily contaminated by free-living rhabditoids from the perianal skin of patients even when collected directly into sterile containers [49]. Free-living environmental rhabditoid larvae may have then been confused with *S. stercoralis* upon culture.

Difficulties in differentiating between the *Strongyloides* species may also have contributed to this assumption. Yamada's study comparing *S. planiceps* to *S. stercoralis* demonstrated the free-living cycle of *S. planiceps* had up to nine generations and confirmed that *S. stercoralis* had only one single generation [44].

7. Implications for Public Health Action

A significant barrier to implementing control programs for strongyloidiasis in endemic communities has been the persistence of an incorrect perception that *S. stercoralis* persists indefinitely in the environment. This misconception that the external free-living cycle is recurrent, and the perceived higher risk of re-infection, appears to have been a barrier to treating asymptomatic persons with chronic strongyloidiasis in endemic communities [50]. Conway, Lindo, Robinson, and Bundy (1995) provided hope for control of strongyloidiasis in endemic areas by restating that the heterogonic free-living cycle has only one single generation, is short-lived in the environment, and has a low transmission rate with a long-lived infection in the human host [46].

Despite the overwhelming evidence for only one external free-living generation, many of the newer life cycle images of *S. stercoralis* in reference texts and websites include a backward arrow to indicate that the external indirect cycle will continue indefinitely in the environment, potentially leading to misunderstandings about the capacity to control *S. stercoralis* in endemic areas.

Access to clean water, footwear, and sanitation has been fundamental to preventing new cases of strongyloidiasis. Treating the human reservoir of infection has achieved success in reducing prevalence and preventing clinical complications in some community studies [30,51–53].

The parasitic adult only produces up to 40 eggs per day. Low and intermittent output of larvae is a major factor for the low sensitivity of faecal testing, especially during the chronic phase of infection. Thus, faecal testing alone cannot be relied on for diagnosis, estimates of prevalence, or determining cure [30,43].

S. stercoralis has been resourceful in survival strategies, evident from both the long-lived autoinfective cycle in human hosts and the amplification of larvae through a single generation of free-living adults. Thus, transmission through other hosts should be considered.

8. Animal Reservoirs of Infection?

The role of reservoir animals in the spread and dissemination of *S. stercoralis* has not been thoroughly considered. It has been established that dogs, cats, and some primates may carry natural infections, but the capacity of these to be transmitted to humans was until recently obscure. Two recent phylogenetic studies of *S. stercoralis* from humans and dogs have been published [54,55]. Both of these papers found two very distinct haplotypes of *S. stercoralis*, one exclusively infecting dogs and a second found to infect dogs and humans interchangeably [54]. The role of domestic and wild dogs, and possibly also domestic cats, in the transmission and maintenance of *S. stercoralis* infection within affected communities warrants further research.

9. Conclusions

Improved understanding of the unique life cycle of *S. stercoralis* will better inform prevention and control strategies to reduce the associated morbidity and mortality caused by this parasite. Breaking the life cycle of any parasite is the key to public health prevention, treatment, and control. Knowledge of the life cycle indicates that this can be done in two ways: first by preventing infection through effective sanitation, hygiene and possibly treatment of dogs, and second by eliminating the parasites in the human host.

The fact that the external life cycle is limited to a maximum of one generation means that there is not an ongoing source of infection in the soil. The infection can only be transmitted when the soil is contaminated by faeces from an infected person, or possibly, infected dogs. The internal autoinfective life cycle ensures indefinite ongoing infection, and this means that infected people are the reservoir of infection, not the soil. This implies that effective treatment of people not only rids them of the morbidity and potential mortality associated with the infection, but also breaks the life cycle.

The increasing prevalence rates of strongyloidiasis and its capacity to kill the human host decades after initial exposure indicates this neglected tropical disease warrants a priority response from health care providers including government and non-government agencies.

Developing strategies such as measuring prevalence, identifying infected populations, providing treatment before clinical complications arise, and reducing the human reservoir of infection in endemic communities are imperative. The possibility of the presence of strains of *S. stercoralis* shared between people and dogs in endemic communities requires further research. A community-led shared effort with a medical, environmental, and veterinary One Health approach to prevention and control of strongyloidiasis may be the best strategy yet to thwart this neglected tropical disease.

Supplementary Materials: The following are available online at www.mdpi.com/2414-6366/3/2/53/s1. Video S1: Video of many *Strongyloides stercoralis* filariform (infective) larvae and one gravid free-living adult female on Koga agar plate culture, demonstrating the rapid, serpentine motility of the filariform larvae. Video S2: Close-up video of gravid free-living adult female *Strongyloides stercoralis* with highly motile filariform larvae and cleaved eggs in the background on Koga agar plate culture, demonstrating numerous eggs within the uterus and distinctive slow motility of this life stage.

Author Contributions: W.P. conceptualized and wrote the first draft with input from R.S.B. and J.A.J. All authors contributed to refining the paper. R.S.B. contributed photos in Figure 2 and movie clips in Supplementary Figures S1 and S2.

Funding: Nil external funding has been received.

Acknowledgments: This paper is dedicated to Rick Speare, who introduced the authors to the unique features and clinical importance of *Strongyloides stercoralis*, and taught us to scientifically question common assumptions. We also acknowledge the feedback on drafts from Jenny Shield, Petra Buttner, and David MacLaren.

Conflicts of Interest: The authors declare no conflict of interest.

Disclaimer: Richard S. Bradbury is co-authoring this paper in his personal capacity and in his capacity as an adjunct academic at Central Queensland University.

References

1. Bisoffi, Z.; Buonfrate, D.; Montresor, A.; Requena-Mendez, A.; Munoz, J.; Krolewiecki, A.J.; Gotuzzo, E.; Mena, M.A.; Chiodini, P.L.; Anselmi, M.; et al. *Strongyloides stercoralis*: A plea for action. *PLoS Negl. Trop. Dis.* **2013**, *7*, e2214. [CrossRef] [PubMed]
2. Genta, R.M. Global prevalence of strongyloidiasis: Critical review with epidemiologic insights into the prevention of disseminated disease. *Rev. Infect. Dis.* **1989**, *11*, 755–767. [CrossRef] [PubMed]
3. Beknazarova, M.; Whiley, H.; Ross, K. Strongyloidiasis: A disease of socioeconomic disadvantage. *Int. J. Environ. Res. Public Health* **2016**, *13*, 517. [CrossRef] [PubMed]

4. Buonfrate, D.; Mena, M.A.; Angheben, A.; Requena-Mendez, A.; Munoz, J.; Gobbi, F.; Albonico, M.; Gotuzzo, E.; Bisoffi, Z.; The COHEMI Project Study Group. Prevalence of strongyloidiasis in Latin America: A systematic review of the literature. *Epidemiol. Infect.* **2015**, *143*, 452–460. [CrossRef] [PubMed]

5. Amor, A.; Rodriguez, E.; Saugar, J.M.; Arroyo, A.; Lopez-Quintana, B.; Abera, B.; Yimer, M.; Yizengaw, E.; Zewdie, D.; Ayehubizu, Z.; et al. High prevalence of *Strongyloides stercoralis* in school-aged children in a rural highland of north-western Ethiopia: The role of intensive diagnostic work-up. *Parasites Vectors* **2016**, *9*, 617. [CrossRef] [PubMed]

6. Vonghachack, Y.; Sayasone, S.; Bouakhasith, D.; Taisayavong, K.; Akkavong, K.; Odermatt, P. Epidemiology of *Strongyloides stercoralis* on Mekong islands in southern Laos. *Acta Trop.* **2015**, *141*, 289–294. [CrossRef] [PubMed]

7. Buonfrate, D.; Angheben, A.; Gobbi, F.; Munoz, J.; Requena-Mendez, A.; Gotuzzo, E.; Mena, M.A.; Bisoffi, Z. Imported strongyloidiasis: Epidemiology, presentations, and treatment. *Curr. Infect. Dis. Rep.* **2012**, *14*, 256–262. [CrossRef] [PubMed]

8. Swanson, S.J.; Phares, C.R.; Mamo, B.; Smith, K.E.; Cetron, M.S.; Stauffer, W.M. Albendazole therapy and enteric parasites in United States-bound refugees. *N. Engl. J. Med.* **2012**, *366*, 1498–1507. [CrossRef] [PubMed]

9. Keiser, J.; Utzinger, J. The drugs we have and the drugs we need against major helminth infections. *Adv. Parasitol.* **2010**, *73*, 197–230. [PubMed]

10. Flannery, G.; White, N. Immunological parameters in northeast Arnhem Land Aborigines: Consequences of changing settlement and lifestyles. In *Urban Ecology and Health in the Third World*; Schell, L.M., Smith, M.T., Bilsborough, A., Eds.; Cambridge University Press: Cambridge, UK, 1993; pp. 202–220.

11. Soulsby, H.M.; Hewagama, S.; Brady, S. Case series of four patients with strongyloides after occupational exposure. *Med. J. Aust.* **2012**, *196*, 444. [CrossRef] [PubMed]

12. Berk, S.L.; Verghese, A.; Alvarez, S.; Hall, K.; Smith, B. Clinical and epidemiologic features of strongyloidiasis. A prospective study in rural Tennessee. *Arch. Intern. Med.* **1987**, *147*, 1257–1261. [CrossRef] [PubMed]

13. Swaminathan, A.T.J.; Wilder-Smith, A.; Schlagenhauf, P.; Thursky, K.; Connor, B.A.; Schwartz, E.; von Sonnenberg, F.; Keystone, J.; O'Brien, D.P. A global study of pathogens and host risk factors associated with infectious gastrointestinal disease in returned international travellers. *J. Infect.* **2009**, *59*, 19–27. [CrossRef] [PubMed]

14. Rahmanian, H.; MacFarlane, A.C.; Rowland, K.E.; Einsiedel, L.J.; Neuhaus, S.J. Seroprevalence of *Strongyloides stercoralis* in a South Australian Vietnam veteran cohort. *Aust. N. Z. J. Public Health* **2015**, *39*, 331–335. [CrossRef] [PubMed]

15. Looss, A. Die wanderung der *Ancylostoma*-und-*Strongyloides*-larven von der haut nach dem darm. In Proceedings of the Comptes Rendus du Sixieme Congres Internationale de Zoologie, Berne, Switzerland, 1905; pp. 225–233.

16. Wilms, M. *Anchylostoma duodenale* und *Anguillula intestinalis*. In *Schmidt's Jahrbücher der in- und Ausländischen Gesammten Medizin*; Wigand: Leipzig/Bonn, Germany, 1897; pp. 256–272.

17. Buonfrate, D.; Requena-Mendez, A.; Angheben, A.; Munoz, J.; Gobbi, F.; Van Den Ende, J.; Bisoffi, Z. Severe strongyloidiasis: A systematic review of case reports. *BMC Infect. Dis.* **2013**, *13*, 78. [CrossRef] [PubMed]

18. Fülleborn, F. Untersuchungen über den infektionsweg bei *Strongyloides* und *Ankylostomum* und die biologie dieser parasiten. *Archiv. Schiffs Trop. Hyg.* **1914**, *18*, 26–80.

19. Grove, D.I. Human strongyloidiasis. *Adv. Parasitol.* **1996**, *38*, 251–309. [PubMed]

20. Schad, G.A. Morphology and life history of *Strongyloides stercoralis*. In *Strongyloidiasis: A Major Roundworm Infection of Man*; Grove, D.I., Ed.; Taylor & Francis: London, UK, 1989; pp. 85–104.

21. Aikens, L.M.; Schad, G.A. Radiolabeling of infective third-stage larvae of *Strongyloides stercoralis* by feeding [75 Se]-selenomethionine-labeled *Escherichia coli* to first- and second-stage larvae. *J. Parasitol.* **1989**, *75*, 735–739. [CrossRef] [PubMed]

22. Schad, G.A.; Aikens, L.M.; Smith, G. *Strongyloides stercoralis*: Is there a canonical migratory route through the host? *J. Parasitol.* **1989**, *75*, 740–749. [CrossRef] [PubMed]

23. Mansfield, L.S.; Alavi, A.; Wortman, J.A.; Schad, G.A. Gamma camera scintigraphy for direct visualization of larval migration in *Strongyloides stercoralis*-infected dogs. *Am. J. Trop. Med. Hyg.* **1995**, *52*, 236–240. [CrossRef] [PubMed]

24. Genta, R.M. Dysregulation of strongyloidiasis: A new hypothesis. *Clin. Microbiol. Rev.* **1992**, *5*, 345–355. [CrossRef] [PubMed]

25. Tsai, Y.T.; Yeh, C.J.; Chen, Y.A.; Chen, Y.W.; Huang, S.F. Bilateral parotid abscesses as the initial presentation of strongyloidiasis in the immunocompetent host. *Head Neck* **2012**, *34*, 1051–1054. [CrossRef] [PubMed]

26. Lai, C.P.; Hsu, Y.H.; Wang, J.H.; Lin, C.M. *Strongyloides stercoralis* infection with bloody pericardial effusion in a non-immunosuppressed patient. *Circ. J.* **2002**, *66*, 613–614. [CrossRef] [PubMed]

27. Mak, D.B. Recurrent bacterial meningitis associated with strongyloides hyperinfection. *Med. J. Aust.* **1993**, *159*, 354. [PubMed]

28. Shimasaki, T.; Chung, H.; Shiiki, S. Five cases of recurrent meningitis associated with chronic strongyloidiasis. *Am. J. Trop. Med. Hyg.* **2015**, *92*, 601–604. [CrossRef] [PubMed]

29. Vandebosch, S.; Mana, F.; Goossens, A.; Urbain, D. *Strongyloides stercoralis* infection associated with repititive bacterial meningitis and SIADH: A case report. *Acta Gastroenterol. Belg.* **2008**, *71*, 413–417. [PubMed]

30. Shield, J.M.; Page, W. Effective diagnostic tests and anthelmintic treatment for *Strongyloides stercoralis* make community control feasible. *P. N. G. Med. J.* **2008**, *51*, 105–119. [PubMed]

31. Gessain, A.; Cassar, O. Epidemiological aspects and world distribution of HTLV-1 Infection. *Front. Microbiol.* **2012**, *3*, 388. [CrossRef] [PubMed]

32. Einsiedel, L.; Fernandes, L. *Strongyloides stercoralis*: A cause of morbidity and mortality for Indigenous people in Central Australia. *Intern. Med. J.* **2008**, *38*, 697–703. [CrossRef] [PubMed]

33. West, B.C.; Wilson, J.P. Subconjunctival corticosteroid therapy complicated by hyperinfective strongyloidiasis. *Am. J. Ophthalmol.* **1980**, *89*, 854–857. [CrossRef]

34. Cummins, R.O.; Suratt, P.M.; Horwitz, D.A. Disseminated *Strongyloides stercoralis* infection. Association with ectopic ACTH syndrome and depressed cell-mediated immunity. *Arch. Intern. Med.* **1978**, *138*, 1005–1006. [CrossRef] [PubMed]

35. Debussche, X.; Toublanc, M.; Camillieri, J.P.; Assan, R. Overwhelming strongyloidiasis in a diabetic patient following ACTH treatment and keto-acidosis. *Diabete Metab.* **1988**, *14*, 294–298. [PubMed]

36. Siddiqui, A.A.; Stanley, C.S.; Skelly, P.J.; Berk, S.L. A cDNA encoding a nuclear hormone receptor of the steroid/thyroid hormone-receptor superfamily from the human parasitic nematode *Strongyloides stercoralis*. *Parasitol. Res.* **2000**, *86*, 24–29. [CrossRef] [PubMed]

37. Albarqi, M.M.; Stoltzfus, J.D.; Pilgrim, A.A.; Nolan, T.J.; Wang, Z.; Kliewer, S.A.; Mangelsdorf, D.J.; Lok, J.B. Regulation of life cycle checkpoints and developmental activation of infective larvae in *Strongyloides stercoralis* by dafachronic acid. *PLoS Pathog.* **2016**, *12*, e1005358. [CrossRef] [PubMed]

38. Patton, J.B.; Bonne-Annee, S.; Deckman, J.; Hess, J.A.; Torigian, A.; Nolan, T.J.; Wang, Z.; Kliewer, S.A.; Durham, A.C.; Lee, J.J.; et al. Methylprednisolone acetate induces, and delta-7-dafachronic acid suppresses, *Strongyloides stercoralis* hyperinfection in NSG mice. *Proc. Natl. Acad. Sci. USA* **2018**, *115*, 204–209. [CrossRef] [PubMed]

39. Little, M.D. Comparative morphology of six species of *Strongyloides* (Nematoda) and redefinition of the genus. *J. Parasitol.* **1966**, *52*, 69–84. [CrossRef] [PubMed]

40. Mati, V.L.; Raso, P.; de Melo, A.L. *Strongyloides stercoralis* infection in marmosets: Replication of complicated and uncomplicated human disease and parasite biology. *Parasites Vectors* **2014**, *7*, 579. [CrossRef] [PubMed]

41. Leighton, P.M.; MacSween, H.M. *Strongyloides stercoralis*: The cause of an urticarial-like eruption of 65 years' duration. *Arch. Intern. Med.* **1990**, *150*, 1747–1748. [CrossRef] [PubMed]

42. Premvati. Studies on *Strongyloides* of primates: 1. Morphology and life history of *Strongyloides fülleborniv* on Linstow, 1905. *Can. J. Zool.* **1958**, *36*, 65–77. [CrossRef]

43. Page, W.; Speare, R. Chronic strongyloidiasis—Don't look and you won't find. *Aust. Fam. Physician* **2016**, *45*, 40–44. [PubMed]

44. Yamada, M.; Matsuda, S.; Nakazawa, M.; Arizono, N. Series-specific differences in heterogonic development of serially transferred free-living generations of *Strongyloides planiceps* and *Strongyloides stercoralis*. *J. Parasitol.* **1991**, *77*, 592–594. [CrossRef] [PubMed]

45. Galliard, H. Recherches sur l'infestation expérimentale à *Strongyloides stercoralis* au Tonkin (XII). *Ann. Parasitol. Hum. Comp.* **1951**, *26*, 201–227. [CrossRef] [PubMed]

46. Conway, D.J.; Lindo, J.F.; Robinson, R.D.; Bundy, D.A. Towards effective control of *Strongyloides stercoralis*. *Parasitol. Today* **1995**, *11*, 420–424. [CrossRef]

47. Van Doorn, H.R.; Koelewijn, R.; Hofwegen, H.; Gilis, H.; Wetsteyn, J.C.; Wismans, P.J.; Sarfati, C.; Vervoort, T.; van Gool, T. Use of enzyme-linked immunosorbent assay and dipstick assay for detection of *Strongyloides stercoralis* infection in humans. *J. Clin. Microbiol.* **2007**, *45*, 438–442. [CrossRef] [PubMed]

48. Speare, R. Identification of species of *Strongyloides*. In *Strongyloidiasis: A Major Roundworm Infection of Man*; Grove, D.I., Ed.; Taylor & Francis: London, UK, 1989; pp. 11–83.

49. Kreis, H.A.; Faust, E.C. Two new species of *Rhabditis (R. macrocera* and *R. clavopapillata)* associated with dogs and monkeys in experimental *Strongyloides* studies. *Trans. Am. Microsc. Soc.* **1933**, *52*, 162–172. [CrossRef]

50. Hudson, B. Strongyloidiasis. *Medical Observer*, 13 March 2012; 41.

51. Page, W.A.; Dempsey, K.; McCarthy, J.S. Utility of serological follow-up of chronic strongyloidiasis after anthelminthic chemotherapy. *Trans. R. Soc. Trop. Med. Hyg.* **2006**, *100*, 1056–1062. [CrossRef] [PubMed]

52. Biggs, B.A.; Caruana, S.; Mihrshahi, S.; Jolley, D.; Leydon, J.; Chea, L.; Nuon, S. Management of chronic strongyloidiasis in immigrants and refugees: Is serologic testing useful? *Am. J. Trop. Med. Hyg.* **2009**, *80*, 788–791. [PubMed]

53. Kearns, T.M.; Currie, B.J.; Cheng, A.C.; McCarthy, J.; Carapetis, J.R.; Holt, D.C.; Page, W.; Shield, J.; Gundjirryirr, R.; Mulholland, E.; et al. *Strongyloides* seroprevalence before and after an ivermectin mass drug administration in a remote Australian Aboriginal community. *PLoS Negl. Trop. Dis.* **2017**, *11*, e0005607. [CrossRef] [PubMed]

54. Nagayasu, E.; Aung, M.; Hortiwakul, T.; Hino, A.; Tanaka, T.; Higashiarakawa, M.; Olia, A.; Taniguchi, T.; Win, S.M.T.; Ohashi, I.; et al. A possible origin population of pathogenic intestinal nematodes, *Strongyloides stercoralis*, unveiled by molecular phylogeny. *Sci. Rep.* **2017**, *7*, 4844. [CrossRef] [PubMed]

55. Jaleta, T.G.; Zhou, S.; Bemm, F.M.; Schar, F.; Khieu, V.; Muth, S.; Odermatt, P.; Lok, J.B.; Streit, A. Different but overlapping populations of *Strongyloides stercoralis* in dogs and humans—Dogs as a possible source for zoonotic strongyloidiasis. *PLoS Negl. Trop. Dis.* **2017**, *11*, e0005752. [CrossRef] [PubMed]

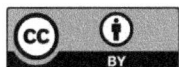

*Tropical Medicine and
Infectious Disease*

MDPI

Review

A Community-Directed Integrated *Strongyloides* Control Program in Queensland, Australia

Adrian Miller [1,*], Elizebeth L. Young [2], Valarie Tye [2], Robert Cody [2], Melody Muscat [3], Vicki Saunders [4], Michelle L. Smith [5], Jenni A. Judd [6] and Rick Speare [7,†]

1   Ellengowan Drive, Charles Darwin University, Darwin 0909, Northern Territory, Australia
2   Woorabinda Multi-Purpose Health Service, Queensland Health, 1 Munns Drive,
     Woorabinda, QLD 4713, Australia; Elizabeth.Young3@health.qld.gov.au (E.L.Y.); adrian.m@gmail.com (V.T.);
     Robert.Cody@health.qld.gov.au (R.C.)
3   Aboriginal and Torres Strait Islander Health, Faculty of Science, Health, Education and Engineering,
     University of the Sunshine Coast, Sippy Downs, QLD 4556, Australia; mmuscat@usc.edu.au
4   Australian Research Alliance for Children and Youth (ARACY), Griffith Criminology Institute,
     Brisbane, QLD 4001, Australia; vickisaunders@bigpond.com
5   School of Health and Exercise Sciences, Faculty of Health and Social Development, University of British
     Columbia, Kelowna, BC V1Y 1V7, Canada; michelle.smith@ubc.ca
6   School of Health Medicine and Applied Sciences, Centre of Indigenous Health Equity Research, Central
     Queensland University, Bundaberg, QLD 4670, Australia; j.judd@cqu.edu.au
7   College of Public Health, Medical and Veterinary Sciences, James Cook University,
     Townsville, QLD 4811, Australia; Rick.Speare@jcu.edu.au
*   Correspondence: adrian.miller@cdu.edu.au; Tel.: +61-8-8946-6060; Fax: +61-8-8946-6064
†   Deceased.

Received: 15 March 2018; Accepted: 27 April 2018; Published: 4 May 2018

Abstract: This paper describes two phases of a community-directed intervention to address strongyloidiasis in the remote Aboriginal community of Woorabinda in central Queensland, Australia. The first phase provides the narrative of a community-driven 'treat-and-test' mass drug administration (MDA) intervention that was co-designed by the Community Health Service and the community. The second phase is a description of the re-engagement of the community in order to disseminate the key factors for success in the previous MDA for *Strongyloides stercoralis*, as this information was not shared or captured in the first phase. During the first phase in 2004, there was a high prevalence of strongyloidiasis (12% faecal examination, 30% serology; n = 944 community members tested) that resulted in increased morbidity and at least one death in the community. Between 2004–2005, the community worked in partnership with the Community Health Service to implement a *S. stercoralis* control program, where all of the residents were treated with oral ivermectin, and repeat doses were given for those with positive *S. stercoralis* serology. The community also developed their own health promotion campaign using locally-made resources targeting relevant environmental health problems and concerns. Ninety-two percent of the community residents participated in the program, and the prevalence of strongyloidiasis at the time of the 'treat-and-test' intervention was 16.6% [95% confidence interval 14.2–19.3]. The cure rate after two doses of ivermectin was 79.8%, based on pre-serology and post-serology tests. The purpose of this paper is to highlight the importance of local Aboriginal leadership and governance and a high level of community involvement in this successful mass drug administration program to address *S. stercoralis*. The commitment required of these leaders was demanding, and involved intense work over a period of several months. Apart from controlling strongyloidiasis, the community also takes pride in having developed and implemented this program. This appears to be the first community-directed *S. stercoralis* control program in Australia, and is an important part of the national story of controlling infectious diseases in Indigenous communities.

Keywords: *Strongyloides stercoralis*; aboriginal; indigenous; soil-transmitted helminths; mass drug administration

1. Background and Introduction

1.1. Background

This paper documents two historical phases of a community-directed *Strongyloides stercoralis* control program. The first phase reports on a community-directed *S. stercoralis* control program in the Indigenous community of Woorabinda, central Queensland Australia. The second phase documents the need to have local Indigenous leadership and direction for community-wide health interventions, and the importance of the researchers having cultural humility. Cultural humility is defined as a lifelong process of self-reflection and self-critique whereby the individual not only learns about another's culture, but one starts with an examination of her/his own beliefs and cultural identities [1]. Cultural humility cannot be collapsed into a single workshop; it is commitment and active engagement in a lifelong process 'that individuals enter on an ongoing basis with patients, communities, colleagues, and with themselves' [1] (p. 118). This paper is a testament to Rick Speare's cultural humility across his research career.

Note that this paper is conspicuously published well after the first phase of this project. Following a strongyloidiasis-related fatality, the first phase originally focused on the clinical outcomes of an ivermectin mass drug administration [MDA] intervention to address *S. stercoralis* in the community. However, while it was evident that ivermectin MDA clearly had a significant effect on decreasing the prevalence of *S. stercoralis* among Woorabinda residents, the real success of this intervention lay in the self-determination of the community and the community health team, who drove the health promotion program to address strongyloidiasis in the community. Without this commitment from the community health team, and their relationships and trust with community members, there would have been little chance of the successful implementation of the ivermectin MDA.

This paper forms part of a new study that explores barriers and enablers to addressing infectious diseases in Indigenous Australian communities. The community voiced their concerns regarding participating in this study, as they felt: (i) they received no feedback from the original study relating to the ivermectin MDA in their community, so the community requested some researchers from James Cook University, in particular Rick Speare, to assist them with making sense of the data from the MDA, and (ii) their story regarding the success of the community-driven approach to addressing the issue of *S. stercoralis* received little attention. In their view, this was the most important aspect of the success of this program.

To address this shortcoming and the failure in communication, the results of the MDA were shared. The community felt that the community health team, in partnership with the community's leadership, was the real success of eradicating *S. stercoralis* in Woorabinda. On the community's invitation, a new research team travelled to Woorabinda to re-engage with community health team in order to capture and share the story of their successful community-driven approach to address this infectious disease, which impacted their community's health and well-being.

1.2. Introduction

Strongyloidiasis is considered one of the most neglected tropical diseases and is estimated to affect over 100 million people worldwide including Indigenous Australians [2,3]. Most cases are chronic, while acute strongyloidiasis is more common in children [4,5]. Chronic strongyloidiasis increases the risk of unpredictable fatal hyperinfection when patients become immunocompromised, malnourished, or immunosuppressed. Hyperinfection can be caused by the administration of corticosteroids to patients with strongyloidiasis [4,5].

In Australia, strongyloidiasis is highly prevalent in Indigenous rural and remote communities, and its management at the individual and community level is sub-optimal [6,7]. For *S. stercoralis*, a prevalence greater than 5% is considered to be hyperendemic, and a public health intervention is required [4,5]. However, although many Indigenous Australian communities appear to have above 5% prevalence, no community-wide control program has been reported. This paper describes the outcome from a community-based intervention to control strongyloidiasis, which was driven by the Aboriginal community in partnership with the community health team.

1.3. Context

Woorabinda is a remote, Aboriginal community that is situated approximately 175 km southwest of Rockhampton in Central Queensland, Australia (24°08′05′ S 149°27′22′ E). Woorabinda is the traditional land of the Wadja and Wadjigal people. In 2005, this small discrete Indigenous community had a population of at least 944, with about 191 western-style houses [8].

In 1996, an initial faecal survey for *S. stercoralis* and review of 130 hospital records indicated an overall prevalence of 5% in the community, with the 5–9-year-old age group having the highest prevalence of infection at 14% [9]. In 2000, the testing of patients presenting to the Woorabinda Multipurpose Health Service showed that at least 12% were positive for *S. stercoralis* on faecal testing, and 30% were positive on serology. In addition, a resident who was referred to a tertiary hospital for treatment of another disease, died from hyperinfection.

The Woorabinda Multipurpose Health Service provided health care to the community through a small hospital run by Queensland Health and an active community health team, the Woorabinda Multipurpose Community Health Team. The majority of the team members were Indigenous Australians with ancestral links to the area, and consisted of an Indigenous nurse, a non-Indigenous nurse, several Aboriginal health workers (AHWs), and local residents employed in various roles.

2. Approach

In the original phase, the Woorabinda Multipurpose Community Health Team, in partnership with the community, decided to initiate and lead a program to control *S. stercoralis* by involving the whole Woorabinda community and using a combination of treatment and prevention strategies. The goal of the program was to reduce the prevalence of *S. stercoralis* by at least 75% (from around an estimated 30% prevalence to less than 7.5%), with complete elimination from Woorabinda being the goal. The objectives were to: (i) implement a treatment program using agreed protocols; (ii) increase community participation in strategies related to the prevention of *S. stercoralis*; and (iii) decrease environmental risk factors contributing to *S. stercoralis* infection. The program was managed by a steering committee that had members from the Woorabinda Health Service, Woorabinda Council, and Central Queensland Public Health Unit; the committee also included community representatives, and other people were co-opted as required. An advisory panel with specific technical expertise assisted this steering committee.

A program work plan was co-developed, and is detailed in Table 1 to show as an example. Awareness-raising and education about *S. stercoralis* were the first components of the project, and only after the community was saturated with information did the treatment and testing stage begin. Community-based health promotion is people-centered and collectivist [10]. This program involved multiple stakeholders and worked across the community, as demonstrated by the engagement with school and environmental health officers, the council, and community health service. Facilitation and ownership of the program by the community assists with problem-solving, builds the capacity of the community, and therefore enhances successful and sustainable programs [11].

Table 1. Woorabinda *S. stercoralis* Control Program Work Plan.

Months After Commencement	Action	Responsibility *
3–4 months	Formation of a steering committee	DON
	Adoption of program plan	Steering committee
	Appointment of personnel to conduct program	DON
	Develop consent forms: ivermectin, albendazole, beta-HCG (test for pregnancy), release of information.	PO/RN
	Develop data collection tools for treatment—paper and electronic	PO/RN
	Develop drug recording systems	PO/RN
	Develop management flow chart	PO/RN
	Develop education and awareness-raising materials	PO/RN
	Collect baseline data results from previous studies conducted in Woorabinda and develop evaluation measures for comparison: (a) Environmental health and household survey; (b) Animal census.	PO
	Environmental health program commences	EHO, EH Coordinator/HW's/Council
	Education and awareness-raising commences	HW
6 months	Pilot of initial treatment	DR/RN/HW
	Review and modification of management flow chart	Steering Committee
	Environmental health program continues	EHO, EH Coordinator/HW's/Council
	Initial serology/treatment of community	DR/RN/HW
	Follow-up of community members not presenting for treatment/re-treatment of positive cases at two weeks	RN/HW
	Education and awareness-raising continues	HW
	Environmental health program continues	EHO, EH Coordinator/HW's/Council
	Analysis of results from initial treatment and report	RN
12–13 months	First follow-up serology and treatment of resistant/positive cases.	DR/RN/HW
	Follow-up community members who have not presented for serology and treatment/resistant cases	RN/HW
	Analysis of results from first follow-up and report	RN
	Second follow-up treatment for resistant cases	DR/RN/HW
	Follow-up community members not presenting for serology and treatment	RN/HW
	Education and awareness raising continues	HW
	Environmental health program continues	EHO, EH Coordinator/HW's/Council
	Analysis of results from second follow-up and report	RN
14 months	Third follow-up serology and treatment	DR/RN/HW
	Follow-up community members not presenting for serology and treatment	RN/HW
	Education and awareness raising continues	HW
	Environmental health program continues	EHO, EH Coordinator/HW's/Council
	Analysis of results from third follow-up and report	RN

Table 1. *Cont.*

Months After Commencement	Action	Responsibility *
	Fourth follow-up serology	DR/RN/HW
	Follow-up community members not presenting for serology and treatment	RN/HW
	Education and awareness raising continues	HW
21–24 months	Environmental health program continues	EHO, EH Coordinator/HW's/Council
	Analysis of results from fourth follow-up and report	RN
	Refer resistant cases to Dr	RN
	Final report and recommendations	RN
	Second yearly review to confirm eradication	Health Service

* DON—Director of Nursing; PO—Project Officer; EHO—Environmental Health Officer; EH Coordinator—Environmental Health Coordinator; DR—Doctor; Council—Local Shire Council; RN—Registered Nurse; HW—Health Worker.

2.1. Community Participation

The Woorabinda Multipurpose Community Health Team worked with stakeholders to develop health education and promotion material to ensure that all of the resources were culturally appropriate and locally relevant. This material focused on explaining *S. stercoralis* and its lifecycle, symptoms of strongyloidiasis, treatment, and prevention of transmission. Female community elders developed several unique health promotion tools, including posters, a comic strip, and Aunty Val's 'Gunna Story' (Figure 1C). In local Aboriginal slang, 'gunna' means faeces. An explanation of the local treatment program and prevention strategies encouraged people to play an active role in stopping the transmission of *S. stercoralis*. These health promotion strategies used a multiple intervention model and included: improvement of defects in sanitation systems by house-to-house inspection, personal hygiene, safe disposal of nappies, wearing shoes, and responsible dog ownership. All of these strategies were in line with the principles of the Ottawa Charter [12], which emphasises that multiple strategies across sectors will assist in improving the health of peoples, groups, communities, and populations. A recent study found that wearing shoes decreased the likelihood of infection of schoolchildren with *S. stercoralis* [13].

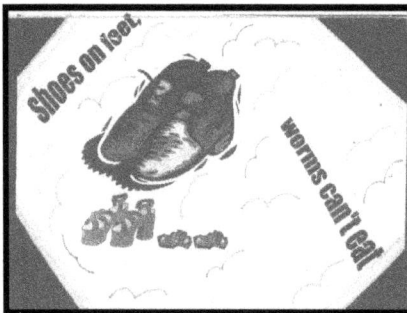

(A)

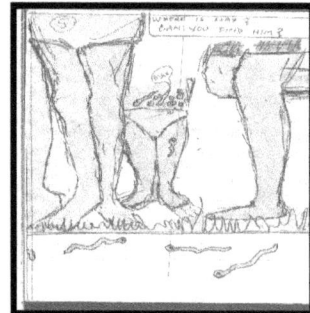

(B)

Figure 1. *Cont.*

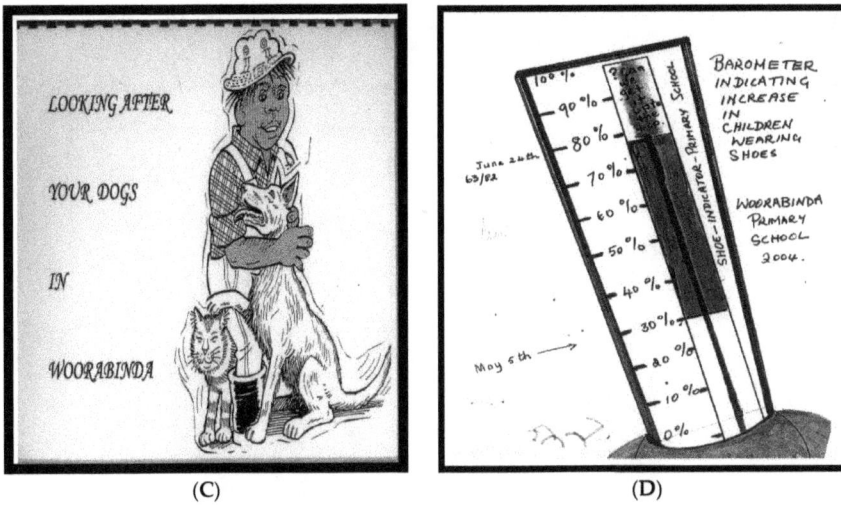

(C)   (D)

Figure 1. Health promotion material developed during the Woorabinda *Strongyloides* control program. (**A**) Poster on protective footwear; (**B**) Jaime and Aunty June's comic strip described the life cycle and transmission of *S. stercoralis*; (**C**) Aunty Val's Gunna Story; (**D**) Shoe barometer.

2.2. Involvement of Primary School Children

Teachers and children at the Woorabinda State Primary School were also actively involved. They developed two very specific items: a shoe barometer that measured the percentage of children wearing shoes to classes (Figure 2), and a *Strongyloides* song that was used on the local radio station, particularly preceding announcements about the control program (Table 2). Health promotion programs are most likely to be effective when they are flexible and responsive to local realities [11].

Table 2. The *Strongyloides* Song Developed and Sung by the Woorabinda State Primary Schoolchildren.

The Strongyloides Song
Words by June Barkworth and adapted by the Woorabinda Schoolchildren. The children and staff of the Woorabinda State School wrote the music. This song was used as a signature tune to herald radio updates on the Strongyloides project.
No, no, no, 'Mr Worm' we don't want you
Travelling through our skin and making us sick,
With boots and shoes on our feet (stamp, stamp)
Blankets on the ground,
We're gon'na stop you from moving around
'Our bodies'
Yes, yes, yes, 'Mr Worm' you have got to go ho, ho, ho, ho,
Go, go, go 'Mr Worm' we're getting tough
You have no place to live in us.
We're gon'na thrash you out, we're gon'na move you on ... ... then
Woorabinda will say that 'Mr Strongyloides' worm is gone.
Yes, yes, yes 'Mr Worm' you have got to go. Ho, ho, ho, ho, ho.

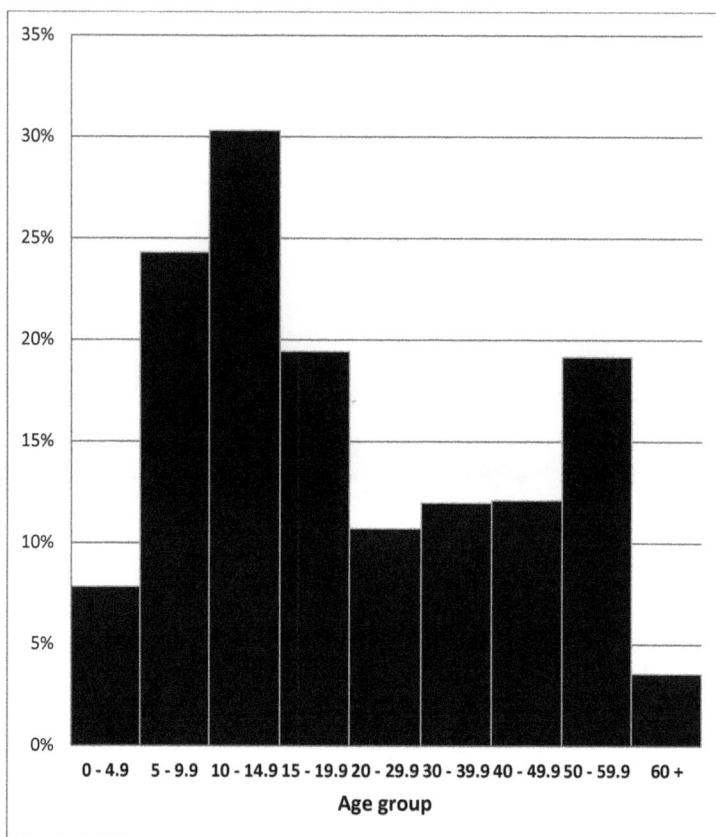

Figure 2. Prevalence of positive *S. stercoralis* serology from an initial survey in phase 1 of the Woorabinda community, July–August 2004.

2.3. Treat-and-Test

All community residents were urged to participate in a 'treat-and-test' survey. Everyone was asked for a sample of blood collected by venipuncture for *S. stercoralis* serology [14], and were treated for *S. stercoralis* at this time. The most effective treatment for *S. stercoralis* is ivermectin [5,15], but ivermectin is not licensed in Australia for treating pregnant women or children with a body weight of less than 15 kg. A less effective alternative option, albendazole, can be used for treatment in the latter category, but was not licensed in Australia for use in pregnant women. The treatment protocol for the Woorabinda program was based on recommendations from the first National Workshop on Strongyloidiasis in September 2001 [16]. This protocol recommended: (1) Children >6 months of age but <10 kg, albendazole: 200 mg daily for three days; (2) Children >6 months of age and 10–15 kg, albendazole: 400 mg daily for three days; and (3) All people except pregnant women >15 kg, ivermectin (Stromectol): 0.2 mg/kg body weight. Women of child-bearing age were offered a pregnancy test prior to treatment with ivermectin. Any person who was subsequently shown to have positive serology for *S. stercoralis* on the initial blood sample was retreated within a month.

2.4. Environmental Risk Factors

Environmental health activities were part of the community-wide program. A housing improvement program as part of a state-wide initiative was operating in Woorabinda using Commonwealth and State government funds. A set of priority areas was developed to address environmental risk factors for *S. stercoralis* in the community. Specific actions included repairing malfunctioning toilets and leaking taps and pipes that could cause areas of persistent damp soil.

2.5. Serological Results

Over a six-week period, 867 people were treated and tested; the group comprised 46% (404/867) males, and 16.6% (144/867) (95% confidence interval 14.2–19.3) had positive serology. The parasite was present in all age groups, with the highest percentage between 5–20 years, with a peak at 10–15 years and a further rise at 50–59 years (Figure 2). The participation rate was approximately 92% (867/944).

Of the participants who tested positive in July and August 2004, 129 were re-tested in February 2005 after treatment, and 103 had reverted to negative: a cure rate of 79.8%. In February 2005, 140 people who had been initially negative for *S. stercoralis* were re-tested, and none had seroconverted over this six-month period, indicating that transmission at Woorabinda appeared to have ceased.

3. Discussion

Most soil transmitted helminth (STH) control programs are driven and managed by health departments, usually from urban centres. Although community-wide control programs for *S. stercoralis* have been advocated since the 1990s [4,17], the only report outside the experimental situation appears to be a Japanese study that monitored and treated a small group of residents on Okinawa, and hence was not a program that engaged the whole community [18]. This Woorabinda program may be the first community-wide program described. It was unusual in that it was initiated, implemented, and managed by the community itself. Woorabinda found the resources—including the funding, person-power, and expertise—that were needed for its successful completion. This was arguably the key factor in achieving a high level of community engagement.

3.1. Impact of the Program

The strategy that was adopted was successful in identifying and treating much of the population. The cure rate after two treatments was high, and transmission of *S. stercoralis* at Woorabinda appeared to have ceased. This is the only description of a successful community-led *S. stercoralis* control program. It appears to be the first to use a 'treat-and-test' strategy where all of the participants were treated initially for *S. stercoralis*, and subsequent management depended on the test result. Although the long-term effect of the program has not been evaluated, the Woorabinda health centre doctor anecdotally reported to the research team that cases of strongyloidiasis are now rare, and strongyloidiasis is no longer considered a public health issue at Woorabinda. Unfortunately, infection with *S. stercoralis* is not notifiable in Australia; hence, the trend in incidence for Woorabinda is unavailable. Making this parasitic infection notifiable is essential for control and elimination [19].

3.2. Local Leadership and Knowledge

The project team used Indigenous and local leadership, with AHW knowledge of the health profile of the local community, the households, and the needs of the community being a very important factor in the success of the mass drug administration program. Additionally, since the AHWs are community members, trust between community members and health staff was high, giving the *S. stercoralis* control program high credibility.

3.3. Big Effort, But Worth It

Members of the health team worked very hard during this program, while still performing their usual work tasks. However, they considered that the effort was worth it, since the disease of concern was controlled, and the health team and the community became united on tackling and solving a significant health problem. Over a decade later, yarns with original members of the health team still reflect their sense of pride in their achievement.

3.4. Knowledge and Understanding of the Parasite

AHWs and other health staff providing information to community members about *S. stercoralis* facilitated the development of localised knowledge and understanding of the parasite. This was contextualised on the community's prior knowledge about hookworm, a STH that had been historically present in the community, but had been eliminated. This allowed the team to develop ways to share new knowledge and understanding about *S. stercoralis* and the benefit of the program. Localised communication strategies were developed and delivered in the form of novel health promotion materials such as a children's song, a children's story in the local language, localised posters, radio advertisements, and a school-based awareness program, which was exemplified by the shoe barometer. The materials developed were a good illustration that in Aboriginal communities, health promotion materials should be localised and humorised [20].

3.5. Development of an Inclusive Governance Model and Skills Development

The team developed a governance model to guide the project, which was a community-driven approach that seconded expert advice at critical points of the program; the steering committee and the advisory panel provided this advice. This approach fostered partnerships between the health and education sectors, researchers, and local government. Strong support for serology tests was provided by Queensland Health laboratory scientists at Rockhampton. AHWs were trained to collect blood (except for infants and babies where phlebotomists were required), and standing orders gave the AHWs authority to administer anthelmintic medications. An implementation protocol with a shared understanding of the commitment required for this program was a core component of the program.

3.6. Aspects to Be Improved

A decrease in the number of people affected meant that momentum for the program to progress to elimination was lost. Although a repeat community-wide survey to document the post-program prevalence of strongyloidiasis would have provided valuable information, owing to lack of further targeted resources, no survey was conducted.

4. Conclusions

This paper illustrates how a community-directed and led *S. stercoralis* control program using a 'treat-and-test' strategy in a remote Australian Aboriginal community brought an outbreak and subsequent high prevalence of strongyloidiasis under control. The use of localised health promotion strategies and materials developed by community members contributed to the program's success, and set out a clear plan for action for other communities needing to address *S. stercoralis*. Since *S. stercoralis* is usually not a health problem in developed countries and is usually associated with poverty, its high prevalence in this community drew attention to the underlying social determinants of health and the need for social solutions, as well as biomedical interventions.

Author Contributions: A.M., J.A.J. and R.S. wrote the paper; E.L.Y., V.T. and R.C. led the mass drug administration, and collected data; R.S. and V.S. analysed the data; V.T. developed and led health promotion resources; M.M. contributed to the paper and lead community engagement; M.L.S. contributed to the paper.

Funding: Aboriginal and Torres Strait Islander Commission, Australian Government.

Acknowledgments: We would like to acknowledge the Aboriginal peoples of the Woorabinda Community and their health workers who dedicated their time and effort in this community program. We would also like to dedicate this paper to the memory of our co-author Emeritus Rick Speare. Rick had a long commitment to improving the health, education and well-being of Aboriginal people and to the research education and development of Aboriginal and Torres Strait Islander scholars. He encouraged the learning of community members and had a long involvement with the Woorabinda community in the nineties. He was many things, a doctor, a vet, a teacher, and a mentor and friend. He spent much of his life understanding *S. stercoralis*, in fact, he wrote his PhD on it. He was committed to lifelong learning and sharing his knowledge and expertise with Aboriginal community people to prevent and manage strongyloidiasis. Finally, an acknowledgement to the late June Barkworth (registered community based nurse, Woorabinda Multi-Purpose Health Service) who led the original phase and William Gulf, Deputy Mayor, Woorabinda Shire Council, who were critical in initiating and driving this MDA.

Ethics and Permissions: All subjects gave their informed consent for inclusion before they participated in the study. The study was conducted in accordance with the Declaration of Helsinki, and the protocol was approved by the Ethics Committee of Queensland Health—Rockhampton Health Services District, Human Research Ethics Committee, 'Woorabinda Strongyloides Eradiation Project Plan 2004', Approval Number 04.06.

Conflicts of Interest: There are no conflicts of interests with any authors.

References

1. Tervalon, M.; Murray-Garcia, J. Cultural humility versus cultural competence: A critical distinction in defining physical training outcomes in multicultural education. *J. Health Care Poor Underser.* **1998**, *9*, 117. [CrossRef]
2. Olsen, A.; van Lieshout, L.; Marti, H.; Polderman, T.; Polman, K.; Steinmann, P.; Stothard, R.; Thybo, S.; Verweij, J.J.; Magnussen, P. Strongyloidiasis—The most neglected of the neglected tropical diseases? *Trans. R. Soc. Trop. Med. Hyg.* **2009**, *103*, 967–972. [CrossRef] [PubMed]
3. Puthiyakunnon, S.; Boddu, S.; Li, Y.; Zhou, X.; Wang, C.; Li, J.; Chen, X. Strongyloidiasis—An insight into its global prevalence and management. *PLoS Negl. Trop. Dis.* **2014**, *8*, e3018. [CrossRef] [PubMed]
4. Shield, J.M.; Page, W. Effective diagnostic tests and anthelmintic treatment for *Strongyloides stercoralis* make community control feasible. *PNG Med. J.* **2008**, *51*, 105–119.
5. Page, W.; Shield, J.; O'Donahoo, F.; Miller, A.; Judd, J.; Speare, R. Strongyloidiasis in Oceania. In *Neglected Tropical Diseases—Oceania*; Loukas, A., Ed.; Springer: Berlin, Germany, 2016; Chapter 3; pp. 69–99.
6. Miller, A.; Smith, M.L.; Judd, J.A.; Speare, R. *Strongyloides stercoralis*: Systematic review of barriers to controlling strongyloidiasis for Australian Indigenous communities. *PLoS Negl. Trop. Dis.* **2014**, *8*, e3141. [CrossRef] [PubMed]
7. Mounsey, K.; Kearns, T.; Rampton, M.; Llewellyn, S.; King, M.; Holt, D.; Currie, B.J.; Andrews, R.; Nutman, T.; McCarthy, J. Use of dried blood spots to define antibody response to the *Strongyloides stercoralis* recombinant antigen NIE. *Acta Trop.* **2014**, *138*, 78–82. [CrossRef] [PubMed]
8. National Regional Profile: Woorabinda Local Government Area. Available online: http://www.abs.gov.au/AUSSTATS/abs@nrp.nsf/Previousproducts/LGA37550Population/People12005-2009?opendocument&tabname=Summary&prodno=LGA37550&issue=2005-2009&num=&view= (accessed on 4 June 2015).
9. Australian Centre for International and Tropical Health and Nutrition (ACITHN). *Environmental Health in Woorabinda: Investigation of Parasite Infections in the Community*; The University of Queensland and Queensland Institute of Medical Research: Brisbane, Australia, 1996.
10. Raeburn, J. *and Rootman, I. People Centered Health Promotion*; John Wiley and Sons: Toronto, ON, Canada, 1998.
11. Judd, J.; Frankish CJ and Moulton, G. Setting Standards in the evaluation of community-based health promotion programs—A unifying approach. *Health Promot. Int. J.* **2001**, *16*, 367–380. [CrossRef]
12. World Health Organization (WHO). Ottawa Charter for Health Promotion. *Health Promot.* **1986**, *1*, 3–5.
13. Khieu, V.; Hattendorf, J.; Schär, F.; Marti, H.; Char, M.C.; Muth, S.; Odermatt, P. *Strongyloides stercoralis* infection and re-infection in a cohort of children in Cambodia. *Parasitol. Int.* **2014**, *63*, 708–712. [CrossRef] [PubMed]
14. Sampson, I.A.; and Grove, D.I. Strongyloidiasis is endemic in another Australian population group: Indochinese immigrants. *Med. J. Aust.* **1987**, *146*, 580–582. [PubMed]

15. Biggs, B.A.; Caruana, S.; Mihrshahi, S.; Jolley, D.; Leydon, J.; Chea, L.; Nuon, S. Management of chronic strongyloidiasis in immigrants and refugees: Is serologic testing useful? *Am. J. Trop. Med. Hyg.* **2009**, *80*, 788–791. [PubMed]

16. Page, W.; Speare, R. Recommendations from the First National Workshop on Strongyloidiasis. Brisbane, 25–26 July 2003. Available online: http://www.tropicalhealthsolutions.com/sites/default/files//uploaded/Recommendations-1NWS.pdf (accessed on 15 March 2018).

17. Conway, D.J.; Lindo, J.F.; Robinson, R.D.; Bundy, D.A.P. Towards effective control of *Strongyloides stercoralis*. *Parasitol. Today* **1995**, *11*, 421–424. [CrossRef]

18. Toma, H.; Shimabukura, I.; Kobayashi, J.; Tasaki, T.; Takara, M.; Sato, Y. Community control studies on *Strongyloides* infection in a model island of Okinawa, Japan. *Southeast Asian J. Trop. Med. Public Health* **2000**, *31*, 383–387. [PubMed]

19. Speare, R.; Miller, A.; Page, W. Strongyloidiasis: A case for notification in Australia? *Med. J. Aust.* **2015**, *202*, 523–524. [CrossRef] [PubMed]

20. Massey, P.D.; Miller, A.; Saggers, S.; Durrheim, D.N.; Speare, R.; Taylor, K.; Pearce, G.; Odo, T.; Broome, J.; Judd, J.; et al. Australian Aboriginal and Torres Strait Islander communities and the development of pandemic influenza containment strategies: Community voices and community control. *Health Policy* **2011**, *103*, 184–190. [CrossRef] [PubMed]

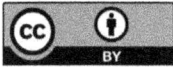

Tropical Medicine and Infectious Disease

MDPI

Review

Argument for Inclusion of Strongyloidiasis in the Australian National Notifiable Disease List

Meruyert Beknazarova [1,*], Harriet Whiley [1], Jenni A. Judd [2], Jennifer Shield [3], Wendy Page [4,5], Adrian Miller [6], Maxine Whittaker [7] and Kirstin Ross [1]

[1] College of Science and Engineering, Flinders University, Bedford Park, SA 5042, Australia; harriet.whiley@flinders.edu.au (H.W.); kirstin.ross@flinders.edu.au (K.R.)
[2] School of Health Medical and Applied Sciences, Centre of Indigenous Health Equity Research, Central Queensland University, Bundaberg, QLD 4670, Australia; j.judd@cqu.edu.au
[3] Department of Pharmacy and Applied Science, La Trobe University, Bendigo, VIC 3552, Australia; j.shield@latrobe.edu.au
[4] Miwatj Health Aboriginal Corporation, Nhulunbuy, NT 0881, Australia; wendy.page@my.jcu.edu.au
[5] Public Health and Tropical Medicine, James Cook University, Cairns, QLD 4870, Australia
[6] Indigenous Research Unit, Griffith University, Nathan, QLD 4111, Australia; adrian.miller@cdu.edu.au
[7] College of Public Health, Medical and Veterinary Sciences, James Cook University, Townsville, QLD 4811, Australia; maxine.whittaker@jcu.edu.au
* Correspondence: mira.beknazarova@flinders.edu.au; Tel.: +61-8-7221-8586

Received: 7 May 2018; Accepted: 31 May 2018; Published: 5 June 2018

Abstract: Strongyloidiasis is an infection caused by the helminth, *Strongyloides stercoralis*. Up to 370 million people are infected with the parasite globally, and it has remained endemic in the Indigenous Australian population for many decades. Strongyloidiasis has been also reported in other Australian populations. Ignorance of this disease has caused unnecessary costs to the government health system, and been detrimental to the Australian people's health. This manuscript addresses the 12 criteria required for a disease to be included in the Australian National Notifiable Disease List (NNDL) under the *National Health Security Act 2007* (Commonwealth). There are six main arguments that provide compelling justification for strongyloidiasis to be made nationally notifiable and added to the Australian NNDL. These are: The disease is important to Indigenous health, and closing the health inequity gap between Indigenous and non-Indigenous Australians is a priority; a public health response is required to detect cases of strongyloidiasis and to establish the true incidence and prevalence of the disease; there is no alternative national surveillance system to gather data on the disease; there are preventive measures with high efficacy and low side effects; data collection is feasible as cases are definable by microscopy, PCR, or serological diagnostics; and achievement of the Sustainable Development Goal (SDG) # 6 on clean water and sanitation.

Keywords: strongyloidiasis; *Strongyloides stercoralis*; notifiable; Australia

---

1. Introduction

Strongyloidiasis is an infection caused by the intestinal and tissue helminth, *Strongyloides stercoralis* [1]. *S. stercoralis* has been estimated to infect up to 370 million people worldwide [2]. In Australia, strongyloidiasis remains endemic in Indigenous populations, infecting communities in Queensland [3], the Northern Territory [4–9], Western Australia [10], northern South Australia [11], and northern New South Wales [12]. Seroprevalence in some communities reaches 60% [4–9,13]. Despite the prevalence and potential for morbidity and mortality posed by this disease, the true incidence in Australia remains unknown [2] as a consequence of both under-diagnosis of the disease and the absence of mechanisms to capture surveillance data [14]. The absence of reliable national data of the geographic extent and rate of transmission of this disease blinds medical and public health professionals attempting to institute effective control. This knowledge gap is not unique to Australia. Schar et al. (2013) noted that adequate information on *S. stercoralis* prevalence is still lacking from many countries, but their review found that the information that does exist points out to it being an infection that must not be neglected. They recommended information needs to be collected in a range of socio-economic and ecological settings and that in many settings the integration of control and treatment of *S. stercoralis* into a holistic helminth control program is warranted [15].

S. stercoralis is a soil-transmitted helminth, infecting a human when infective stage larvae penetrate the skin, enter the circulation, and subsequently travel to the lungs via the blood, from where it is swallowed into the gut [16]. This is the traditional ordered pathway, though evidence exists that random migration through the body to reach the intestine is also likely, even in primary infection [17–19]. A free-living phase of the parasitic life cycle occurs in the soil after host defaecation in the open, but this can only last one generation, and thus a soil reservoir of the parasite is not a factor in long-term control after implementation. Symptoms are protean, including respiratory, gastrointestinal, and skin disorders [18,20]. Unlike most other soil-transmitted helminth infections, *S. stercoralis* larvae can persist indefinitely inside the host through asexual reproduction by parthenogenesis and subsequent autoinfection [21,22].

After initial infection, there is a rapid increase in numbers as the result of an autoinfective burst [23]. This causes acute disease. This typically abates in immunocompetent people, becoming asymptomatic, or mildly symptomatic, often mimicking the symptoms of other diseases [9,24]. Due to its peculiar autoinfective nature, disease is often lifelong and a single remaining larva of *S. stercoralis* post-treatment can cause recrudescence of disease. In immunocompetent persons, the disease is chronic and long-lasting. In immunocompromised/immunosuppressed persons, or those receiving corticosteroid treatment, the infection may transform to a hyperinfective or disseminated disease syndrome, with up to 90% mortality [16,25–29].

Strongyloides is typically found in tropical and subtropical zones, but is mainly associated with areas of low socioeconomic status as a consequence of inadequate sanitary conditions [30]. This is supported by evidence of strongyloidiasis being found in desert communities [6,11]. Strongyloidiasis is described as the most neglected of the Neglected Tropical Diseases (NTDs) [14], and it is important to make strongyloidiasis notifiable so that epidemiological and prevalence data can be obtained to inform appropriate strategies for controlling the disease.

2. The Australian National Notifiable Disease Surveillance System (NNDSS)

The Quarantine Act (NSW) of 1832 was the first legislative document to cover public health issues and included mandatory reporting of diseases to local health authorities in Australia [31]. The Communicable Disease Network Australia (CDNA) was established in 1989 to enhance national communicable disease surveillance reporting to the then National Public Health Partnership (NPHP) [32]. In 2006, NPHP split into the Australian Health Protection Committee (AHPC) and the Australian Health Development Committee (AHDC). CDNA now operates under the AHPC.

The Australian National Notifiable Diseases Surveillance System (NNDSS) was first introduced in 1990 and serves as a platform to collate and report data on nationally-approved notifiable diseases from all jurisdictions to the Commonwealth [32,33]. The National Notifiable Disease List (NNDL) was created in 2008 under the National Health Security Act 2007 (Commonwealth), a document that contains a list of notifiable communicable diseases to the NNDSS.

3. Criteria for Inclusion on the National Notifiable Disease List

To determine whether a disease should be notifiable, there are currently 12 criteria against which a disease is ranked. These criteria were established by the CDNA in 2014 [32]. Table 1 presents an assessment of strongyloidiasis against each of these criteria. A score of 28 (if conservative estimates are used) to 30 (if less conservative estimates are used) was calculated for strongyloidiasis based on

CDNA descriptors. The CDNA criteria state that if a disease scores less than 15, national notification is not recommended; if it falls between 15 to 25, national notification is to be considered further; and if it is higher than 25, national notification is recommended. As such, even with a conservative estimate of 28, strongyloidiasis fulfils the requirements for national notification to be recommended [32]. The criteria can be found at: (http://www.health.gov.au/internet/main/publishing.nsf/Content/8DF6148BCAC589D6CA257EE5001D0DF7/$File/Protocol-change-NNDL.pdf).

Based on Table 1 there are six key arguments for making strongyloidiasis notifiable:

- The disease is important to Indigenous health, and closing the health inequity gap between Indigenous and non-Indigenous Australians is a priority.
- A public health response is required to detect cases of strongyloidiasis and to establish the true incidence and prevalence of the disease.
- There is no alternative national surveillance system to gather data on the disease.
- There are preventive measures with high efficacy and low side effects.
- Data collection is feasible as cases are definable by microscopy, PCR, or serological diagnostics.
- Achievement of the Sustainable Development Goal (SDG) # 6 on clean water and sanitation.

4. Prevalence of Strongyloidiasis in Australia

Strongyloidiasis may have been present in Australia prior to the arrival of Europeans. Due to improvements in sanitation and healthcare, it is no longer typically seen in non-Indigenous Australian communities [34], but remains a major health problem for Indigenous communities, particularly in remote areas. Despite its long-term persistence in Australia, it is difficult to determine the true distribution and prevalence of the disease. The first confirmed reports of strongyloidiasis in Australia date back to the early 1900s in north Queensland [35–37]. The first reports of it specifically affecting Aboriginal communities (in Atherton Tablelands) date back to the early 1900s, at which time it was noted to affect Aboriginal people at almost 30 times that of non-Aboriginal [34]. To date, infection-related mortality rate in Indigenous people is much higher compared with that in non-Indigenous population. Strongyloidiasis is one of the causes of deaths [38]. Current estimates of strongyloidiasis incidence are limited and based on opportunistic testing in hotspot areas and diagnostic pathology laboratory data [39]. The former is biased towards high prevalence communities and the latter towards subjects with easy access to healthcare and laboratory services and having sufficiently symptomatic disease to require diagnostic evaluation. There is also no standard detection method available. A study conducted in north Queensland in 2006 showed a strongyloidiasis prevalence in Indigenous and non-Indigenous populations of 24% and 10% respectively [40]. An epidemiological study with Aboriginal communities in Northern Australia conducted over 2010–2011 showed a strongyloidiasis seroprevalence of 21% [7]. Overall, based on studies completed in different localized endemic areas from 1980 to 2010, strongyloidiasis prevalence is estimated to range from 2% to 41% based on faecal microscopy surveys [3,5,10,41] and from 5% to 60% based on serology survey tests [42,43]. Furthermore, infected people are known to live elsewhere in Australia apart from endemic areas [44].

Strongyloidiasis also affects other populations. GeoSentinel Surveillance Network site holds a database for returned international travelers with infectious gastrointestinal disease. Based on analysis of their international database during the period 1996–2005, *S. stercoralis* was rated the fifth most common pathogen [45]. Screening and treatment is now policy for refugees coming to Australia. However, screening has not yet been introduced to policy or systems for endemic Aboriginal communities in Australia. Immigrants and refugees from South East Asia also have high prevalence rates, as do returned travelers [20,46]. In a South Australian study, 11.6% of Vietnam veterans tested seropositive for *S. stercoralis* [47]. Four non-Indigenous cases of strongyloidiasis acquired through occupational exposure were reported in Central Australia [44].

Table 1. *Strongyloides stercoralis* against 12 criteria for NNDL assessment.

#	Criterion	Score	Notes on Strongyloidiasis
	Priority setting		
1	Necessity for public health response	2/4 = case reporting important for detecting outbreaks that require investigating or contacts require routine intervention	A public health response and immediate intervention is required based on the following; 1. Inadequate hygiene and sanitary conditions are the main factors for human strongyloidiasis. A person can get infected when coming into contact with or near infected human or dog faeces. In low socioeconomic status communities, such as some Indigenous communities, sanitation conditions present a high risk for strongyloidiasis transmission, contamination, re-infection, and recurrence [30]. Therefore, it is crucial to get a public health response to create and maintain adequate sanitary and hygiene conditions in the communities to prevent the disease. Culturally comprehensive health education for understanding the nature of infectious diseases and how they are transmitted is fundamental for maintaining hygienic conditions [48]. 2. There is the opportunity to highlight environmental health role in the public health response. There is an opportunity to make a difference in endemic communities and specific families/communities with high need targeting the SDG # 6 on clean water and sanitation. 3. Interventions programs such as targeted mass drug administration (MDA) have shown to be very effective in reducing the reservoir of human infection, and need to be implemented regularly on a local and national level in endemic communities [7]. 4. Another intervention program in an endemic Indigenous community incorporated *S. stercoralis* screening into the adult health check, and positive cases were treated and followed up. This selective chemotherapy intervention resulted in a decreased risk of potentially fatal hyperinfection and decreased prevalence in the community [13,49]. 5. Strongyloidiasis has been shown to prevent weight gain in children, and therefore it is critical to identify and treat *S. stercoralis* infection to avoid intervention by social services. This intervention can result in child removal from parents into care if the child shows signs of malnutrition [49]. An environmental health response to geographic hot spots would also bring in the SDG # 6 on clean water and sanitation.
2	Utility and significance of notification for prevention programs	1/4 = Need to establish burden of illness for monitoring or research purposes/priority setting	The geographic prevalence of *S. stercoralis* within Australia is essential to understand and map the hotspots. Notification and establishing the true burden of infection will improve monitoring, prevention and research, for assessing the effectiveness of prevention and control programs at the local and regional levels. Currently, there are no true disability-adjusted life years (DALYs) identified for strongyloidiasis, mainly because of poor estimates of disease prevalence.
3	Vaccine preventability	0/4 = No vaccine available	No vaccine available

Table 1. *Cont.*

#	Criterion	Score	Notes on Strongyloidiasis
4	Importance for Indigenous health	4/4 = Very high	Strongyloidiasis is endemic in the Indigenous population, affecting up to 60% of the population in some remote communities. Strongyloidiasis has been and continues to be an issue in the Australian Indigenous population, causing unnecessary morbidity and mortality in all age groups [39]. Many in the Australian Indigenous population, as a result of socioeconomic conditions and compromised/suppressed immunity due to chronic disease, are unusually susceptible to both acute strongyloidiasis, and life-threatening disseminated and/or hyperinfective strongyloidiasis.
5	Emerging or re-emerging disease	2/4 = slowly re-emerging or increasing incidence/prevalence disease over the past 5 years	Strongyloidiasis has been called 'the most neglected of Neglected Tropical Diseases' [14]. Cases have been reported since the early 1900s. The literature shows that the prevalence of the disease trend declined following mass drug administration (MDA) of ivermectin (2010) and albendazole (1995) in these communities [7,13]. However, the disease has never been eliminated and tends to reappear [5,41]. The disease has been neglected, and the real prevalence of the disease is underestimated due to lack of disease surveillance. Due to the unique autoinfective cycle of *S. stercoralis*, chronic strongyloidiasis lasts for a lifetime if not effectively diagnosed and treated. Cases of hyperinfection and iatrogenic fatal dissemination are predicted to increase as the infected populations age and are at a higher risk of being immunosuppressed. Corticosteroids have been considered a factor in 65% of fatalities from hyperinfection [50]. Another factor contributing to this emerging disease status with increasing cases of severe, complicated strongyloidiasis, has been the lack of awareness of strongyloidiasis in medical personnel who have been trained in Australia.
6	Communicability and potential for outbreaks	2/4 = Medium	There is a potential for outbreaks in poor-infrastructure settings with low sanitary and hygiene conditions, which together produce a high risk for strongyloidiasis transmission from person to person via faecal-skin and faecal-oral routes [51].
7	Severity and socioeconomic impact	1/4 = low severity and socioeconomic impacts in chronic strongyloidiasis (strongyloidiasis in healthy person) or 2/4 = medium severity and socioeconomic impacts in disseminated or hyperinfective strongyloidiasis	In healthy people, chronic strongyloidiasis may have only mild, intermittent, and non-specific symptoms. However, the autoinfection feature of this helminth and parthenogenesis, allows single larvae reproducing within the host leading to a chronic, long-lasting disease. If not diagnosed and treated, the disease can take a more serious form as the person becomes immunocompromised/immunosuppressed, with an often-fatal outcome. A case fatality rate of almost 90% has been reported [6]. Strongyloidiasis presents unnecessary cost to the health systems, as strongyloidiasis is both preventable and treatable if diagnosed early, and in the chronic stage. The diagnostic and treatment costs, including selective chemotherapy, targeted MDA and water, sanitation and hygiene (WASH) have been estimated in previous research and shown to be affordable [52,53]. It was estimated in US citizens that presumptive preventive intervention would decrease DALYs caused by intestinal parasites, including *Strongyloides*, by up to 1976- saving USD 16.4 million [54].

Table 1. *Cont.*

#	Criterion	Score	Notes on Strongyloidiasis
8	Preventability	4/4 = preventive measure with high efficacy/low side effects/high acceptability and uptake	Adequate sanitary and hygiene conditions including safe water supply, proper toileting and hygiene facilities would provide long term sustainable prevention and elimination of strongyloidiasis [51]. This should be combined with health education and research to determine the gold standard for strongyloidiasis diagnosis. Treatment of chronic strongyloidiasis prevents hyperinfection. Currently, ivermectin is the drug of first choice to treat human strongyloidiasis, followed by albendazole [55]. Ivermectin and albendazole, given according to therapeutic guidelines for strongyloidiasis [41], have been shown to eliminate the disease in 70% to 85% of those with chronic strongyloidiasis. Both drugs have negligible side effects. Ivermectin requires only one to two administrations. Albendazole requires two courses of daily doses for three days. A single dose is ineffective [7,13].
9	Level of public concern and/or political interest	2/4 = low to medium public concern or political interest or 3/4 = medium to high public concern or political interest	Strongyloidiasis is an overlooked, neglected disease [14]. However, when people are made aware of the disease, there is high public concern. This is illustrated by a recently published article on strongyloidiasis in 'The Conversation' which received a large number of responses by the general public showing their interest and concern about the disease [56]. Closing the Gap (the health inequity gap between Indigenous and non-Indigenous Australians) is a high priority in mainstream Australia [57]. The fact that locally-acquired infection in Australia is almost exclusively seen in Indigenous communities should be of great public and political concern.
Feasibility of collection			
10	A case is definable	4/4 = Case has an acceptable laboratory definition with or without a clinical definition	A strongyloidiasis case is definable and we propose to notify strongyloidiasis by the laboratories based on positive serology or parasitological diagnosis [58]. In disseminated and hyperinfective strongyloidiasis, faecal examination has higher sensitivity due to large numbers of viable larvae and the patient is usually in a hospital setting at the time of diagnosis. In immunocompetent persons, chronic strongyloidiasis might not always be detected by microscopy due to low and irregular larval load, and serology has the highest sensitivity and is recommended [29].
11	Data completeness is likely to be acceptable	2/4 = Data represent a proportion of community cases with a known undercount	Data on the prevalence of strongyloidiasis is limited. Studies suggest that up to 60% of the population in Indigenous rural or remote communities is infected with strongyloidiasis. A study in North Queensland found that 10% of the non-Indigenous population has strongyloidiasis [40]. It is believed that the disease is likely to be more widespread in Australia that the current data suggest.
12	Alternative surveillance mechanisms	4/4 = No alternative surveillance mechanisms in place.	There is no surveillance mechanism available to monitor and report on strongyloidiasis.

Total score: 28–30.

It is difficult to estimate mortality rates associated with strongyloidiasis as it is responsible for several fatal clinical manifestations, each of which may be attributed to other causes [59]. For example, during hyperinfective strongyloidiasis, larvae migrate from the gastrointestinal system to other organs, transporting enteric bacteria with them. This can result in community-acquired septicaemia or meningitis, or local sepsis, which are then registered as cause of death on death certificates, despite the underlying cause of death being strongyloidiasis [6]. Additionally, acute strongyloidiasis can also cause severe gastrointestinal (intestinal obstruction), or respiratory (pulmonary strongyloidiasis) disease that can be potentially fatal if the strongyloidiasis is not diagnosed and treated [60–62].

5. Socioeconomic Impact Caused by Strongyloidiasis

Due to the chronic nature of most NTDs, their burden is usually estimated using disability-adjusted life years (DALYs) lost. One DALY equals one year of life lost by a healthy person due to a disease. A study in the United States of America compared the costs and benefits of no preventive intervention and preventive intervention of 1996 people that were at risk of intestinal parasite infections, including *S. stercoralis* [54]. Preventive intervention included presumptive treatment with 400 mg of albendazole daily for five days and data was analyzed using a decision-analysis model. It was estimated that presumptive preventive intervention against human parasites would decrease DALYs by 1976 and save up to 16.4 million USD. While it is difficult to estimate treatment efficacy for an individual parasite due to complexity of the tests used in this study, strongyloidiasis was shown to cause the highest number of deaths and hospitalization costs [54]. Notably, DALYs do not describe the complete story of harmful consequences of strongyloidiasis, such as an economic impact from productivity loses, and social impact on individuals and the community [63]. DALYs are also not appropriate to use when estimating the burden of strongyloidiasis due to the underestimated prevalence and in cases of asymptomatic strongyloidiasis.

Under-diagnosis, under-treatment, and a neglected approach to this disease cause chronic strongyloidiasis cases to develop, which is costly to the health system with expensive imaging and investigations being undertaken before diagnosis. Currently, effective treatment of strongyloidiasis is available and available information technology can be used to establish a notification database. Health promotion and community engagement are also required and need to be incorporated into public health and population health strategies, which can make a difference in disease detection and treatment and ultimately, closing the gap.

6. Recommendation to Make Strongyloidiasis a Notifiable Disease

Notifiable disease data are collected to estimate the prevalence of the disease, identify hotspots of infection, and determine any susceptible populations. These data will then be used by the public health institutions and authorities to implement prevention and control measures and/or interventions at local, regional, and national levels. Notification of the disease allows estimates of the effectiveness of the treatment and/or control strategies that would result in a systematic evidence-based approach to addressing this public health issue [64]. Strongyloidiasis represents a chronic, possibly widespread, potentially debilitating, and life-threatening disease endemic in Australia, which affects Indigenous communities and new Australian populations at a rate far in excess of the general population. Extra-intestinal strongyloidiasis is now listed as a notifiable disease by the Centre for Disease Control in the Northern Territory. The logical next step of national notification, and thus registration, of cases of strongyloidiasis would allow public health authorities the critical information they need to implement relevant prevention, control actions, and regulations.

Globally, it has been noted that strongyloidiasis is an underreported disease and information on at-risk and affected populations is missing [15]. This review found that information on incidence is virtually non-existent, and without this information we lack insight into 'how often and how quickly people are re-infected after successful treatment', 'how often first-time infections are sustained over a longer period', and knowledge of risks for infection for children and adults is missing. They argued for supporting longitudinal studies, especially at a community level, to address these knowledge gaps about an important infectious disease.

There is a compelling justification for strongyloidiasis to be made notifiable in order to establish prevalence data, identify the most severely affected regions and groups and subsequently implement and monitor public health interventions to control this important disease. Based on this, it is recommended that strongyloidiasis is made nationally notifiable and added to the Australian NNDL as a matter of priority.

Author Contributions: M.B. conceived in a review design, put the ideas together, and drafted the manuscript. H.W. and K.R. provided academic input to the draft. K.R., J.J., J.S. and W.P. provided their extensive knowledge and expertise of the topic to the manuscript. A.M. and M.W. provided their knowledge to some aspects of the manuscript. M.B. incorporated all the authors' comments, K.R. reviewed the final version of the manuscript. All authors approved the final manuscript.

Acknowledgments: The work has been supported by the Australian Government Research Training Program Scholarship. Authors received no funds to publish in open access.

Conflicts of Interest: The authors declare no conflict of interest.

Dedication: The authors would like to dedicate this work to Emeritus Professor Rick Speare. He spent much of his life understanding *S. stercoralis*, preventing and managing strongyloidiasis in Indigenous communities. He argued for inclusion of strongyloidiasis to the Australian National Notifiable Disease List as means of controlling the disease.

References and Note

1. Grove, D.I. *Strongyloidiasis: A Major Roundworm Infection of Man*; Taylor and Francis Ltd.: London, UK, 1989.
2. Bisoffi, Z.; Buonfrate, D.; Montresor, A.; Requena-Méndez, A.; Muñoz, J.; Krolewiecki, A.J.; Gotuzzo, E.; Mena, M.A.; Chiodini, P.L.; Anselmi, M. *Strongyloides stercoralis*: A plea for action. *PLoS Negl. Trop. Dis.* **2013**, *7*, e2214. [CrossRef] [PubMed]
3. Prociv, P.; Luke, R. Observations on strongyloidiasis in Queensland Aboriginal communities. *Med. J. Aust.* **1993**, *158*, 160–163. [PubMed]
4. Mounsey, K.; Kearns, T.; Rampton, M.; Llewellyn, S.; King, M.; Holt, D.; Currie, B.J.; Andrews, R.; Nutman, T.; McCarthy, J. Use of dried blood spots to define antibody response to the *Strongyloides stercoralis* recombinant antigen NIE. *Acta Trop.* **2014**, *138*, 78–82. [CrossRef] [PubMed]
5. Shield, J.; Aland, K.; Kearns, T.; Gongdjalk, G.; Holt, D.; Currie, B.; Prociv, P. Intestinal parasites of children and adults in a remote Aboriginal community of the Northern Territory, Australia, 1994–1996. *West. Pac. Surveill. Response J.* **2015**, *6*, 44–51. [CrossRef]
6. Einsiedel, L.; Fernandes, L. *Strongyloides stercoralis*: A cause of morbidity and mortality for Indigenous people in central Australia. *Int. Med. J.* **2008**, *38*, 697–703. [CrossRef] [PubMed]
7. Kearns, T.M.; Currie, B.J.; Cheng, A.C.; McCarthy, J.; Carapetis, J.R.; Holt, D.C.; Page, W.; Shield, J.; Gundjirryirr, R.; Mulholland, E. *Strongyloides* seroprevalence before and after an ivermectin mass drug administration in a remote Australian Aboriginal community. *PLoS Negl. Trop. Dis.* **2017**, *11*, e0005607. [CrossRef] [PubMed]
8. Flannery, G.; White, N.; Flannery, G.; White, N. Immunological parameters in northeast Arnhem Land Aborigines: Consequences of changing settlement patterns and lifestyles. In *Urban Ecology and Health in the Third World*; Schell, L.M., Smith, M., Bilsborough, A., Eds.; Cambridge University Press: Cambridge, UK, 1993; pp. 202–220.
9. Johnston, F.H.; Morris, P.S.; Speare, R.; McCarthy, J.; Currie, B.; Ewald, D.; Page, W.; Dempsey, K. Strongyloidiasis: A review of the evidence for Australian practitioners. *Aust. J. Rural Health* **2005**, *13*, 247–254. [CrossRef] [PubMed]
10. Jones, H.I. Intestinal parasite infections in Western Australian Aborigines. *Med. J. Aust.* **1980**, *2*, 375–380. [PubMed]
11. Einsiedel, L.; Spelman, T.; Goeman, E.; Cassar, O.; Arundell, M.; Gessain, A. Clinical associations of human t-lymphotropic virus type 1 infection in an Indigenous Australian population. *PLoS Negl. Trop. Dis.* **2014**, *8*, e2643. [CrossRef] [PubMed]

12. Walker-Smith, J.; McMillan, B.; Middleton, A.; Robertson, S.; Hopcroft, A. Strongyloidiasis causing small-bowel obstruction in an Aboriginal infant. *Med. J. Aust.* **1969**, 1263–1265.

13. Page, W.A.; Dempsey, K.; McCarthy, J.S. Utility of serological follow-up of chronic strongyloidiasis after anthelminthic chemotherapy. *Trans. R. Soc. Trop. Med. Hyg.* **2006**, *100*, 1056–1062. [CrossRef] [PubMed]

14. Olsen, A.; van Lieshout, L.; Marti, H.; Polderman, T.; Polman, K.; Steinmann, P.; Stothard, R.; Thybo, S.; Verweij, J.J.; Magnussen, P. Strongyloidiasis—The most neglected of the neglected tropical diseases? *Trans. R. Soc. Trop. Med. Hyg.* **2009**, *103*, 967–972. [CrossRef] [PubMed]

15. Schär, F.; Trostdorf, U.; Giardina, F.; Khieu, V.; Muth, S.; Marti, H.; Vounatsou, P.; Odermatt, P. *Strongyloides stercoralis*: Global distribution and risk factors. *PLoS Negl. Trop. Dis.* **2013**, *7*, e2288. [CrossRef] [PubMed]

16. Ericsson, C.D.; Steffen, R.; Siddiqui, A.A.; Berk, S.L. Diagnosis of *Strongyloides stercoralis* infection. *Clin. Infect. Dis.* **2001**, *33*, 1040–1047.

17. Schad, G.; Aikens, L.M.; Smith, G. *Strongyloides stercoralis*: Is there a canonical migratory route through the host? *J. Parasitol.* **1989**, *75*, 740–749. [CrossRef] [PubMed]

18. Grove, D.I. Human strongyloidiasis. *Adv. Parasit.* **1995**, *38*, 251–309.

19. Mansfield, L.S.; Alavi, A.; Wortman, J.A.; Schad, G.A. Gamma camera scintigraphy for direct visualization of larval migration in *Strongyloides stercoralis*-infected dogs. *Am. J. Trop. Med. Hyg.* **1995**, *52*, 236–240. [CrossRef] [PubMed]

20. Caruana, S.R.; Kelly, H.A.; Ngeow, J.Y.; Ryan, N.J.; Bennett, C.M.; Chea, L.; Nuon, S.; Bak, N.; Skull, S.A.; Biggs, B.A. Undiagnosed and potentially lethal parasite infections among immigrants and refugees in Australia. *J. Travel Med.* **2006**, *13*, 233–239. [CrossRef] [PubMed]

21. Streit, A. Reproduction in *Strongyloides* (nematoda): A life between sex and parthenogenesis. *Parasitology* **2008**, *135*, 285–294. [CrossRef] [PubMed]

22. Greiner, K.; Bettencourt, J.; Semolic, C. Strongyloidiasis: A review and update by case example. *Clin. Lab. Sci.* **2008**, *21*, 82–88. [PubMed]

23. Schad, G.; Thompson, F.; Talham, G.; Holt, D.; Nolan, T.; Ashton, F.; Lange, A.; Bhopale, V. Barren female *Strongyloides stercoralis* from occult chronic infections are rejuvenated by transfer to parasite-naïve recipient hosts and give rise to an autoinfective burst. *J. Parasitol.* **1997**, *83*, 785–791. [CrossRef] [PubMed]

24. Montes, M.; Sawhney, C.; Barros, N. *Strongyloides stercoralis*: There but not seen. *Curr. Opin. Infect. Dis.* **2010**, *23*, 500–504. [CrossRef] [PubMed]

25. Croker, C.; Reporter, R.; Redelings, M.; Mascola, L. Strongyloidiasis-related deaths in the United States, 1991–2006. *Am. J. Trop. Med. Hyg.* **2010**, *83*, 422–426. [CrossRef] [PubMed]

26. Fardet, L.; Généreau, T.; Poirot, J.L.; Guidet, B.; Kettaneh, A.; Cabane, J. Severe strongyloidiasis in corticosteroid-treated patients: Case series and literature review. *J. Infect.* **2007**, *54*, 18–27. [CrossRef] [PubMed]

27. Marcos, L.A.; Terashima, A.; DuPont, H.L.; Gotuzzo, E. *Strongyloides* hyperinfection syndrome: An emerging global infectious disease. *Trans. R. Soc. Trop. Med. Hyg.* **2008**, *102*, 314–318. [CrossRef] [PubMed]

28. Igra-Siegman, Y.; Kapila, R.; Sen, P.; Kaminski, Z.C.; Louria, D.B. Syndrome of hyperinfection with *Strongyloides stercoralis*. *Rev. Infect. Dis.* **1981**, *3*, 397–407. [CrossRef] [PubMed]

29. Page, W.; Speare, R. Chronic strongyloidiasis—Don't look and you won't find. *Aust. Fam. Phys.* **2016**, *45*, 40–44.

30. Beknazarova, M.; Whiley, H.; Ross, K. Strongyloidiasis: A disease of socioeconomic disadvantage. *Int. J. Environ. Res. Public Health* **2016**, *13*, 517. [CrossRef] [PubMed]

31. New South Wales. The quarantine act 1832. In *No 16a*, 1832.

32. Australian Government Department of Health. Australian National Notifiable Diseases and Case Definitions. Available online: http://www.health.gov.au/casedefinitions (accessed on 7 May 2018).

33. Miller, M.; Deeble, M.; Roche, P.; Spencer, J. Evaluation of Australia's national notifiable disease surveillance system. *Commun. Dis. Intell. Q. Rep.* **2004**, *28*, 311–323. [PubMed]

34. Heydon, G.; Green, A. Some worm infestations of man in Australia. *Med. J. Aust.* **1931**, *1*, 619–628.

35. Johnston, T.H. A census of the endoparasites recorded as occurring in Queensland, arranged under their hosts. *Proc. R. Soc. Qld.* **1916**, *28*, 31–79.

36. Nicoll, W. The conditions of life in tropical Australia. *Epidemiol. Infect.* **1917**, *16*, 269–290. [CrossRef]

37. Willis, H.H. A note on the value of oil of chenopodium in the treatment of *Strongyloides* infection. *Med. J. Aust.* **1920**, *16*, 379–380.

38. Einsiedel, L.J.; Fernandes, L.A.; Woodman, R.J. Racial disparities in infection-related mortality at Alice Springs Hospital, Central Australia, 2000–2005. *Med. J. Aust.* **2008**, *188*, 568–571. [PubMed]

39. Page, W.; Shield, J.; O'Donahoo, F.; Miller, A.; Judd, J.; Speare, R. Strongyloidiasis in Oceania. In *Neglected Tropical Diseases-Oceania*; Loukas, A., Ed.; Springer: Berlin, Germany, 2016; pp. 69–99.
40. Eager, T. *Strongyloides* in Kuranda—An overview since 2006. In Proceedings of the Annals of the ACTM, 6th National Workshop on Strongyloidiasis, Pullman Reef Hotel, Cairns, Australia, 14 July 2011.
41. Holt, D.C.; Shield, J.; Harris, T.M.; Mounsey, K.E.; Aland, K.; McCarthy, J.S.; Currie, B.J.; Kearns, T.M. Soil-transmitted helminths in children in a remote Aboriginal community in the Northern Territory: Hookworm is rare but *Strongyloides stercoralis* and *Trichuris trichiura* persist. *Trop. Med. Infect. Dis.* **2017**, 2, 51. [CrossRef]
42. Sampson, I.; Smith, D.; MacKenzie, B. Serological diagnosis of *Strongyloides stercoralis* infection. In Proceedings of the 2nd National Workshop on Strongyloidiasis, Royal Brisbane Hospital, Herston, Australia, 25–26 June 2003.
43. Miller, A.; Young, E.L.; Tye, V.; Cody, R.; Muscat, M.; Saunders, V.; Smith, M.L.; Judd, J.A.; Speare, R. A community-directed integrated *Strongyloides* control program in Queensland, Australia. *Trop. Med. Infect. Dis.* **2018**, 3, 48. [CrossRef]
44. Soulsby, H.M.; Hewagama, S.; Brady, S. Case series of four patients with *Strongyloides* after occupational exposure. *Med. J. Aust.* **2012**, 196, 444. [CrossRef] [PubMed]
45. Swaminathan, A.; Torresi, J.; Schlagenhauf, P.; Thursky, K.; Wilder-Smith, A.; Connor, B.A.; Schwartz, E.; Keystone, J.; O'Brien, D.P. A global study of pathogens and host risk factors associated with infectious gastrointestinal disease in returned international travellers. *J. Infect.* **2009**, 59, 19–27. [CrossRef] [PubMed]
46. De Silva, S.; Saykao, P.; Kelly, H.; MacIntyre, C.; Ryan, N.; Leydon, J.; Biggs, B. Chronic *Strongyloides stercoralis* infection in Laotian immigrants and refugees 7–20 years after resettlement in Australia. *Epidemiol. Infect.* **2002**, 128, 439–444. [CrossRef] [PubMed]
47. Rahmanian, H.; MacFarlane, A.C.; Rowland, K.E.; Einsiedel, L.J.; Neuhaus, S.J. Seroprevalence of *Strongyloides stercoralis* in a South Australian Vietnam veteran cohort. *Aust. N. Z. J. Publ. Health* **2015**, 39, 331–335. [CrossRef] [PubMed]
48. Shield, J.M.; Kearns, T.M.; Garngulkpuy, J.; Walpulay, L.; Gundjirryirr, R.; Bundhala, L.; Djarpanbuluwuy, V.; Andrews, R.M.; Judd, J. Cross-cultural, Aboriginal language, discovery education for health literacy and informed consent in a remote Aboriginal community in the Northern Territory, Australia. *Trop. Med. Infect. Dis.* **2018**, 3, 15. [CrossRef]
49. Fearon, D.; Wilson, A. Developing a protocol for the diagnosis and management of *Strongyloides* infections in paediatric patients in central Australia. In Proceedings of the 12th National Workshop on Strongyloidiasis, Charles Darwin University, Darwin, Australia, 23 September 2017.
50. Genta, R.M. Dysregulation of strongyloidiasis: A new hypothesis. *Clin. Microbiol. Rev.* **1992**, 5, 345–355. [CrossRef] [PubMed]
51. Grove, D.I. Strongyloidiasis: Is it transmitted from husband to wife? *Br. J. Vener. Dis.* **1982**, 58, 271–272. [CrossRef] [PubMed]
52. Gordon, C.A.; Kurscheid, J.; Jones, M.K.; Gray, D.J.; McManus, D.P. Soil-transmitted helminths in tropical Australia and Asia. *Trop. Med. Infect. Dis.* **2017**, 2, 56. [CrossRef]
53. Beknazarova, M.; Whiley, H.; Ross, K. Mass drug administration for the prevention of human strongyloidiasis should consider concomitant treatment of dogs. *PLoS Negl. Trop. Dis.* **2017**, 11, e0005735. [CrossRef] [PubMed]
54. Muennig, P.; Pallin, D.; Sell, R.L.; Chan, M.S. The cost effectiveness of strategies for the treatment of intestinal parasites in immigrants. *New Engl. J. Med.* **1999**, 340, 773–779. [CrossRef] [PubMed]
55. Henriquez-Camacho, C.; Gotuzzo, E.; Echevarria, J.; White, A.C., Jr.; Terashima, A.; Samalvides, F.; Pérez-Molina, J.A.; Plana, M.N. Ivermectin versus albendazole or thiabendazole for *Strongyloides stercoralis* infection. *Cochrane Database Syst. Rev.* **2016**, 1, 1–36. [CrossRef] [PubMed]
56. Whiley, H.; Ross, K.; Beknazarova, M. Strongyloidiasis Is a Deadly Worm Infecting Many Australians, yet Hardly Anybody Had Heard of It. *The Conversation*, 5 September 2017. Available online: https://theconversation.com/strongyloidiasis-is-a-deadly-worm-infecting-many-australians-yet-hardly-anybody-has-heard-of-it-81687 (accessed on 7 May 2018).
57. Hoy, W.E. 'Closing the gap' by 2030: Aspiration versus reality in Indigenous health. *Med. J. Aust.* **2009**, 190, 542–544. [PubMed]

58. Speare, R.; Miller, A.; Page, W.A. Strongyloidiasis: A case for notification in Australia? *Med. J. Aust.* **2015**, *202*, 523–524. [CrossRef] [PubMed]

59. Hutchinson, P. Strongyloidiasis: an investigation into prevalence. In Proceedings of the 2nd National Workshop on Strongyloidiasis, Royal Brisbane Hospital, Herston, Australia, 25–26 June 2003.

60. Shields, A.M.; Goderya, R.; Atta, M.; Sinha, P. *Strongyloides stercoralis* hyperinfection presenting as subacute small bowel obstruction following immunosuppressive chemotherapy for multiple myeloma. *BMJ Case Rep.* **2014**. [CrossRef] [PubMed]

61. Mukerjee, C.M.; Carrick, J.; Walker, J.C.; Woods, R.L. Pulmonary strongyloidiasis presenting as chronic bronchitis leading to interlobular septal fibrosis and cured by treatment. *Respirology* **2003**, *8*, 536–540. [CrossRef] [PubMed]

62. Byard, R.; Bourne, A.; Matthews, N.; Henning, P.; Roberton, D.; Goldwater, P. Pulmonary strongyloidiasis in a child diagnosed on open lung biopsy. *Surg. Pathol.* **1993**, *5*, 55–62.

63. Hotez, P.J.; Alvarado, M.; Basáñez, M.G.; Bolliger, I.; Bourne, R.; Boussinesq, M.; Brooker, S.J.; Brown, A.S.; Buckle, G.; Budke, C.M. The global burden of disease study 2010: Interpretation and implications for the neglected tropical diseases. *PLoS Negl. Trop. Dis.* **2014**, *8*, e2865. [CrossRef] [PubMed]

64. Speare, R. Criteria for notifiability status for strongyloidiasis. In Proceedings of the Annals of the ACTM, 6th National Workshop on Strongyloidiasis, Pullman Reef Hotel, Cairns, Australia, 14 July 2011.

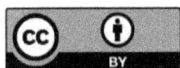

Tropical Medicine and
Infectious Disease

MDPI

Article

Immunisation Rates of Medical Students at a Tropical Queensland University

Erin Fergus [1],*, Richard Speare [2],† and Clare Heal [1]

[1]   School of Medicine and Dentistry, James Cook University, Mackay 4740, Australia; clare.heal@jcu.edu.au
[2]   Anton Brent Centre for Health System Strengthening, James Cook University, Townsville 4811, Australia
*   Correspondence: erin.fergus@my.jcu.edu.au; Tel.: +61-431-987-578
†   Deceased.

Received: 25 April 2018; Accepted: 15 May 2018; Published: 23 May 2018

Abstract: Although medical students are at risk of contracting and transmitting communicable diseases, previous studies have demonstrated sub-optimal medical student immunity. The objective of this research was to determine the documented immunity of medical students at James Cook University to important vaccine-preventable diseases. An anonymous online survey was administered thrice in 2014, using questions with categories of immunity to determine documented evidence of immunity, as well as closed-ended questions about attitudes towards the importance of vaccination. Of the 1158 medical students targeted via survey, 289 responses were included in the study (response rate 25%), of which 19 (6.6%) had documented evidence of immunity to all of the vaccine-preventable diseases surveyed. Proof of immunity was 38.4% for seasonal influenza, 47.1% for pertussis, 52.2% for measles, 38.8% for varicella, 43.7% for hepatitis A, and 95.1% for hepatitis B (the only mandatory vaccination for this population). The vast majority of students agreed on the importance of vaccination for personal protection (98.3%) and patient protection (95.9%). In conclusion, medical students have sub-optimal evidence of immunity to important vaccine-preventable diseases. Student attitudes regarding the importance of occupational vaccination are inconsistent with their level of immunity. The findings of this study were used to prompt health service and educational providers to consider their duty of care to manage the serious risks posed by occupational communicable diseases.

Keywords: medical students; healthcare students; immunisation; vaccination; occupational diseases; infection control

1. Introduction

Immunisation of medical students is an important infection control strategy, one that is strongly recommended by leading international public health advisory bodies [1,2]. Clinical guidelines for vaccination decision-making in Australia have been developed by the Australian Technical Advisory Group on Immunisation. Occupational vaccination recommendations from this group state that healthcare workers and students should ensure immunity to hepatitis B, seasonal influenza, measles, mumps, rubella, pertussis, and varicella. Additionally, those who work in remote Indigenous communities or with Indigenous children should be vaccinated against hepatitis A [3]. Adherence to these recommendations is mandated variably across Australian health services and universities—there is no national legislated requirement for occupational vaccination. For Australian-born medical students, many of these vaccinations would have been provided through a government-subsidised childhood immunisation scheme. However, for adults who are not in high-risk medical populations, any additional vaccines are the financial responsibility of the individual [3]. Private health insurance providers in Australia are not required to reimburse for vaccine-related expenses.

Despite the strength of occupational vaccination recommendations, medical students consistently have sub-optimal immunity to vaccine-preventable diseases, as was highlighted in a recent review of the literature on vaccine coverage among healthcare students [4]. The only published Australian research on medical student immunity was undertaken between 2002 and 2005 at the University of New South Wales. Using questionnaires and serological testing, the authors concluded that a significant proportion of first-year medical students were not immune to important vaccine-preventable diseases [5].

The primary objective of this study was to determine the documented immunity of medical students at a tropical Queensland university to important vaccine-preventable diseases. The findings were used to inform health service and educational providers about the adequacy of their current immunisation policies.

2. Organisational Context

Medical students at James Cook University, Queensland, Australia, are enrolled in a six-year undergraduate degree. Clinical exposure commences in first year and increases proportionally with progress through the course. Students in years one, two, and three are considered 'pre-clinical', receiving most of their education (including patient interaction) within the university environment. Students in years four, five, and six are in their 'clinical' years of medical school; the majority of their teaching takes place in hospitals. The main medicine campus is in Townsville, with other centres located across Northern Australia in Cairns, Mackay, and Darwin. Medical students are financially responsible for their immunisation-related expenses. They are sometimes included in Queensland Health staff vaccination initiatives, but not in all facilities. As per James Cook University and Queensland Health policy at the time of this research in 2014, healthcare students were required to provide proof of seroconversion to hepatitis B. The remainder of the immunisation schedule was recommended but not mandatory. These policies have since been updated [6,7].

3. Materials and Methods

An anonymous online survey was administered to medical students at James Cook University. The questions in the survey were specifically designed to ascertain history of documented immunity to important vaccine-preventable diseases (influenza, pertussis, measles, varicella, hepatitis A, and hepatitis B). These diseases were selected based on their significant potential for nosocomial transmission in this medical student population. Categories were used to define immunisation status, using proof of immunity guidelines from the Australian Immunisation Handbook and the Centers for Disease Control and Prevention [1,3]. Figure 1 demonstrates the use of this category system. Included in the survey were questions about socio-demographic variables. There were also two closed-ended questions about student attitudes towards the importance of occupational vaccination.

The survey was piloted on a group of ten final-year medical students. Emails were sent to medical students enrolled in all six years on three occasions during July and August 2014. A hyperlink directed students to the information statement and informed consent document, followed by the survey. The hyperlink was also posted on social media and promoted by the James Cook University Medical Students Association. This study was approved by the Human Research Ethics Committee at James Cook University (approval number H5664).

Data was collected by SurveyMonkey (www.surveymonkey.com) and analysed using SPSS for Windows, version 22.0 (IBM, New York, NY, USA). Incomplete responses were removed from the data set prior to analysis. Students who were 'unsure' of their vaccination status were grouped with the unvaccinated students for further analysis. Those who were unable to seroconvert to hepatitis B were considered immune, given that in the years after vaccination up to 60% of people lose detectable antibody but not protection [8]. Data were rigorously examined for error. Descriptive analyses were employed. Pearson's chi-square tests were used to investigate for statistically significant relationships between immune status and the independent variables (age, gender, nationality, year level group, and campus). Frequency tables were used to determine completeness of student vaccine coverage. Pearson's chi-square tests were used again to investigate for significant associations between completeness of vaccination and the independent variables.

> Q10. Select the option that describes your immunity to measles.
> - I am immune to measles (go to Q11)
> - I am not immune to measles (go to Q13)
> - I am unsure if I am immune to measles (go to Q13)
>
> Q11. There are several ways that a person can become immune to measles. These are listed below. Select the option/s that best describes how you obtained your measles immunity.
> - I have received two doses of a measles-containing vaccine
> - I have had serological tests that show I am immune to measles
> - I have had measles
> - I was born before 1966, therefore it can be presumed that I have acquired immunity to measles
>
> Q12. You have indicated that you are immune to measles. If required, could you provide written documentation to prove your immunity to measles?
> - Yes
> - No

Figure 1. Use of categories to define measles immunity.

4. Results

Of 1158 enrolled medical students, 289 students (25%) across the four James Cook University medicine campuses completed the survey (33 surveys that were only partially completed were not included). The majority of students were aged between 18 and 24 (86.5%), were female (68.9%), and had grown up in Australia (82.7%). When compared to the demographic profile of the James Cook University medical student population in 2014, the sample is well matched in terms of year level group distribution; however, females are over-represented in the sample population (Table 1).

Table 1. Demographic profile of the sample population compared with the James Cook University (JCU) medical student population in 2014.

Student Demographics	Sample Population (*n* = 289)	JCU Medical Students (*n* = 1158)	Difference (%)
Females	199 (68.9%)	669 (57.7%)	11.2%
Pre-clinical students	150 (51.9%)	635 (54.8%)	−2.9%
First year	48 (16.6%)	219 (18.9%)	−2.3%
Second year	47 (16.2%)	220 (19%)	−2.8%
Third year	55 (19%)	196 (16.9%)	2.1%
Clinical students	139 (48.1%)	523 (45.2%)	2.9%
Fourth year	38 (13.1%)	170 (14.7%)	−1.6%
Fifth year	47 (16.3%)	191 (16.5%)	−0.2%
Sixth year	54 (18.7%)	162 (14%)	4.7%

The mandatory hepatitis B vaccine had the highest rate of documented immunity at 95%, while measles was 52.2% and all other vaccines surveyed were less than 50% (Tables 2 and 3). There was a statistically significant association between influenza immunity and medical student seniority—54.7% of clinical students received the influenza vaccine in 2014, compared to 23.3% of pre-clinical students ($p < 0.001$). Pre-clinical or clinical year level group did not predict immunity to pertussis, measles, varicella, hepatitis A, or hepatitis B (Table 4). There were no statistically significant associations between immunity to any of the diseases and student age, gender, campus, or nationality ($p > 0.05$).

Notably, the majority of students perceived vaccination as important for their personal protection (11.1% agree, 87.2% strongly agree); as well as for patient protection (11.8% agree, 84.1% strongly agree).

Table 2. Rates of self-reported seasonal influenza vaccination among medical students.

Disease	Vaccination Status		
	Vaccinated	Not Vaccinated	Unsure If Vaccinated
Seasonal influenza (2013)	113 (39.1%)	172 (59.5%)	4 (1.4%)
Seasonal influenza (2014)	111 (38.4%)	176 (60.9%)	2 (0.7%)

Table 3. Rates of documented immunity to selected vaccine-preventable diseases among medical students.

Disease	Immunisation Status			
	Immune with Proof	Immune without Proof	Not Immune	Unsure of Status
Pertussis	136 (47.1%)	48 (16.6%)	33 (11.4%)	72 (24.9%)
Measles	151 (52.2%)	69 (23.9%)	4 (1.4%)	65 (22.5%)
Varicella	112 (38.8%)	114 (39.4%)	8 (2.8%)	55 (19%)
Hepatitis A	126 (43.7%)	33 (11.4%)	38 (13.1%)	92 (31.8%)
Hepatitis B	275 (95.1%) [1]	10 (3.5%)	1 (0.3%) [2]	3 (1%)

[1] Nine respondents (3.1%) unable to seroconvert; [2] one respondent (0.3%) with active hepatitis B infection.

Table 4. Rates of documented immunity among year level groups.

Disease	Proportion of Students with Evidence of Immunity		
	Pre-Clinical Medical Students (*n* = 150)	Clinical Medical Students (*n* = 139)	*p*-Value
Influenza	23.3%	54.7%	<0.001
Pertussis	48%	46%	0.739
Measles	48.7%	56.1%	0.205
Varicella	38.7%	38.8%	0.975
Hepatitis A	41.3%	46%	0.420
Hepatitis B	96%	94.2%	0.487

The proportion of students with documented immunity to all of the diseases surveyed was 6.6% (19/289). The remaining 93.4% of respondents would fulfil criteria for one or more catch-up immunisations. Administration of 823 vaccination catch-up schedules for individual diseases would be recommended to the students surveyed: an average of 3.05 per survey respondent. There were no statistically significant associations between comprehensiveness of vaccine coverage and year level group, age, gender, campus, or nationality (*p* > 0.05).

5. Discussion

The majority of medical students (93.4%) in this study were assessed as needing at least one vaccine. This suggests that there is significant vulnerability to communicable disease among this population, with resultant public health implications for hospital staff and patients and the university community. This population's strong belief in the importance of occupational vaccination is inconsistent with their low levels of immunity, suggesting that there is a need for research into other factors that influence medical student vaccination uptake.

Catch-up immunisations were recommended for 74% of medical students in a paediatric hospital in Basel, Switzerland [9], which is comparable to the findings of this study. Similarly, less than 30% of medical and nursing students in an Athenian study were in full compliance with recommended vaccinations [10]. In this study, documented immunity to recommended vaccines was lower than that demonstrated in Lille, France—72.7% of the French medical students had proof of immunity to pertussis, 78% had proof of immunity to measles, and 78.9% had proof of immunity to varicella [11]. Hepatitis B immunity was documented in 91.8% of French healthcare students, which is similar to our findings [12]. Among medical students studying at James Cook University, there was no statistically significant difference in immunity between those who grew up in Australia and those who grew up in other parts of the world. There was also no difference between the medical school campuses. These negative findings serve to reiterate that sub-optimal medical student immunity is not limited by geographic boundaries.

The rates of influenza vaccine uptake in this study were higher than the rates observed among medical students in Strasbourg, Warsaw, and Teheran (29.7%, 15.2%, and 4.7%, respectively) [13]. Sub-optimal influenza vaccination in other healthcare worker populations sets a poor example for medical students. A review of the literature pertaining to seasonal influenza vaccination among Australian hospital healthcare workers found that rates ranged from 16.3% to 58.7% (29% to 53% for physicians) [14]. The majority of studies into healthcare worker immunity have focused on seasonal influenza, but there is research that has demonstrated poor Australian healthcare worker compliance with recommended vaccination schedules [15]. These findings suggest that doctors may be poor vaccination role models for medical students.

In this study, medical students in their clinical years were more likely to be vaccinated against seasonal influenza than their more junior pre-clinical colleagues. There are several potential explanations for this finding. Knowledge, specifically regarding disease severity and vaccine safety, has previously been identified as an important determinant of medical student immunization behaviour [13,16,17]. Higher rates of influenza immunity in more senior students could therefore be attributed to acquisition of knowledge during medical school. However, year level was not associated with increased immunity to any of the other diseases surveyed. This could suggest a difference in the way that influenza teaching is delivered. Alternatively, it is possible that clinical medical students are more often opportunistically included in seasonal staff vaccination clinics during their hospital and community placements.

The levels of documented hepatitis B immunity among North Queensland medical students are high, which is attributable to the mandatory government and university requirement to be immune to this disease. Interestingly, documented hepatitis A immunity was similar to the other diseases surveyed, despite it not being included in the Australian childhood vaccination schedule. Hepatitis A vaccination is routinely recommended to travellers, thus the holiday patterns of medical students may be impacting their vaccination behaviour (other potential influences, although admittedly less likely, include the desire to safely consume raw oysters and semi-dried tomatoes [18,19]). Another explanation is that North Queensland medical students have responded to the recommendation that all healthcare workers and students practising in Indigenous Australian communities have immunity to hepatitis A. Nevertheless, this seems less likely, given the generally poor uptake of the non-mandatory vaccinations in this population.

The rate of self-reported immunity to pertussis was higher in this study than in the general Australian adult population. In the 2009 Adult Vaccination Survey, conducted by the Australian Institute of Health and Welfare, 11.3% of respondents reported being vaccinated against pertussis as an adult or adolescent. The Adult Vaccination Survey also noted that only 18.9% of adult Australians received the free pandemic (H1N1) influenza vaccine in 2009 [20]. Rates of seasonal influenza uptake in this medical student population were similar to those reported in Australian adults in 2014 (39%); however, the students fared more favourably when compared to younger Australian adults (24% influenza vaccine uptake in those aged 18–24 years; 23% in those aged 25–34 years) [21].

The first limitation of this study is the low survey response rate (25%), although the year level distribution of the sample population is well matched to the known demographic characteristics of the James Cook University medical student population. A second limitation of this study is its reliance on self-reporting of immunisation status (due to resource and funding constraints that precluded collection of serological data). However, it is recognised that the most important requirement for assessment of vaccination status is to have written documentation of vaccination, and for most diseases, there are no adverse events associated with re-vaccination of adults [3]. Thus, the category system specifically requesting documented proof of immunity that was utilised in this study should be considered an acceptable method of confirming vaccination history when serological data is unavailable.

6. Outcomes and Recommendations

This study highlighted the important need to address the vaccination rates of medical students, a population who, theoretically, should be extremely motivated to ensure their immunity to common vaccine-preventable diseases. Shortly following the acquisition of these survey results, qualitative research was undertaken on this medical student population to identify the determinants of their vaccination behaviour. Strategies to improve immunity were identified and published [22]. The vaccination policy for healthcare students at James Cook University has subsequently been updated since these results were provided to the organisation in 2014—prior to clinical exposure, students are now required to provide proof of immunity to measles, mumps, rubella, varicella, and pertussis, in addition to hepatitis B [23]. There has also been a medical student-led influenza vaccination campaign, which received national acclaim in 2017 [24]. Future research efforts could focus on exploring the impact of mandatory vaccination on medical student beliefs and behaviours.

It is evident that medical students cannot be relied upon to ensure their own immunity. Other health service and educational providers must reflect on their current immunisation policies and take action in order to protect the health of their students and the wider community.

Author Contributions: E.F. conceived and designed the experiment with assistance from R.S. and C.H.; E.F. performed the experiments and analysed the data; E.F. prepared the original manuscript, with editing and analysis from R.S. and C.H.

Funding: This research was funded by a medical honours grant from James Cook University, grant number JCU-QLD-416461. The funding sponsor had no role in the design of the study; in the collection, analyses, or interpretation of data; in the writing of the manuscript, or in the decision to publish the results.

Acknowledgments: This paper is dedicated to Emeritus Professor Richard Speare. The idea to investigate immunisation in our own backyard was sparked during a lecture Rick gave, and his mentorship, wisdom, and enthusiasm were invaluable throughout this research. We are honoured to have worked with Rick. We are grateful for the statistical support of Peter O'Rourke from the QIMR Berghofer Medical Research Institute.

Conflicts of Interest: The authors declare no conflict of interest. E.F. was a final-year medical student at James Cook University in 2014 when this research was undertaken. R.S. and C.H. hold/have held research and teaching positions at James Cook University.

References

1. Shefer, A.; Atkinson, W.; Friedman, C.; Kuhar, D.T.; Mootrey, G.; Bialek, S.R. Immunization of health-care personnel: Recommendations of the advisory committee on immunization practices. *MMWR Recomm. Rep.* **2011**, *60*, 1–45.

2. World Health Organization. *Summary of WHO Position Papers—Immunization of Health Care Workers*; World Health Organization: Geneva, Switzerland, 2017.

3. Australian Technical Advisory Group on Immunisation. *The Australian Immunisation Handbook*, 10th ed.; Australian Government Department of Health: Canberra, Australia, 2013.

4. Loulergue, P.; Launay, O. Vaccinations among medical and nursing students: Coverage and opportunities. *Vaccine* **2014**, *32*, 4855–4859. [CrossRef] [PubMed]

5. Torda, A.J. Vaccination and screening of medical students: Results of a student health initiative. *Med. J. Aust.* **2008**, *189*, 484–486. [PubMed]

6. Queensland Health. *Guideline for the Vaccination of Health Care Workers*; Queensland Government: Brisbane, Australia, 2012; p. 6.

7. James Cook University. *Faculty of Medicine, Health and Molecular Sciences Infectious Diseases Policy*; James Cook University: Douglas, Australia, 2008.

8. Centers for Disease Control and Prevention. *Epidemiology and Prevention of Vaccine-Preventable Diseases*, 13rd ed.; Public Health Foundation: Washington, DC, USA, 2015.

9. Baer, G.; Bonhoeffer, J.; Schaad, U.B.; Heininger, U. Seroprevalence and immunization history of selected vaccine preventable diseases in medical students. *Vaccine* **2005**, *23*, 2016–2020. [CrossRef] [PubMed]

10. Pavlopoulou, I.D.; Daikos, G.L.; Tzivaras, A.; Bozas, E.; Kosmidis, C.; Tsoumakas, C.; Theodoridou, M. Medical and nursing students with sub-optimal protective immunity against vaccine-preventable diseases. *Infect. Control Hosp. Epidemiol.* **2009**, *30*, 1006–1011. [CrossRef] [PubMed]

11. Faure, E.; Cortot, C.; Gosset, D.; Cordonnier, A.; Deruelle, P.; Guery, B. Vaccinal status of healthcare students in Lille. *Med. Mal. Infect.* **2013**, *43*, 114–117. [CrossRef] [PubMed]

12. Loulergue, P.; Fonteneau, L.; Armengaud, J.-B.; Momcilovic, S.; Levy-Brühl, D.; Launay, O.; Guthmann, J.P. Vaccine coverage of healthcare students in hospitals of the Paris region in 2009: The Studyvax Survey. *Vaccine* **2013**, *31*, 2835–2838. [CrossRef] [PubMed]

13. Machowicz, R.; Wyszomirski, T.; Ciechanska, J.; Mahboobi, N.; Wnekowicz, E.; Obrowski, M.; Zycinska, K.; Zielonka, T.M. Knowledge, attitudes, and influenza vaccination of medical students in Warsaw, Strasbourg, and Teheran. *Eur. J. Med. Res.* **2010**, *15*, 235. [PubMed]

14. Seale, H.; Macintyre, C.R. Seasonal influenza vaccination in Australian hospital health care workers: A review. *Med. J. Aust.* **2011**, *195*, 336–338. [CrossRef] [PubMed]

15. Murray, S.B.; Skull, S.A. Poor health care worker vaccination coverage and knowledge of vaccination recommendations in a tertiary Australia hospital. *Aust. N. Z. J. Public Health* **2002**, *26*, 65–68. [CrossRef] [PubMed]

16. Martinello, R.A.; Jones, L.; Topal, J.E. Correlation between healthcare workers' knowledge of influenza vaccine and vaccine receipt. *Infect. Control Hosp. Epidemiol.* **2003**, *24*, 845–847. [CrossRef] [PubMed]

17. Betsch, C.; Wicker, S. E-health use, vaccination knowledge and perception of own risk: Drivers of vaccination uptake in medical students. *Vaccine* **2012**, *30*, 1143–1148. [CrossRef] [PubMed]

18. Conaty, S.; Bird, P.; Bell, G.; Kraa, E.; Grohmann, G.; McAnulty, J.M. Hepatitis A in New South Wales, Australia, from consumption of oysters: The first reported outbreak. *Epidemiol. Infect.* **2000**, *124*, 121–130. [CrossRef] [PubMed]

19. Donnan, E.J.; Fielding, J.E.; Gregory, J.E.; Lalor, K.; Rowe, S.; Goldsmith, P.; Antoniou, M.; Fullerton, K.E.; Knope, K.; Copland, J.G.; et al. A multistate outbreak of hepatitis A associated with semidried tomatoes in Australia, 2009. *Clin. Infect. Dis.* **2012**, *54*, 775–781. [CrossRef] [PubMed]

20. Australian Institute of Health and Welfare. *2009 Adult Vaccination Survey: Summary Results*; Australian Institute of Health and Welfare: Canberra, Australia, 2011.

21. Department of Health. *Newspoll Omnibus Survey on Adult Flu Vaccinations: Summary Report*; Australian Government: Canberra, Australia, 2014.

22. Fergus, E.; Speare, R.; Heal, C. Developing strategies to increase the immunity of medical students at an Australian university. *Vac. Rep.* **2016**, *6*, 56–61. [CrossRef]

23. James Cook University. *Division of Tropical Health and Medicine Health Record and Immunisation Form*; James Cook University: Douglas, Australia, 2018.

24. Australian Medical Students' Association. 2017 AMSA Awards Recipients. Available online: https://drive.google.com/file/d/0B2U6a-o2UvDQMFNncWQ0bnlldnc/view (accessed on 25 April 2018).

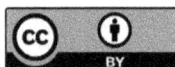

Tropical Medicine and
Infectious Disease

MDPI

Review

The History of Bancroftian Lymphatic Filariasis in Australasia and Oceania: Is There a Threat of Re-Occurrence in Mainland Australia?

Catherine A. Gordon [1,*], Malcolm K. Jones [2] and Donald P. McManus [1]

[1] Molecular Parasitology Laboratory, QIMR Berghofer Medical Research Institute, Brisbane, QLD 4006, Australia; Don.McManus@qimrberghofer.edu.au
[2] School of Veterinary Science, University of Queensland, Brisbane, QLD 4072, Australia; m.jones@uq.edu.au
* Correspondence: Catherine.Gordon@qimrberghofer.edu.au; Tel.: +61-7-3845-3069

Received: 26 April 2018; Accepted: 31 May 2018; Published: 4 June 2018

Abstract: Lymphatic filariasis (LF) infects an estimated 120 million people worldwide, with a further 856 million considered at risk of infection and requiring preventative chemotherapy. The majority of LF infections are caused by *Wuchereria bancrofti*, named in honour of the Australian physician Joseph Bancroft, with the remainder due to *Brugia malayi* and *B. timori*. Infection with LF through the bite of an infected mosquito, can lead to the development of the condition known as elephantiasis, where swelling due to oedema leads to loss of function in the affected area and thickening of the skin, 'like an elephant'. LF has previously been endemic in Australia, although currently, no autochthonous cases occur there. Human immigration to Australia from LF-endemic countries, including those close to Australia, and the presence of susceptible mosquitoes that can act as suitable vectors, heighten the possibility of the reintroduction of LF into this country. In this review, we examine the history of LF in Australia and Oceania and weigh up the potential risk of its re-occurrence on mainland Australia.

Keywords: *Wuchereria bancrofti*; lymphatic filariasis; elephantiasis

---

1. Introduction

Lymphatic filariasis (LF), also known as Bancroftian filariasis or elephantiasis—due to swelling often in the lower limbs and genitals, upper limbs, and other areas of the body—is part of Australian history, with father and son, Dr. Joseph and Dr. Thomas Bancroft, two pre-eminent physicians and parasitologists, integral to the elucidation of the life-cycle of the human parasitic roundworm causing the disease. The causative agent of Bancroftian filariasis is a spirurid nematode *Wuchereria bancrofti*, named in honour of Joseph Bancroft and of Dr. Otto Wucherer, who was based in Brazil [1].

The earliest evidence of LF comes from Egypt, with a statue of Pharaoh Mentuhotep II (2055–2004 BC) depicting swollen limbs, which are characteristic of the disease (Figure 1) [2], while artefacts from around 500 AD in West Africa also display scrotal swelling. The earliest written record of elephantiasis comes from the Ebers Papyrus (1550 BC) in Egypt [3]. The Greek medical writer, Celsus (30 BC–50 AD), also wrote about elephantiasis [3], the term as used then referring to both LF and leprosy [2], which can also present as elephantiasis due to the thickening of skin 'like an elephant'. In later times, ancient Greek and Roman writers began referring to leprosy as 'elephantiasis graecorum' and LF as 'elephantiasis arabum' [2]. Similar descriptions of LF were provided by Chinese, Indian, Persian, and Arabian physicians from this time (500–600 AD). A Dutch merchant, Jan Huyghen van Linschoten, wrote of individuals in the Indian state of Goa (1588–1592) having 'one of their legs and one foot from the knee downwards as thick as an elephant's leg', almost certainly describing LF [2].

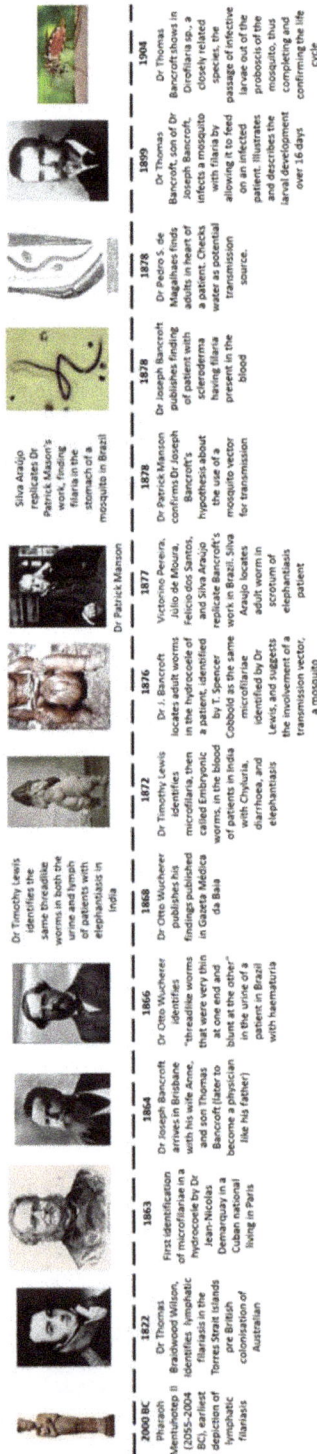

Figure 1. Timeline of Bancroftian filariasis showing the earliest known record in the form of a statue of Pharaoh Mentuhotep II (2055–2004) and through to the elucidation of the lifecycle finalised in 1904 by Dr. Thomas Bancroft.

2000 BC Pharaoh Mentuhotep II (2055–2004 BC), earliest depiction of lymphatic filariasis

1822 Dr Thomas Braidwood Wilson, identifies lymphatic filariasis in the Torres Strait Islands pre British colonisation of Australian

1863 First identification of microfilariae in a hydrocoele by Dr Jean-Nicolas Demarquay in a Cuban national living in Paris

1864 Dr Joseph Bancroft arrives in Brisbane with his wife, Anne, and son Thomas Bancroft (later to become a physician like his father)

1866 Dr Otto Wucherer identifies "threadlike worms that were very thin at one end and blunt at the other" in the urine of a patient in Brazil with haematuria

1868 Dr Otto Wucherer publishes his findings in Gazeta Médica da Baia

1872 Dr Timothy Lewis identifies microfilariae, then called Embryonic worms, in the blood of patients in India with Chyluria, diarrhoea, and elephantiasis

Dr Timothy Lewis identifies the same threadlike worms in both the urine and lymph of patients with elephantiasis in India

1876 Dr J. Bancroft locates adult worms in the hydrocoele of a patient, identified by T. Spencer Cobbold as the same microfilariae identified by Dr Lewis, and suggests the involvement of a transmission vector, a mosquito

1877 Victorino Pereira, Júlio de Moura, Felício dos Santos, and Silva Araujo replicate Bancroft's work in Brazil. Silva Araujo locates adult worm in scrotum of elephantiasis patient

Silva Araujo replicates Dr Patrick Mason's work, finding filaria in the stomach of a mosquito in Brazil

Dr Patrick Manson

1878 Dr Patrick Manson confirms Dr Joseph Bancroft's hypothesis about the use of a mosquito vector for transmission

1878 Dr Joseph Bancroft publishes of patient with scleroderma having filaria present in the blood

1878 Dr Pedro S. de Magalhaes finds adults in heart of a patient. Checks water as potential transmission source.

1899 Dr Thomas Bancroft, son of Dr Joseph Bancroft, infects a mosquito with filaria by allowing it to feed on an infected patient. Illustrates and describes the larval development over 16 days

1904 Dr Thomas Bancroft shows in Dirofilaria sp. a closely related species, the passage of infective larvae out of the proboscis of the mosquito, thus completing and confirming the life cycle

Currently, there are 856 million people in 52 countries worldwide that are at risk of infection with the three species of nematodes which cause LF, including *W. bancrofti*, which accounts for 90% of LF cases [4], and *Brugia malayi* and *B. timori*, which are responsible for the remainder [5]. There are a number of other filarial nematodes, including zoonotic species, which can also cause infections in humans but do not present as LF [6]. In this review, we will be concentrating primarily on *W. bancrofti* only due to our focus on Oceania and the Pacific, where *Brugia* species are less common. *Brugia* species will only be referred to in areas where they are co-endemic with *W. bancrofti*.

In Australia, LF has been recorded historically along the eastern coast, extending from the Northern Rivers area of New South Wales to Far North Queensland and the islands of the Torres Strait (Figure 2). A focus was recorded for Brisbane, the capital city of the state of Queensland, where Bancroft practiced medicine [7]. Autochthonous cases have not been described since 1956 [8] in Australia, but returned travelers and service personnel, as well as immigrants and refugees, are a potential source of LF [6,9]. Our closest Pacific neighbours, Papua New Guinea (PNG) and Indonesia, remain endemic and could be the source of potential new cases and new invasive mosquito species capable of transmitting the disease.

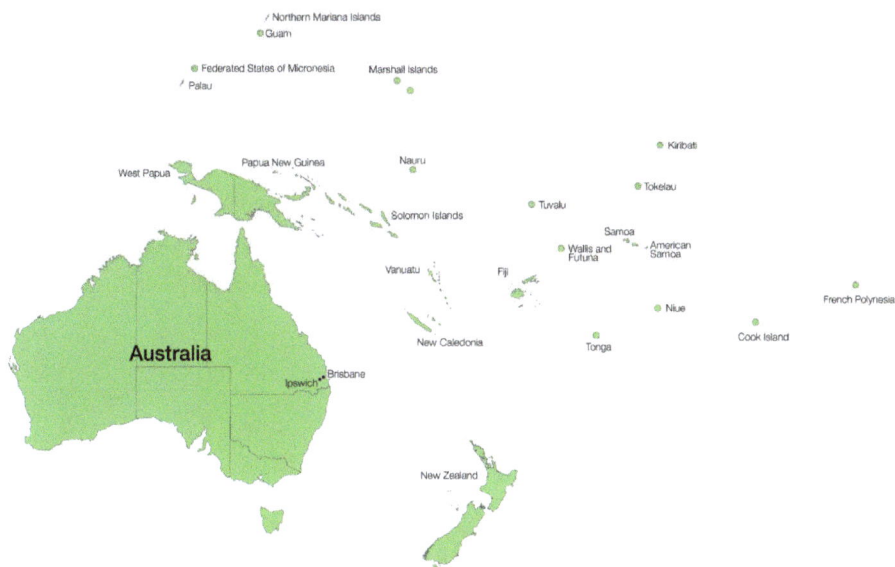

Figure 2. Location of the Islands present in Oceania and the Pacific referred to in this review.

There are an estimated 2.7 million cases of LF in Oceania, accounting for 2% of the global disease burden due to this disease, although this figure comes from only one report of national data in PNG [10]. However, this may be an overestimate as prevalence varies greatly by village and province [11]. Utilising the Global Program for Elimination of Lymphatic Filariasis (GPELF) criteria, 4.81 million individuals in PNG live in endemic districts [11]. In the 2016 progress report, the number of people requiring preventative chemotherapy was 14.7 million in 11 countries of the Western Pacific [12]. While autochthonous cases of LF no longer occur in Australia, research has continued at Australian research institutes and Universities, notably at James Cook University, where the late Professor Rick Speare, whom this special issue is commemorating, was heavily involved in filariasis studies. Primarily this work revolved around diagnostics and the status of LF in PNG, which will be considered further later.

The GPELF elimination strategy has two components. The first is to achieve transmission interruption, whereby the infection is not spread to new individuals, and the second is to control morbidity by alleviating the suffering of those who are or have previously been infected. When we talk of elimination in this paper, we refer to this definition by the WHO GPELF program [13].

2. Lifecycle

Although explored more fully below, the life-cycle is presented here. *Wuchereria bancrofti*, the causative agent of Bancroftian LF worldwide, requires two hosts to complete its life cycle; the human host, in which sexual reproduction occurs and the mosquito host, where maturation of L1 larvae to the infective L3 stage occurs (Figure 3) [14].

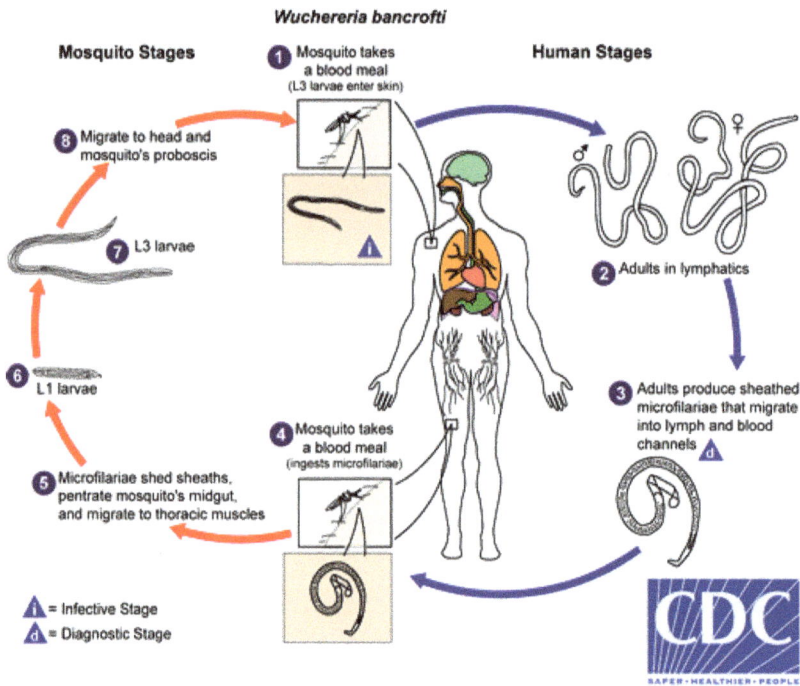

Figure 3. Life cycle of *Wuchereria bancrofti*. Image courtesy of the Centers for Disease Control and Prevention [14].

Adult worms sexually reproduce in the lymphatic system of an infected human. The adult females produce microfilariae (mf) which migrate into the blood. The mf are then taken up by a mosquito as it takes a blood meal and the mf mature into L1 larvae through to the infective L3s, which are deposited on to the skin of the human host during mosquito feeding [14] (Figure 3). It takes roughly 12 months for adult worms to mature and begin producing mf.

3. Disease

The pathology which manifests in the human host is varied, and a small proportion of long-term chronic cases can develop to the state that is referred to as elephantiasis, in reference to the swelling and thickening of the skin that can occur as a result of infection. Lymphedema, lymphangitis, lymphadenitis, funiculitis, cellulitis, chyluria, and hydrocele, swelling of the scrotum, and recurrent episodes of acute dermato-lymphangio-adenitis (ADLA) can also occur. There is a range of rare inflammatory and obstructive manifestations, including arthritis and myositis, pericardial effusion, and pericarditis. Development to overt clinical disease can take many years despite the presence of large numbers of mf in the blood, while individuals showing overt disease may have very low mf. This may be due to the adult worms no longer reproducing, which occurs after five years, single sex infections, adult worms still maturing, or as a result of the host immune response clearing infection [15].

The most common acute clinical manifestation is filarial fever, and the most common chronic manifestation is scrotal hydrocele [2]. Filarial fevers can occur without any other symptoms of LF infection and are due to toxins and allergens released by the parasite and secondary bacterial infection. Filarial fever begins with rigor and tremor, persisting for 1–3 h, and may be associated with congestion. Vomiting during an attack is symptomatic of retroperitoneal lymphatic involvement [2]. Scrotal hydrocele is a swelling in the scrotum that occurs when fluid collects around the testes and may or may not be preceded by other symptoms of LF infection, such as funiculitis [2]. In some cases, hydrocele will disappear following LF treatment or it may grow and progress. Treatment with doxycycline may cause a reduction in the size of smaller hydroceles, which is not seen with drugs used in mass drug administration (MDA). In general, large hydroceles require surgery [2].

In the years following infection while external symptoms may be low, considerable internal changes can be occurring, which may be responsible for the later overt physical disease symptoms, should they occur at all. The presence of adult worms is associated with the dilation of lymph vessels, lymphangiectasia [16]. This effect can be seen in areas of the lymph system where the adult worms are not physically present, which indicates that secretory/excretory parasite products may be present and have a more systemic effect [16]. The Gram-negative endosymbiont bacterium *Wolbachia* may also play a role in disease and contribute to inflammation following the death of adult worms and the subsequent release of the bacteria into the blood and lymph [16]. Patients who go on to develop lymphedema may also have a genetic predisposition, with lymphedema occurring in family groups [17]. However, clustering in family groups may be due to environmental conditions predisposing towards LF infection. Individuals with lymphedema in a Haitian study had higher levels of filarial antigens compared to those who did not have lymphedema [17], although this could be due to other factors, including disease stage.

ADLA can occur due to the death of adult worms, which can result in nodules or lesions in lymphatic vessels, or due to secondary bacterial infection, primarily by streptococci, which cause fissuring and loss of skin integrity [16,18,19]. During ADLA attacks, bacteria can be found in the blood and lymph [17]. Secondary infections tend to become more common as lymphedema progresses; however, they can be mediated by limb hygiene measures, which have been shown to help prevent ADLA attacks [20]. Fungal infections may help precipitate ADLA attacks by providing entry points for bacteria [18]. ADLA is an important step in the progression to lymphedema and elephantiasis, with an initial ADLA attack preceding and precipitating lymphedema, and subsequent ADLA attacks causing worsening lymphedema [18]. Additional ADLA symptoms include fever, chills, headache, vomiting, pain in the affected area, and vomiting. Severe cases can lead to toxaemia, altered senses, and urinary incontinence.

Tropical pulmonary eosinophilia (TPE) syndrome is also associated with filarial infection, although it is quite rare, with less than 1% of infections thought to lead to TPE [21]. The main symptoms include cough, shortness of breath, and wheezing, which may lead to long-term respiratory defects due to scarring of the lungs, resulting in restrictive and obstructive pulmonary abnormalities [21]. TPE occurs as a result of hypersensitivity to the filarial antigens of *W. bancrofti* and *Brugia* species, although it may also be due, in some cases, to zoonotic filarial infections as well [21]. TPE may occur in infected individuals due to sensitivity to the filarial antigen, which may trigger asthma [19].

4. Diagnosis

The two most common forms of diagnostic procedures for *W. bancrofti* detection are peripheral blood smears to identify mf, and antigen detection assays that test for parasite antigens in peripheral blood; there are no antigen detection tests for *Brugia* spp. [22]. Other diagnostic tests include antibody-based assays, DNA detection by polymerase chain reaction (PCR)-based assays, and mf membrane filtration. The most common antigen detection test currently employed in control programs is the filariasis immunochromatographic test (ICT) which was developed for field application. Both the ICT and mf detection have been employed in the 1998-launched WHO Pacific Programme to Eliminate LF (PacELF), the Pacific arm of the Global Programme, which aims to eliminate LF as a public health problem by 2020. The ICT has been replaced in the program with the filariasis test strip (FTS) diagnostic. One of the complications with mf detection is the nocturnality of *W. bancrofti*, necessitating that blood is drawn at night in order to provide the best opportunity to pick up the larvae [23]. In the Pacific, however, the strain of *W. bancrofti* that occurs does not demonstrate nocturnality [8]. The mf have difficulty passing through peripheral capillaries and are only seen in the peripheral blood at night, when they have the greatest activity [23]. During the day, when they are less active, they are unable to pass through the capillaries due to the reduction in their activity levels [23]. The advantage of immunodiagnostic procedures, both for antigen and antibody detection, is that blood can be drawn at any time. Circulating cell-free DNA (cfDNA) would also be detectable at any time, although night blood will contain larvae, thereby providing more DNA for detection, resulting in increased sensitivity [24,25].

4.1. ICT Antigen Test

The ICT antigen test, previously sold as the BinaxNOW Filariasis card test, was developed in 1997 by an Australian company (ICT diagnostics; New South Wales) and is a rapid test that detects soluble antigens of *W. bancrofti* circulating in the blood [26,27]. The test can be performed in the field and a result is obtained in 5–15 min; no preparation of blood or serum is required [26]. The ICT is in the form of a card with two pads, one of which is for the addition of serum (50 μL) and the other for a kit reagent. The card is then closed and the result viewed through a 'window' in the card. A positive result shows as a line underneath a control line [26]. Initial studies suggested that the test was 100% specific and highly sensitive [26], but there is evidence of cross-reactivity of the test with antigens from the related filarial species *Loa loa* in Africa [28,29]. In areas where *W. bancrofti* is the only filarial nematode present, this does not pose a problem, but when multiple filarial species are present, this will impact on the prevalence and distribution results. This test has been phased out and is no longer available. It has been replaced by the filariasis test strip (FTS) [30].

4.2. Filariasis Test Strip (FTS)

The ICT was used widely in the beginning of the GPELF but has been replaced by the FTS. Like the ICT, the FTS is a point-of-care test that detects *W. bancrofti* antigens. The test comes as a kit containing a test strip, work tray, and micropipette [31]. The micropipette is used to collect 75 μL of blood from a fingerprick. The blood is applied to the sample pad on the strip and left for 10 min, before the result is ready to be read. To be valid, the control line must be present. A valid positive result is two lines appearing, one control and one test. A valid negative result will only show the control line. The FTS was developed by Alere, the same company that manufactured the ICT, and was funded by a Bill and Melinda Gates Foundation grant [32]. In comparisons of the two tests, there was 99% agreement, while the FTS was more sensitive at lower antigen levels [31,32]. In addition to higher sensitivity at low antigen levels, the FTS is cheaper and has a longer shelf life [31].

4.3. Blood Smears (mf Detection)

Blood smears detect mf in the blood of an infected patient. As mentioned above, mf may not be present in patients with overt disease for a number of reasons, including single sex infections, the death of adult worms, adult worms no longer reproducing, or immature worms [15]. There are two types of blood smear that can be performed; a thick smear and a thin smear, and usually multiple slides are prepared to enhance the chances of finding the mf. Slides are stained with Giemsa to facilitate detection. Three-line thick smears are recommended for LF detection and involve three lines of blood of approximately 20 μL each placed horizontally next to each other on the slide and stained with

Giemsa [8,15]. Blood can also be filtered through a membrane (3 μm pore size) and the membrane examined directly, although this is discouraged due to potential infection from aerosolised blood as it is forced through the membrane [15]. Concentration methods such as the Kontt's or modified Knott's technique are safer and allow for screening larger volumes of blood [15,19].

4.4. Other Diagnostic Methods

While the ICT and blood smears are the most common procedures used, there are a number of other available diagnostic tests including molecular- and serological-based assays. Serological tests include ELISA and CELISA (Cellabs Pty Ltd., Manly, Australia), an assay developed in Australia at James Cook University [33], which have been validated using dried blood spots (DBS) as well as the usual serum samples. The CELISA is also sold by TropBio (James Cook University, Townsville, Australia) as the Og4C3 antigen test which is considered a gold standard test for mf detection [34]. Og34C filter paper combined with ELISA has been shown to be more sensitive than ICT in a trial in PNG [35]. DBS have also been utilised for the DNA detection of LF by PCR [36].

Wolbachia levels in infected humans can be used to monitor the effect of drugs against adult worms, with levels reducing after the adults are killed [37,38].

5. Prevention and Treatment

One of the best methods of thwarting the spread of a vector-borne disease involves targeting the vector, so as to prevent the mosquito from biting but also as a general mosquito population control measure. Methods used to prevent biting include the application of a personal repellent and the use of treated or untreated bed nets [39,40]. Mosquitoes generally need to bite a person upwards of several thousand times before LF infection occurs [15,41]; this is unlike malaria and other blood-borne pathogens, where infection can occur after far fewer bites. Studies in areas before and after the introduction of bednets have shown a reduction in mf prevalence in surveyed mosquitoes, indicating a decrease in LF transmission by mosquitoes through the introduction of bednets [40].

Treatment for LF is currently under the remit of mass drug administration (MDA). The WHO states that MDA should be undertaken in endemic areas and include everybody over two years old, except for pregnant women and those who are unwell [42]. To eliminate LF, multiple rounds of MDA should be undertaken annually, for a period of at least five years. This time frame was chosen as this is the expected reproductive lifespan of adult filarial worms in infected humans [42]. As chemotherapy has limited effects on the adult worms, it is possible to retain adults post-treatment that become less reproductively active until five to six years of age, at which stage they are considered reproductively inactive [43–45]. It is thus possible to be infected with adult worms that are no longer producing mf, but will be positive by serology. Previously, the main drug regimens in MDA was a combination of diethylcarbamazine citrate (DEC) with albendazole, albendazole alone, or a combination of ivermectin with albendazole [13,37]. In 2017, this was updated to a recommended three-drug treatment known as IDA, a combination of ivermectin, diethylcarbamazine citrate, and albendazole [46]. It is thought that the use of IDA drug combination will accelerate the global elimination of LF. More recent studies have indicated doxycycline and rifampicin, antibiotics that target *Wolbachia* spp., as a potential treatment, with high adult worm killing in patients given these drugs [43]. However, as doxycycline is an anti-malaria drug, it is unlikely to be approved for use in malaria-endemic areas due to the high potential for drug resistance exhibited by *Plasmodium* spp. parasites. MDA treatment has also been shown to reverse sub-clinical pathology in children [16].

ADLA can be treated with antibiotics to clear bacterial infection, bed rest, elevating the affected limb, and paracetamol [18,20]. Further attacks can be prevented by practicing hygiene and washing of the affected limb with soap daily, and treating any skin injuries quickly and appropriately with antibiotic ointments. Keeping the skin dry and using antifungal creams can prevent the development of fungal infections, which can provide entry of bacteria. The extent of lymphedema will determine how effective this treatment can be in preventing ADLA attacks due to the difficulty in washing deep skin folds, particularly with thickened, pitting skin which occurs in higher grades of lymphedema [18].

Lymphodema can be treated by bandaging or stocking, limb elevation at night, exercise of the affected limb, massage, intermittent pneumatic compression of the affected limb, heat therapy, and surgery [18,47].

6. History of LF in Australia

The work of unravelling the lifecycle of LF relied on observations of a number of physicians and parasitologists over many years (Figure 1). In 1863, the surgeon Jean-Nicolas Demarquay observed mf from a hydrocele of an infected Cuban national living in Paris [48]. This observation was followed in 1866 by the identification of threadlike worms in the urine of a patient by Dr. Otto Wucherer, working in the Brazilian state of Bahia [1,48,49]. Wucherer published his findings in the *Gazeta Médica da Bahia*, a journal not widely distributed at the time, and his important discoveries were not read by many others in the field, particularly in Europe. When Dr. Joseph Bancroft, working as physician in what is now the central business district of Brisbane, Australia, sent mf to Dr. T.S. Cobbold, working in the UK, via Dr. William Roberts, in 1874, who subsequently published his findings, calling the parasite *Filaria bancrofti*, it was without knowledge of the prior discovery by Dr. Wucherer (Figure 1) [50].

There was a divide between the Brazilian researchers and those in Europe, with the former taking aspects of European medicine deemed important for Brazil, but who were also keen to identify and deal with distinctive problems of health in tropical areas. There was also a divide between the older and younger generations within Brazil in how to deal with the many pressing health issues. This led to the founding of the Tropicalistas, a group initially made up of 14 physicians practicing in Brazil, and later known as the Bahian Tropical School, although no formal teaching occurred [51]. The group was dedicated to practicing and discussing modern medicine and its application to the tropical diseases that affected the poor in Brazil. Among the initial members were Otto Wucherer, John Paterson, and Jose Francisco da Silva Lima, who were at the forefront of the movement, and who helped propel a reformation of medical knowledge in Brazil, and indeed tropical diseases in general [49,51]. The *Gazeta Medica da Bahia* was published by the Tropicalistas to disseminate information and research findings [51], but as an essentially local publication, it had limited visibility outside of Brazil.

6.1. Natural History in Australia

Wuchereria bancrofti (variously called *Filaria bancrofti* by T. S. Cobbold in 1876, and *Filaria sanguinis hominis* by P. Manson in 1878; *W. bancrofti* was not formalised until 1921) was initially found in Australia in the Torres Strait by T. B. Wilson in 1822 [7]. There are no known records, either written, in art, or in oral traditions of Australian Aboriginals (present in Australia for >40,000 years), for elephantiasis occurring on mainland Australia prior to colonisation by the British. It is possible that it was present at least in the Torres Strait due to the closeness of these islands to PNG and the movement of people between them. The first report of LF in the Torres Strait was made in 1822 [7]. A review of human filariasis in Australia published in 1986 suggested that LF in this country may have originated from PNG and was brought across to the Torres Strait by the movement of people between these islands. Further introduction of LF was facilitated by the immigration of individuals from LF-endemic areas, namely India, China, and the Pacific Islands [7,52]. British expatriates living in India invariably brought their Indian servants with them when emigrating to Australia, while Chinese immigrants began arriving in greater numbers from 1851 to the early 1900s with the advent of the Australian gold rush. Pacific Islanders were recruited as indentured labourers from 1863 to work on farms in tropical areas. From 1884 to 1901, these workers were restricted to working in tropical and sub-tropical localities unless they had been in the colony for more than five years [7]. Thus, there were individuals from endemic areas, and presumably infected with LF, if it is accepted that LF was not present in mainland Australia prior to the 1800s, living and working in an environment that had high populations of mosquitoes capable of transmitting LF—an environment eminently conducive to the transmission of LF.

There was some debate as to which of these groups of immigrants were responsible for bringing LF into Australia. Between 1853–1862, around 50 Chinese men were hospitalised with what was termed leprosy; however, Joseph Bancroft was of the opinion that some of these patients may have been misdiagnosed or also carried LF [7,53]. Salter, however, argued that the distribution of LF in tropical areas of Australia indicated that Pacific Islanders, restricted to these areas, were the source of transmission [7]. It is generally accepted now that LF was initially introduced from China in the 1850s, and again in 1861 when Pacific Island indentured labourers were introduced, and reintroduced from both locations over the next few decades [7,52].

In south-east Queensland, Brisbane appeared to be a focus of infection, with 40 cases recorded between 1891–1893, and a further 60 from 1898–1903. There was a noted seasonal variation, with a higher number of mf observed in the blood during summer. This is likely due to seasonal variation in mosquito populations, with higher rainfall in summer providing more breeding sites for mosquitoes. The higher numbers of mf in summer are therefore due to the repeated biting of mosquitoes due to the increased population of mosquitoes in the summer months [7]. A survey that was performed on 600 patients admitted to the Brisbane General hospital in 1904 identified a 15% prevalence of mf [7,8]. Subsequent surveys at the hospital in 1908 identified a prevalence of 10.8% (n = 1200), 11.5% in 1910, and 5% in 1911 [7,8]. Between 1922–1924, a more comprehensive survey, incorporating patients from northern Queensland as well as Brisbane, was performed. The highest number of examined individuals were from Brisbane, where the highest prevalence of mf of 3.6% was recorded, followed by Rockhampton, a city in central Queensland, where a prevalence of 3.4% was reported [54]. Certainly, LF was a major problem in Queensland and northern NSW at this time. Interestingly, one of the highest prevalences in the Brisbane area was from Stradbroke Island Aborigines with 4.4% infected (n = 45), and Purga Aboriginal Mission with 5.1% infected (n = 39) [54]. The high prevalence in these indigenous communities was more likely due to the presence of high populations of mosquitoes resulting from the high number of mosquito breeding sites in these areas, rather than evidence of LF present in Aboriginal individuals prior to colonisation.

The prevalence of LF began decreasing in surveys from the late 1930s onwards, with a 0% (n = 228) prevalence of mf in patients from Brisbane General Hospital in 1938, although in 1944, a prevalence of 6.7% (n = 252) was recorded in the mental health hospital, Goodna. However, by 1949, the prevalence had fallen to 3.9%. Between 1937 and 1956, there were 56 admissions for LF, but all were negative for mf, indicating an old infection with no reproduction occurring [8]. The last active cases identified were in 1937 with two Australian Aboriginals being mf-positive sometime between 1949 and 1956 from islands in the Torres Strait, and a Mackay man in 1956 who had high numbers of mf [7,8].

In addition to the islands of the Torres Strait, Australia also has two other island territories. These are the Territory of Cocos (Keeling) (population 544), and Christmas Island (population 1843), both in the Indian Ocean. Christmas Island is closer to Indonesia (350 km) than Australia (1550 km). LF has not been recorded in either island group, but the closeness of Christmas Island to Indonesia, which is endemic for LF, may provide a potential source of infection. *Culex* mosquitoes capable of transmitting LF are present on the island.

6.2. Discovery of the Adult Parasites

Closer to south-east Queensland, where Dr. Joseph Bancroft was practicing medicine, the first reports of mf (the only known life-cycle stage at this time) in the area came from Dr. John Mullen, who described a case of chyluria (a rare condition in which lymphatic fluid leaks into the kidneys and turns the urine milky white) in Fortitude Valley, Brisbane, and by Dr. Thomas Rowlands, who in 1874 identified mf in the urine of a patient in Ipswich, a city to the west of Brisbane [7,55]. In 1874, Bancroft began isolating the mf from the blood of patients, which he subsequently preserved and sent to Dr. Roberts in Manchester and later, when the initial samples were destroyed in the post, to T. S.

Cobbold, who identified the mf as well as an egg capsule, hypothesising that the adult worms must live in the human host [56,57]. Subsequently, Bancroft isolated female adult worms from a lymphatic abscess, and later from the hydrocele of a patient (1877), sending them to T. S. Cobbold, who published the finding in 1877 [56–58], naming them *Filaria bancrofti*. Dr. Bancroft's discovery of the adult worms only preceded the same discovery by Lewis in India by seven months, and by de Silva Araujo in Brazil by nine months [7]. Discovery of a complete male adult specimen did not occur until 1888, although fragments had been found as early as 1879 [55,59].

6.3. Discovering the Vector

Bancroft wondered how such parasites living in the blood might be transmitted and hypothesised the involvement of a mosquito vector, a hypothesis also put forward by Manson [50]. To explore this idea further, he took an infected patient to his home, 'Kelvin Grove', named after the gardens of the same name in Glasgow, and later used as the name of the suburb of Brisbane in which Bancroft lived. Bancroft allowed *Aedes vigilax* mosquitoes to feed on the patient. It is not stated explicitly that mf were recovered from the mosquitoes by Bancroft, but in a letter to Cobbold, Manson was able to find mf in the stomach of mosquitoes in his own experiments. Despite the use of *A. vigilax* in Bancroft'sexperiment, *C. quinquefasciatus* (*Culex fatigans*) appears to have been the main transmitter of LF historically in Australia, although *A. aegypti* was also present in Brisbane at this time [7,60,61]. Initially, it was believed that the mosquito transported mf picked up from the blood of an infected individual to water, where the mf presumably matured and were ingested with water, thus infecting the human host. Elucidation of the role of the mosquito as a vector transmitting the mf to humans, rather than merely as a means to transport the mf to water, was only fully completed by Joseph's son, Thomas Bancroft, in 1901.

Elucidation of the transmission of LF by a mosquito took a number of years of research by both Sir Patrick Manson and Dr. Thomas Bancroft. Thomas Bancroft was initially skeptical about the mosquito as a vector, but nonetheless set out to reproduce Manson's work. Some of the issues regarding experimentation on mosquitoes as hosts were due to misconceptions, including that these insects only fed once [62]. As Thomas states, 'It never occurred to us that our mosquitoes wanted to be fed, consequently they died of starvation about the sixth day, and before the filariae had developed sufficiently' [7,62,63]. While residing in Burpengary, to the north of Brisbane, Thomas Bancroft corresponded with Manson regarding development of the filarial worms and continued research on the mosquito as a vector. To this end, using a grant from the British Medical Association, he employed a young servant, infected with LF, to be bitten by mosquitoes and found that it took 16–17 days for the larvae to mature. At this stage (1899), it was still considered by many, including Thomas Bancroft and Manson, that the mosquitoes merely introduced the filariae to water, and that LF was transmitted by drinking contaminated water [52,62,64]. Shortly after showing that the filariae died after only a few hours in water, Thomas Bancroft explored the idea that infection was due to swallowing an infected mosquito, before deciding that the filariae might gain access to the human blood stream during the act of feeding: 'It has occurred to me that the young filariae may gain entrance to the human host whilst mosquitoes bearing them are in the act of biting. The entrance of warm blood into the mosquito may excite the young larvae, causing them pass down the proboscis into the human skin' [7,62,63]. In 1901, Thomas Bancroft then demonstrated the presence of filariae in the proboscis of the mosquito [61], thereby implicating mosquitoes in the direct transmission of filariae to humans through feeding.

7. Epidemiology

Both Joseph and Thomas Bancroft were highly vocal in advocating control measures for LF. Joseph Bancroft was primarily concerned with water safety and preventing mosquitoes laying eggs in water by closing rainwater tanks, or boiling or filtering water, while Thomas Bancroft promoted the use of mosquito nets, particularly for infected individuals [61,65]. A number of mosquito control measures were eventually undertaken, including the destruction or screening of containers, improved drainage, the destruction of breeding areas, and fish stocking. These control measures were undertaken in 1911 by the Brisbane City Council (BCC), which had, at the time, only been recently amalgamated from several smaller authorities [60]. The BCC was given responsibility for mosquito control by the State of Queensland. Between 1900 and 1910, active transmission occurred near the General Hospital in Brisbane (now the Royal Brisbane and Women's Hospital in the suburb of Herston), where there was both a concentration of infected patients and breeding sites for *C. quinquefasciatus*. Once mosquito control measures began to impact the number of mosquitoes present, transmission was reduced and, eventually, LF was eliminated [7].

LF continues, however, to be a persistent public health problem outside of Australia, and research into LF has continued in Australian research institutes and universities including, as earlier indicated, at James Cook University and the laboratory of the late Dr. Rick Speare [47,66–71]. The most recent LF cases identified in Australia have all been in immigrants, refugees, and returned travelers coming from endemic areas [9], while the last recorded case of locally-acquired LF was in Mackay in 1956 [7].

8. Current LF Prevalence in Oceania

In 1997, the highest recorded prevalence of LF worldwide (29.11%, 1.80 million) was in the Pacific Islands, including the Cook Islands, Fiji, French Polynesia, Guam, Kiribati, Marshall Islands, Micronesia, Nauru, New Caledonia, Niue, Palau Islands, PNG, Solomon Islands, Tonga, Tuvalu, Vanuatu, and Western Samoa [72] (Figure 2), although the highest number of infections occur in Asia (62.35 million) and Africa (50.57 million). Many of the Pacific nations are part of PacELF, which has been highly successful, and many of the Pacific countries previously endemic for LF are now well on the way to the goal of elimination by 2020, with current prevalences well below 1%.

8.1. Active Transmission

8.1.1. Papua New Guinea (PNG)

PNG is the closest neighbouring country to Australia (Figure 2); historically, it was endemic for LF prior to the British colonisation of Australia, and continues to be endemic. As already mentioned, James Cook University has been involved over the past two decades in the elimination of LF and is designated as a WHO collaborating center for the control of LF, recently expanded to include soil-transmitted helminths (STH) and other neglected tropical diseases [73].

There are limited available reports of the current LF prevalence levels in PNG. A research study in 14 villages in Dreikikir district, utilising diethylcarbamazine and/or ivermectin, as part of an MDA, reduced the prevalence from 47% (*n* = 797) in 1994 to 1% (*n* = 750) in 1998, showing that MDA might be sufficient for causing transmission interruption in areas with low to moderate endemicity [74]. A more recent study investigating the mosquito vectors, specifically *Anopheles* species, used volunteers from an endemic village to determine the level of uptake of mf by mosquitoes [75]. Individuals from the village were screened and LF antigen-positive individuals were requested to provide a blood sample, which was subsequently examined for mf and then used to feed mosquitoes in the laboratory [75]. The mosquitoes were dissected and examined for mf [75]. All three *Anopheles* species utilised in the study proved efficient in the uptake of mf [75]. A comprehensive literature review showed LF prevalences of 30.4–64.7% for the period 1983–1992, 30.1–56.9% for the period 1993–2000, and 7.8–12.8% for the period 2003–2011, indicating a downward trend in the most recent time period [11]. The same study estimated the at-risk population resident in the endemic areas to be 4.81 million (70.4%).

Research programs in PNG have also included examining the use of insecticide-treated bednets in order to help prevent transmission [40]. A study that investigated the effect of bednets in reducing the incidence of LF infection in three PNG villages found a large reduction in mf prevalence in mosquitoes after bednets were introduced. In 1998, after five years of MDA, the prevalence was reduced to 3.7–10.8%. Prior to the introduction of bednets, the human prevalence was 23.7–38.6%, emphasising that ongoing mosquito control is as essential for elimination as chemotherapy [40]. Mf prevalence in *Anopheles punctulatus* mosquitoes decreased from 1.8 to 0.4% after the bednets were distributed; however, MDA was also occurring in the villages, which would also account for the lower mf uptake by mosquitoes as there should have been less live mf in treated individuals [40]. The benefit of the nets was primarily reflected in a decrease in reported bites from 6.4–61.3 to 1.1–9.4 bites per day.

It is clear that the prevalence of LF has been considerably reduced from initially very high levels in PNG, likely as a result of MDA and mosquito control [76–78]. PNG joined the PacELF program in 2005. Initial baseline prevalence in 2006 in six provinces ranged from 28.36% in Bougainville to 32.71% in East New Britain. There was one province, Oro, where prevalence at the baseline was significantly lower than the other provinces, at 1.26%. Since then, MDA has been carried out initially in all six provinces, before being reduced to five provinces in 2010–2013 [79]. In concert with MDA, diethylcarbamazine-medicated salt was also introduced in some areas [19,79]. Previously medicated salt had been used successfully in China, India, and Tanzania for LF control. In PNG, however, it faced some problems as most salt for cooking was acquired from cooking food in sea water and local health workers had been trying to reduce salt intake for heart health [19].

8.1.2. The Indonesian Province of Papua (Originally Irian Jaya)

Western New Guinea (WNG), also known as Papua (formerly Indonesian Irian Jaya) and West Papua, is located at the western end of the island of New Guinea, with the eastern end of the island being PNG (Figure 2). WNG was annexed by Indonesia in 1962 and is the only Indonesian territory to be situated in Oceania. It has been included in this review, despite being nominally part of South East Asia rather than the Pacific group, due to its closeness to Australia and PNG, sharing of a land border with the latter, and its similarity in terms of the environment. Historically, *W. bancrofti* was highly prevalent in WNG, particularly in prisoners in FakFak during the Second World War—likely due to the concentration of infected persons and the presence of susceptible mosquitoes [8]. As of 2012, an estimated 113.2 million individuals required treatment for LF in Indonesia [80].

The three species that cause human LF (*B. malayi*, *B. timori*, *W. bancrofti*) occur in Indonesia, and LF cases occur in all provinces; WNG has some of the highest rates of LF in Indonesia [81]. There are few contemporary manuscripts detailing prevalence in West Papua, although filariasis is still highly prevalent elsewhere in Indonesia [82]. In 2009, Papua had the third highest incidence of LF with 1158 recorded cases [83], while in 2015, West Papua had 1244 cases, followed by Papua with 1184 [84]. Clinical cases actually increased in Indonesia between 2000 and 2009, although this was likely due to increased awareness and active searching for the disease, particularly after 2002, when the national LF program commenced [83,85]. Between 2010 and 2015, the number of clinical cases remained fairly consistent (11,969–13,032), although there was an overall increase in infected individuals, including a high peak of nearly 15,000 cases, indicating that it is still of high public health importance there [84]. Indonesia is part of the global initiative to eliminate LF by 2020 and undertakes annual MDAs (of five to six rounds yearly) and mosquito control in an effort to achieve this goal [85]. There have been some implementation and compliance issues concerning the MDAs, with an average coverage of 39.4% in 2010, increasing to 73.9% in 2014, before decreasing slightly to 69.5% in 2015 [81,84]. Low compliance is due to a number of reasons, including asymptomatic infections with individuals considering treatment to be unnecessary, the fear of side effects (including among pregnant women), taking too many drugs, the lack of trust towards those distributing the drugs, infrastructure problems, the reliability of databases, and the poor training and competence of health workers [81,85,86].

8.1.3. Timor-Leste (East Timor)

Timor-Leste is a small island nation in South East Asia to the north of Australia and makes up half of the island of Timor (Figure 2). It has been included in this review due to its closeness to Australia, and also due to the presence of Australian peacekeepers during 1999–2002. This was in accordance with United Nations resolutions to assure safety and civil order after a referendum was conducted for the East Timorese to vote for independence from Indonesia, which annexed the country in 1975, prior to which Timor was under the control of Portugal. The vote was ultimately overwhelming in favour of independence, after which violent clashes occurred, stirred up by pro-Indonesian militia. At this stage, a UN peacekeeping force was introduced and this was largely made up of Australian soldiers.

Two agents of LF, *Brugia timori* and *W. bancrofti*, occur in Timor-Leste, both of which are nocturnally periodic. The earliest study on LF in Timor-Leste occurred in 1958 and recorded a prevalence of 2% (*n* = 3350) for a species described then as *B. malayi*—later classified as *B. timori*. Blood was also collected at night from 48 individuals, finding a prevalence of 10.4% [8].

In the mid 1960s, the two forms of filariasis in Timor were identified and separated. It was at this time that the *Brugia* species in Timor was acknowledged to be different morphologically to the usual *B. malayi* and was called the 'Timor mf'. At the same time, the presence of *W. bancrofti* was also confirmed.

In 1964, a survey recorded a prevalence of 7.4% for *B. malayi* (*timori*) only infections, 2.6% *W. bancrofti* only, and 1.7% were infected with both species [8]. Later studies in the 70s, and more recently in 2002, confirmed that while *W. bancrofti* accounted for 90% of LF cases worldwide, in Timor-Leste, the dominant species is actually *B. timori*. In 2007, the prevalence of LF was 2.6% (*n* = 3461), although the prevalence may have been underreported due to the low sensitivity of the diagnostic procedure used, involving antibody detection in urine.

A more recent national survey (2011–2012) conducted by the Timor-Leste government in conjunction with AusAID and WHO, examined blood samples taken from fingerpricks for the prevalence of mf, and recorded a prevalence of 17.5% for *B. timori*. This survey covered 13 districts, collecting 2164 blood samples [87]. Prevalence was high in all villages, with the lowest recorded prevalence being 10.3%, and a number of children <5 years of age were seropositive, indicating that high transmission rates were still occurring. Indeed, prevalence was higher in nearly all villages in 2012, compared with the national survey results in 2002. This may have been due to an increased number of samples collected in 2012 and actual bias in the sample collection [87].

Serology undertaken on Australian soldiers involved in the peacekeeping mission from 1999–2002 indicated that they were certainly exposed to filarial nematodes, although all were asymptomatic, and it was unclear if any had progressed to an established or patent infection [88].

8.1.4. Samoa (Formerly Western Samoa)

Samoa is comprised of two islands to the north-east of Australia (Figure 2), with a third island, American Samoa, under the control of the USA, lying close by. The earliest reports of elephantiasis in Samoa were made in 1878, noting the 'frequent occurrence' of patients with lymphoedema in the legs and genitals [8]. In 1923, the earliest recorded prevalence survey for LF identified an mf prevalence of 28.7% (*n* = 4294) and an elephantiasis prevalence of 2.7%. By 1945, these prevalences had not changed significantly (mf 19.2–24.1%, 3.6% elephantiasis). The first LF control program was instigated in 1965 as part of a pilot study by the WHO and UNICEF and comprised DEC chemotherapy weekly for six weeks, followed by monthly treatments for 12 months [8]. The coverage for this was 21% of the population and reduced the mf rate from 19.06% pre-treatment to 1.63% post-treatment. A second round of chemotherapy, comprising monthly doses for 12 months in 1973, further reduced the prevalence to 0.11%; there was a slight increase in the mf prevalence from completion of the first control program to 2.26% [8].

Samoa has been part of PacELF since 2001, when the country prevalence was 2.62%, although two areas had prevalences between 3.05–7.35% determined using ICT [79]. By 2006, the prevalence had been reduced to 0.36%. Despite the low prevalence, active transmission may still be occurring, as evidenced by a case of LF identified in 2011 in Australia in a Samoan man who had recently visited Samoa and presented with swelling in the right leg and scrotum [9]. However, it can take many years for overt symptoms to occur so it is unclear if he may have been infected from an earlier visit or if he had lived in Samoa as a child.

American Samoa joined PacELF in 1999; the baseline prevalence of 16.50% was reduced to 2.3% by 2007 after seven rounds of MDA [79]. A final round of MDA commenced in 2009, with active surveillance after this [79]. A study utilising serum samples collected in 2010 found a prevalence of 0.75–3.2% (>128 units, >32 units respectively) by the Og4C3 antigen ELISA, and 8.1% by Wb123 antibody ELISA [89]. Hotspots of transmission were identified in that study and a follow-up in 2014 confirmed that active transmission was still occurring [90].

8.2. Active Surveillance

8.2.1. New Caledonia

The French territory of New Caledonia is a collection of islands that lie 1201 km east of Australia in the Pacific Ocean (Figure 2). LF has been endemic there since at least the 18th century, when the prevalence was as high as 59% in some villages [8]. In a survey of 382 individuals in 1999, 33.5% were seropositive for LF and 3.7% had mf present on blood smear examination. Two patients had clinical manifestations suggestive of LF, but neither had mf and only one was seropositive [91]. A more recent cross sectional survey in 2013 tested 1035 individuals and found a seroprevalence of 0.62% [92]. As two of the seropositive patients had never travelled outside of New Caledonia, it was considered that low-level transmission might be occurring. However, no mf were found in either patient and PCR was negative, which may indicate an earlier or past infection, or an immature infection [92]. Certainly, follow-up would be recommended.

8.2.2. Tuvalu (Formerly Ellice Islands)

Tuvalu is a group of islands halfway between Australia and Hawaii in the Pacific Ocean (Figure 2). In 1923, when the islands were known as the Ellice Islands, an mf prevalence of 46% was reported in 1169 volunteers; in 1945, a smaller survey of 258 individuals found a prevalence of 34.1% [8].

Tuvalu joined the PacELF program in 1999. At the onset of MDA, implemented from 2001–2005, the baseline prevalence was 22.30%; this was reduced to 3.4% in 2007–2008 [79].

8.2.3. Micronesia

Micronesia is a collection of thousands of islands to the north of Australia (Figure 2). Micronesia comprises five sovereign nations, the Federated States of Micronesia (FSM), Palau, Kiribati, Marshall Islands, and Nauru, as well as three United States of America territories—Northern Mariana Islands, Guam, and Wake Island. Seemingly, LF has historically been of low prevalence or non-endemic on these islands [8]. Of the U.S.A. territories, Guam has had no reported incidence, whereas in the Mariana Islands, 13.5% (*n* = 243) of individuals had mf on blood smears; however, the parasite was only found on one of the islands and has been considered non-endemic since the start of the PacELF [79]. Only two islands in the Marshall Island group have historical LF data, with mf prevalence in individuals being 1% and 3.6%. Palau had a reported mf rate of 12.6% in 1967, which was reduced to 0.3% after MDA in 1970 [8]. Nauru, now considered to be non-endemic for LF, had a historical prevalence of 36.1% in 1933 [8].

The FSM were thought to be non-endemic for LF after MDA in the 1970's. In 2002, a survey of 50 children in a remote atoll of FSM identified 38% as being seropositive. A follow-up survey in the following year also examined adults (*n* = 253), finding 38% seropositivity in the whole community and an mf prevalence of 22% [93]. Transmission was obviously still active at this site, reinforcing the need to continue surveillance in at risk areas. At the time, the local inhabitants reported an increase in the mosquito population, which may have accounted for the increase in LF transmission—although LF still had to be present in the community for transmission to occur; as a result, the local residents embarked on mosquito control themselves [93].

The following nations and territories in Micronesia are still implementing or require targeted treatment according to the Pacific Technical Report by the WHO [79]: Palau, FMR, Marshall Islands, and Kiribati. All other nations and territories are considered non-endemic for LF.

8.2.4. Fiji

Fiji lies to the east of Australia and comprises more than 300 islands (Figure 2). Historical reports of LF in Fiji began in 1876 when elephantiasis was common amongst Fijians, particularly those who lived in marshy areas [8]. In 1905, the prevalence of mf in the blood of individuals was recorded as 25.7% (*n* = 608), and in 1912, there was a prevalence of 27.1% (*n* = 1320), indicating high-level transmission [8]. This continued through to 1944, when the largest survey undertaken to that point identified a prevalence of 14.2% (*n* = 57,888). Vector control began in 1961, with a pilot study finding a reduction in mf prevalence from 12.1% to 2.7% after its commencement in the area [8].

Fiji has participated in ongoing MDA since joining the PacELF in 2001. Baseline prevalence for PacELF by antigen detection in 2001 was 15.17%, reducing to 9.50% in 2007 post-MDA which involved five yearly rounds of chemotherapy. The mf prevalence in 2007 was 1.40% [79]. The uptake of chemotherapy has been very successful in Fiji, with coverage in 2012 being 94% [79,94].

8.3. Elimination Achieved

8.3.1. Solomon Islands

The Solomon Islands lie to the north-east of Australia (Figure 2) and have a history of LF, although the disease is considered eliminated today—possibly as an added benefit of mosquito control for malaria eradication. A single case of elephantiasis, reported in 2011, was thought to have been acquired some years earlier and not as a result of active transmission [71]. Surveillance of villages near where the patient lived found only one other person positive for LF, but no mf were detected [71].

The highest prevalence of LF in the Solomon Islands was recorded in 1945 and ranged from 10.2–31.5% by village, which was similar to the 28.5% prevalence recorded in 1965 [8]. During the 1960s and 1970s, there were several attempts made at controlling the malaria vector, *Anopheles farauti*, which would have impacted LF transmission as it is also a vector of LF. Treated bednets were introduced in 1992 and more recent measures have included indoor residual spraying. While malaria is still endemic in the Solomon Islands, vector control for malaria has seemingly resulted in the elimination of LF.

8.3.2. Republic of Vanuatu

Vanuatu is an Island group comprising around 80 islands that lie to the north of New Caledonia and 1750 km east of Australia (Figure 2). Vanuatu was originally known as the New Hebrides, so named by Captain James Cook, and was managed by the French and British before becoming an independent country in 1980.

MDA was implemented in 2000 by the Ministry of Health with the aim of eliminating LF as a public health problem by 2004, when the MDA was targeted to cease if prevalence was <1% [95,96]. Historical reports of LF in Vanuatu are scarce and likely grouped together with reports from the New Hebrides. In 1927, the reported prevalence was 31% (*n* = 318) [95,96]. A survey was performed in 1998, two years prior to the commencement of MDA, and again in 2002, two years after the commencement of MDA as part of PacELF. The follow-up survey in the 2002 study focused on the four provinces with the highest prevalence at baseline and examined blood from 572 individuals. Seroprevalence in 1998 was 22% compared to 8% in 2002, and mf prevalence was 11% in 1998 and 0.8% in 2002 [95]. These dropped further in a 2005/6 survey to a seropositivity of 0.16% and 0% mf prevalence [96]. The most recent survey in 2012 reported only two cases. Surveillance is ongoing to ensure that the transmission of LF is no longer occurring [97]. Vanuatu is therefore well on the way to declaring the elimination of LF. In addition to MDA, bednets are utilised to prevent not only LF, but also malaria, which is prevalent. An additional component is health education, which appeared to ameliorate many of the concerns causing poor MDA compliance in other pacific countries [95]; MDA compliance ranged from 75.5–81.5% over the five years of the MDA (2000–2004) [96]. As of 2016, LF is considered to have been eliminated from Vanuatu [98].

8.3.3. Tonga

Tonga lies to the east of Australia and is made up of 170 islands in the Pacific Ocean (Figure 2). The first report of LF in Tonga was that by Captain James Cook in 1785, who noted the occurrence of elephantiasis (described as the swelling of legs, arms, and scrotum). In 1896, the prevalence ranged from 20–46.9%, depending on the location, and in 1965, ranged from 28.2 to 49.6% [8]. At the beginning of the PacELF program in 2000, the prevalence was 2.7%, which was reduced to 0.38% in 2006. Elimination of LF from Tonga was declared in 2017 [98].

8.3.4. Cook Islands

The Cook Islands comprise 15 islands in the South Pacific (Figure 2) and have historically had a very high prevalence of LF. In 1925–1926, the mf prevalence ranged from 26% and 54.8% across the islands. High prevalence continued through to 1949 when the recorded prevalence was still as high as 42.5%. MDA commenced in 1969 on Aitutaki and was expanded thereafter, reducing the prevalence to 0.2% in 1971 [8]. In 1999, the Cook Islands joined PacELF; the prevalence then of LF by ICT as part of PacELF was 8.60% and in 2007, the prevalence by ICT was 0.33% after yearly multiple rounds of MDA, with only two islands returning positive results. These islands were targeted with further MDA. Elimination was declared in 2016, although active surveillance continues [79,98].

8.3.5. Niue

Niue (current population 1624) is a small self-governing state in association with New Zealand to the east of Tonga and south of American Samoa (Figure 2). In 1954, there was an mf prevalence of 22.1% ($n = 748$), after which MDA commenced and in 1956, the prevalence had beenreduced to 2.9% ($n = 2791$) [8]. In 1972, a second MDA program was implemented, prior to which the prevalence was 16.3% [8]. Niue joined the PacELF program in 1999, when the prevalence was reported as being 3.12%. Surveys after four years of MDA recorded a prevalence of 0.23%. As of 2016, LF was considered eliminated from Niue [98].

9. Immigration to Australia

In 2016, the top ten countries from which individuals emigrated to Australia were, in order of highest to lowest number, the UK, New Zealand, China, India, the Philippines, Vietnam, Italy, South Africa, Malaysia, and Germany [99]. Of these, India, the Philippines, and Vietnam are endemic for LF, while Malaysia and China have eliminated the disease. South-East Asia, which includes the Philippines and Vietnam, as well as other countries with relatively high rates of migration to Australia, such as Cambodia and Myanmar, account for roughly 15 million cases of LF [80]. As of 2012, 41.7 million individuals required treatment in Myanmar for LF, 29.4 million in the Philippines, and 73,495 in Thailand, while Vietnam is under surveillance and approaching elimination [80]. Health screening of immigrants and refugees into Australia does not include testing for LF. Thus, it is likely that cases without obvious symptoms or physical manifestations will not be identified upon entry to Australia. As LF is not a notifiable disease, it is unclear how many cases of LF have been brought into Australia by immigrants, refugees, and returned travelers. Relatively recent cases of LF diagnosed in Australia have been contracted in Myanmar, India, and Samoa [9].

10. Mosquito Hosts for LF

10.1. Host Species and Distribution in Australia (Including Islands of the Torres Strait)

There are a number of mosquito genera capable of transmitting LF, including species from the genera *Culex, Anopheles, Mansonia*, and *Aedes*. *Aedes aegypti* transmits dengue in North Queensland and can also transmit LF, although early reports of mosquito LF transmitting efficacy initially indicated that it was not involved [8,100]. Thomas Bancroft first identified *Ae. aegypti* as a vector in the transmission of dengue in 1906 in Brisbane. Dengue was only eradicated from Brisbane in 1948 [60]. Dengue is now not endemic in Australia and outbreaks are generally due to an infected person (or infected mosquito) entering the country. In 2017 [101], there were three outbreaks of dengue in North Queensland, with a total of nine confirmed cases. There have been larger outbreaks since 2000, with nearly 900 cases recorded between 2003 and 2004, and 890 cases between 2008–2009 [102]. These outbreaks indicate that this is a still a large problem despite ongoing mosquito spraying and community education towards reducing the habitats of *Ae. aegypti*. The *Ae. aegypti* mosquito breeds in water containers close to houses, including pot bases, birdbaths, and puddles of water in tarpaulins, which help bring the mosquito into contact with humans to transmit diseases [103]. This mosquito species was largely removed from Brisbane in the early 1900s due to advances in water supply, namely, the introduction of a large water reservoir that reduced the number of water tanks, and council ordinances that rainwater tanks needed to be covered with all openings covered in mesh, therefore reducing breeding sites for mosquitoes [7,60].

There are a number of *Aedes, Anopheles*, and *Culex* species present in Australia, and a single species of *Mansonia*. The vector status of many of these species is unknown, but many bite humans only rarely and are therefore unlikely to be vectors; other species primarily inhabit swamps and bushland, which would reduce their effectiveness in transmitting LF or other vector-borne diseases.

C. quinquefasciatus is capable of transmitting LF and is also present in Australia; unlike *Ae. aegypti*, which is now restricted to Queensland although previously found in NSW, *C. quinquefasciatus* is present in all states and territories of Australia [104]. Historically, this mosquito, which has a very broad range and is present worldwide, was the main transmitter of LF, although it may have been quite inefficient in this regard, which may have contributed to the eventual elimination of LF in Australia [7,8]. Its breeding habitats include ditches, drains, and septic tanks and it is common in urban areas with poor drainage and sanitation [105]. Other species capable of transmitting LF present in Australia are: *An. bancroftii* (which may also be capable of transmitting malaria), *An. farauti, An. amictus, Ae. kochi, Ae. vigilax, M. uniformis, C. annulirostris*, and *C. bitaeniorhynchus*. *Aedes albopictus*, an invasive mosquito species not native to Australia, has previously been introduced into the islands of the Torres Strait [106] and mainland Australia [107], and has also become established in Asia, Europe, Africa, and the Americas. *Aedes albopictus* is an important mosquito species due to its successful establishment in many parts of the world and its ability to act as a vector of both LF and dengue. This mosquito is no longer present in Australia due to successful control programs. However, it is still present in PNG and Indonesia, and thus colonisation could potentially occur in the future if mosquito control programs are halted.

10.2. Vector Competence—Are Some Species Better Than Others at Transmitting LF

Transmission of LF is quite inefficient, with upwards of several hundred to thousands of infective bites required for transmission to occur [108]. Different mosquito species also have varying efficiencies and in general, there is lower vector efficiency observed in the Pacific and Oceania than observed in Africa [108]. In early studies in Tanzania and Liberia, where the vectors were *C. quinquefasciatus* and *An. gambiae* in Tanzania and *An. gambiae* only in Liberia, upwards of 11,000 infective bites were required to induce microfilaraemia. The lowest number of bites was 269, also in Tanzania. In comparison, the highest required number of bites in Asia/the Pacific was 67,568 infective bites in Fiji (*Ae. polynesiensis*), followed closely by 57,803 in Indonesia (*C. quinquefasciatus*). The lowest number was 142 in Malaysia, where the infective species was *B. malayi* (*Mansonia* spp.) [108]. A factor that could greatly influence this is that the mf are not injected into the blood as is the case in malaria, but are introduced onto the skin, with the mf then making their way into the bite wound and thus into the blood [14]. The skin is a generally harsh environment for micro-organisms to survive in; it can be quite dry, and secretes substances which can cause the skin to become more acidic and also damage or cause death. Therefore, transmission is less straight forward than occurs with vector-borne pathogens that are injected directly into the blood.

Some mosquito species are more efficient at transmitting LF than others. Vector competency relies on the uptake of mf from the infected human host, development in the mosquito to the infective L3 larvae, and transmitting those infective larvae to humans [109–113]. Certain species of mosquito are able to transmit parasites from humans harbouring low levels of mf, whereas other species can only transmit when high numbers of mf are present; paradoxically, very high levels of mf have been associated with the early death of mosquitoes [109,114]. The mf can also demonstrate nocturnality [115]; thus, mosquitoes taking a blood meal during the day are likely to encounter low parasitaemia which, depending on the mosquito species and when they are active, may limit transmission. There is a strain of *W. bancrofti* in the South Pacific which does not appear to exhibit nocturnal periodicity and mf can be found at any time of the day [8]. Additionally, the time of day that the infected mosquito is feeding will affect when mf can be seen in the blood, with peak mf levels in the blood observed during the peak biting periods of the mosquitoes [116]. While some mosquitoes are classified as day biters, there is often peak biting in the early morning and evening, such as the case with *Ae. polynesiensis*. Some mosquito species do not feed on or bite humans, whereas other species that do bite humans will have varying degrees of 'ferocity', with some species giving more bites than others. *Ae. Polynesiensis* is considered a good vector of LF [117,118], likely due to a number of factors, including its high biting frequency, compared with other mosquitoes [118]. A high biting frequency will decrease the time required for infection to occur.

Anopheles spp. mosquitos cause injury to mf during uptake due to foregut apertures, which are less developed in *Culex* and *Aedes* spp. Mosquitoes, resulting in less damage to mf [111,112,114]. *Anopheles* spp. mosquitos also need to ingest high numbers of mf for gut penetration and subsequent development of the larvae to L3. However, results on mf uptake and damage vary between species, geographical location, and study design. A study on the vector competency of *Anopheles* species in PNG showed a considerable difference in ingested mf between *An. punctulatus* (4.2–23.7%), *An. farauti s. s.* (mf prevalence in *Anopheles punctulatus* 8.6%), and *An. hinesorum* (61.9–100%) at low and high density exposures, respectively [75]. The mf recovered from mosquitos were examined for damage during uptake, although *An. hinesorum* mf were only examined in low-intensity infections. As a proportion, more mf were damaged in low-intensity infections. *An. punctulatus* had the highest proportion of damaged mf in low-intensity infections, but the proportions of damaged mf were similar between *An. punctulatus* and *An. farauti* in medium and high intensity infections [75]. *An. farauti* exhibited low survivorship in direct correlation to the intensity of infection—in high intensity infections, survivorship of the mosquito was very low, with only 20% surviving to 14 days post-infection; survivorship was not examined in the other species [75]. The filarial vector competency of *Ae. aegypti* is linked to the age of the mosquito, with older mosquitoes being less efficient in transmitting filarial nematodes, although frequent blood meals can reverse this trend [119].

As indicated in older studies, it appears that *C. quinquefasciatus* is a poor vector for LF, which may have helped with the elimination of LF from Australia. However, it is possible that there are geographic differences between the mosquito species which may cause variation in LF-transmitting ability. One study compared *Ae. aegypti* and Haitian *C. quinquefasciatus* and found a much higher uptake of mf and development to L3 larvae in the former species, which had been considered a poor vector in older studies [100,104].

Climate and Potential Spread of Mosquito Vectors in Australia

Based on climate modelling (2000–2009), the eastern seaboard of Australia would provide suitable habitats for *Ae. albopictus*, while future predictions for climate change in Australia indicate a wider suitable range for both *Ae. albopictus* and *Ae. aegypti*, which were previously present in NSW, WA, and the NT [60,107,120]. In Europe, climate change has already impacted the transmission of vector-borne diseases by expanding tropical and subtropical zones and this has led to increases in the survivability zones for insect vectors, particularly mosquitoes. This has resulted in the spread of *Dirofilaria* species, zoonotic filarial nematodes which utilise mosquitoes as transmission vectors, into new areas in Europe [6]. Other species capable of transmitting LF are already present in Australia, such as *C. quinquefasciatus*, and *An. farauti*, which is a vector of LF in Papua New Guinea [11]. The introduction from outside Australia of *Ae. polynesiensis*, a competent LF vector, would be of concern. This mosquito is exclusively tropical, and climate change may increase its viable range in Australia. It is therefore important to prevent its spread, particularly as it can also act as a vector for dengue, chikungunya, and Ross River viruses [121–123].

11. Conclusions

LF appears not to have been endemic on mainland Australia prior to European colonisation, but was present in the islands of the Torres Strait, and was thought to be introduced several times by immigrants from China and the Pacific Islands. Relevant mosquito species that can transmit LF are present in all states of Australia. Immigration will continue to be a concern for the importation of new diseases including mosquito-transmitted infections such as dengue and chikungunya, as well as LF. Current control measures in North Queensland against *Ae. aegypti* for dengue, and in Brisbane against marsh mosquitoes, will likely benefit any future need for the control of LF as well. LF is a very poorly-transmitted disease, requiring the presence of a highly concentrated population of infected individuals for successful spread. The absence of a competent mosquito host such as *Ae. polynesiensis*, also reduces the risk for re-introduction to Australia. It is therefore very unlikely that LF will ever become re-established in Australia, with only sporadic reports of infections in returned travelers and, more likely, in immigrants and refugees from endemic areas.

The main area of risk to Australia for the re-introduction of LF remains the Torres Strait islands, which lie very close to endemic PNG in the north and mainland Australia in the south. There is already concern for the importation of other diseases such as TB from PNG via the Torres Strait [124]. However, MDA and mosquito control in PNG have also reduced the prevalence of LF there, thus decreasing the likelihood of re-introduction to the islands of the Torres Strait.

The potential for the re-introduction of LF onto the Australian mainland seems remote. As LF caused by *W. bancrofti* can be readily treated with DEC, ivermectin, or albendazole, and coupled with the ongoing, highly successful mosquito control efforts against dengue and other mosquito-borne viruses, it seems very unlikely that LF would regain a foothold on the Australian mainland. Monitoring in the Torres Strait, however, should occur as the risk of infection introduced from PNG remains a threat, albeit at a low level.

Author Contributions: C.A.G. wrote the first draft of the manuscript, C.A.G., D.P.M., and M.K.J. contributed to editing and rewrites. All authors have read and approved the final paper.

Conflicts of Interest: The authors declare no conflict of interest.

References

1. Angus, B.M.; Cannon, L.R.G.; Adlard, R.D. *Parasitology and the Queensland Museum with Biographical Notes on Collectors*; Queensland Museum: Queensland, Austrialia, 2007; Volume 53.
2. Goel, T.C.; Goel, A. *Lymphatic Filariasis*; Springer Nature: Singapore, 2016.
3. Hajdu, S.I. Elephantiasis. *Ann. Clin. Lab. Sci.* **2002**, *32*, 207–209. [PubMed]

4.   Small, S.T.; Ramesh, A.; Bun, K.; Reimer, L.; Thomsen, E.; Baea, M.; Bockarie, M.J.; Siba, P.; Kazura, J.W.; Tisch, D.J.; et al. Population genetics of the filarial worm *Wuchereria bancrofti* in a post-treatment region of Papua New Guinea: Insights into diversity and life history. *PLoS Negl. Trop. Dis.* **2013**, *7*, e2308. [CrossRef] [PubMed]

5.   WHO. Lymphatic Filariasis. Available online: http://www.who.int/mediacentre/factsheets/fs102/en/ (accessed on 25 January 2018).

6.   Gordon, C.A.; McManus, D.P.; Jones, M.K.; Gray, D.J.; Gobert, G.N. The increase of exotic zoonotic helminth infections: The impact of urbanization, climate change and globalization. *Adv. Parasitol.* **2016**, *91*, 311–397. [CrossRef] [PubMed]

7.   Boreham, P.F.L.; Marks, E.N. Human filariasis in Australia: Introduction, investigation and elimination. *R. Soc. Qld.* **1986**, *97*, 23–52.

8.   Sasa, M. *Human Filariasis*; Univeristy of Tokyo Press: Tokyo, Japan, 1976.

9.   Jeremiah, C.J.; Aboltins, C.A.; Stanley, P.A. Lymphatic filariasis in Australia: An update on presentation, diagnosis and treatment. *Med. J. Aust.* **2011**, *194*, 655–657. [PubMed]

10. Kline, K.; McCarthy, J.S.; Pearson, M.; Loukas, A.; Hotez, P.J. Neglected tropical diseases of Oceania: Review of their prevalence, distribution, and opportunities for control. *PLoS Negl. Trop. Dis.* **2013**, *7*, e1755. [CrossRef] [PubMed]

11. Graves, P.M.; Makita, L.; Susapu, M.; Brady, M.A.; Melrose, W.; Capuano, C.; Zhang, Z.; Dapeng, L.; Ozaki, M.; Reeve, D.; et al. Lymphatic filariasis in Papua New Guinea: Distribution at district level and impact of mass drug administration, 1980 to 2011. *Parasit. Vectors* **2013**, *6*, 7. [CrossRef] [PubMed]

12. WHO. Summary of global update on preventive chemotherapy implementation in 2016: Crossing the billion. *Wkly. Epidemiol. Rec.* **2017**, *92*, 589–609.

13. WHO. Global Programme to Eliminate Lymphatic Filariasis. Available online: http://www.who.int/lymphatic_filariasis/elimination-programme/en/ (accessed on 25 January 2018).

14. CDC. Biology—Life Cycle of *Wuchereria bancrofti*. Available online: https://www.cdc.gov/parasites/lymphaticfilariasis/biology_w_bancrofti.html (accessed on 1 February 2018).

15. Joseph, H.; Speare, R.; Melrose, W. Laboratory diagnosis of lymphatic filariasis in Australia: Available tools and interpretation. *Aust. J. Med. Sci.* **2012**, *33*, 2–9.

16. Shenoy, R.K.; Bockarie, M.J. Lymphatic filariasis in children: Clinical features, infection burdens and future prospects for elimination. *Parasitology* **2011**, *138*, 1559–1568. [CrossRef] [PubMed]

17. Lammie, P.J.; Cuenco, K.T.; Punkosdy, G.A. The pathogenesis of filarial lymphedema: Is it the worm or is it the host? *Ann. N. Y. Acad. Sci.* **2002**, *979*, 131–142; discussion 188–196. [CrossRef] [PubMed]

18. Shenoy, R.K. Clinical and pathological aspects of filarial lymphedema and its management. *Korean J. Parasitol.* **2008**, *46*, 119–125. [CrossRef] [PubMed]

19. Melrose, W.D. Lymphatic filariasis: New insights into an old disease. *Int. J. Parasitol.* **2002**, *32*, 947–960. [CrossRef]

20. Stocks, M.E.; Freeman, M.C.; Addiss, D.G. The effect of hygiene-based lymphedema management in lymphatic filariasis-endemic areas: A systematic review and meta-analysis. *PLoS Negl. Trop. Dis.* **2015**, *9*, e0004171. [CrossRef] [PubMed]

21. Mullerpattan, J.B.; Udwadia, Z.F.; Udwadia, F.E. Tropical pulmonary eosinophilia—A review. *Indian J. Med. Res.* **2013**, *138*, 295–302. [PubMed]

22. Melrose, W.; Rahmah, N. Use of Brugia rapid dipstick and ICT test to map distribution of lymphatic filariasis in the Democratic Republic of Timor-Leste. *Southeast Asian J. Trop. Med. Public Health* **2006**, *37*, 22–25. [PubMed]

23. Knott, J. The periodicity of the microfilaria of *Wuchereria bancrofti*. Preliminary report of some injection experiments. *Trans. R. Soc. Trop. Med. Hyg.* **1935**, *29*, 59–64. [CrossRef]

24. Jongthawin, J.; Intapan, P.M.; Lulitanond, V.; Sanpool, O.; Thanchomnang, T.; Sadaow, L.; Maleewong, W. Detection and quantification of *Wuchereria bancrofti* and *Brugia malayi* DNA in blood samples and mosquitoes using duplex droplet digital polymerase chain reaction. *Parasitol. Res.* **2016**, *115*, 2967–2972. [CrossRef] [PubMed]

25. Weerakoon, K.G.; McManus, D.P. Cell-free DNA as a diagnostic tool for human parasitic infections. *Trends Parasitol.* **2016**, *32*, 378–391. [CrossRef] [PubMed]

26. Weil, G.J.; Lammie, P.J.; Weiss, N. The ICT filariasis test: A rapid-format antigen test for diagnosis of bancroftian filariasis. *Parasitol. Today* **1997**, *13*, 401–404. [CrossRef]

27. Weil, G.J.; Liftis, F. Identification and partial characterisation of a parasite antigen in sera from humans infected with *Wuchereria bancrofti. J. Immunol.* **1987**, *138*, 3035–3041. [PubMed]

28. Wanji, S.; Amvongo-Adjia, N.; Njouendou, A.J.; Kengne-Ouafo, J.A.; Ndongmo, W.P.; Fombad, F.F.; Koudou, B.; Enyong, P.A.; Bockarie, M. Further evidence of the cross-reactivity of the Binax NOW filariasis ICT cards to non-*Wuchereria bancrofti* filariae: Experimental studies with *Loa loa* and *Onchocerca ochengi*. *Parasit. Vectors* **2016**, *9*, 267. [CrossRef] [PubMed]

29. Wanji, S.; Amvongo-Adjia, N.; Koudou, B.; Njouendou, A.J.; Chounna Ndongmo, P.W.; Kengne-Ouafo, J.A.; Datchoua-Poutcheu, F.R.; Fovennso, B.A.; Tayong, D.B.; Fombad, F.F.; et al. Cross-Reactivity of filariasis ICT Cards in areas of contrasting endemicity of *Loa loa* and *Mansonella perstans* in Cameroon: Implications for shrinking of the lymphatic filariasis map in the central African region. *PLoS Negl. Trop. Dis.* **2015**, *9*, e0004184. [CrossRef] [PubMed]

30. WHO. Improved Availability of New Test to Enhance Global Lymphatic Filariasis Elimination. Available online: http://www.who.int/neglected_diseases/news/new_test_enhance_global_lf_elimination/en/ (accessed on 25 May 2018).

31. Weil, G.J.; Curtis, K.C.; Fakoli, L.; Fischer, K.; Gankpala, L.; Lammie, P.J.; Majewski, A.C.; Pelletreau, S.; Won, K.Y.; Bolay, F.K.; et al. Laboratory and field evaluation of a new rapid test for detecting *Wuchereria bancrofti* antigen in human blood. *Am. J. Trop. Med. Hyg.* **2013**, *89*, 11–15. [CrossRef] [PubMed]

32. WHO. *Strengthening the Assessment of Lymphatic Filariasis Transmission and Documenting the Achievement of Elimination*; WHO: Geneva, Switzerland, 2014.

33. Masson, J.; Douglass, J.; Roineau, M.; Aye, K.M.; Htwe, K.M.; Warner, J.; Graves, P.M. Relative performance and predictive values of plasma and dried blood spots with filter paper sampling techniques and dilutions of the lymphatic filariasis Og4C3 antigen ELISA for samples from Myanmar. *Trop. Med. Infect. Dis.* **2017**, *2*, 7. [CrossRef]

34. El-Moamly, A.A.; El-Sweify, M.A.; Hafez, M.A. Using the AD12-ICT rapid-format test to detect *Wuchereria bancrofti* circulating antigens in comparison to Og4C3-ELISA and nucleopore membrane filtration and microscopy techniques. *Parasitol. Res.* **2012**, *111*, 1379–1383. [CrossRef] [PubMed]

35. Reeve, D.; Melrose, W. Evaluation of the Og34C filter paper technique in lymphatic filariasis prevalence studies. *Lymphology* **2014**, *47*, 65–72. [PubMed]

36. Supali, T.; Ismid, I.S.; Wibowo, H.; Djuardi, Y.; Majawati, E.; Ginanjar, P.; Fischer, P. Estimation of the prevalence of lymphatic filariasis by a pool screen PCR assay using blood spots collected on filter paper. *Trans. R. Soc. Trop. Med. Hyg.* **2006**, *100*, 753–759. [CrossRef] [PubMed]

37. Debrah, A.Y.; Mand, S.; Marfo-Debrekyei, Y.; Batsa, L.; Pfarr, K.; Buttner, M.; Adjei, O.; Buttner, D.; Hoerauf, A. Macrofilaricidal effect of 4 weeks of treatment with doxycycline on *Wuchereria bancrofti. Trop. Med. Int. Health* **2007**, *12*, 1433–1441. [CrossRef] [PubMed]

38. Turba, M.E.; Zambon, E.; Zannoni, A.; Russo, S.; Gentilini, F. Detection of *Wolbachia* DNA in blood for diagnosing filaria-associated syndromes in cats. *J. Clin. Microbiol.* **2012**, *50*, 2624–2630. [CrossRef] [PubMed]

39. Bockarie, M.J.; Tavul, L.; Kastens, W.; Michael, E.; Kazura, J.W. Impact of untreated bednets on prevalence of *Wuchereria bancrofti* transmitted by *Anopheles farauti* in Papua New Guinea. *Med. Vet. Entomol.* **2002**, *16*, 116–119. [CrossRef] [PubMed]

40. Reimer, L.J.; Thomsen, E.K.; Tisch, D.J.; Henry-Halldin, C.N.; Zimmerman, P.A.; Baea, M.E.; Dagoro, H.; Susapu, M.; Hetzel, M.W.; Bockarie, M.J.; et al. Insecticidal bed nets and filariasis transmission in Papua New Guinea. *N. Engl. J. Med.* **2013**, *369*, 745–753. [CrossRef] [PubMed]

41. Anderson, N.W.; Klein, D.M.; Dornink, S.M.; Jespersen, D.J.; Kubofcik, J.; Nutman, T.B.; Merrigan, S.D.; Couturier, M.R.; Theel, E.S. Comparison of three immunoassays for detection of antibodies to *Strongyloides stercoralis. Clin. Vaccine Immunol.* **2014**, *21*, 732–736. [CrossRef] [PubMed]

42. Ichimori, K. MDA-lymphatic filariasis. *Trop. Med. Health* **2014**, *42*, 21–24. [CrossRef] [PubMed]

43. Debrah, A.Y.; Mand, S.; Marfo-Debrekyei, Y.; Batsa, L.; Albers, A.; Specht, S.; Klarmann, U.; Pfarr, K.; Adjei, O.; Hoerauf, A. Macrofilaricidal activity in *Wuchereria bancrofti* after 2 weeks treatment with a combination of rifampicin plus doxycycline. *J. Parasitol. Res.* **2011**, *2011*, 201617. [CrossRef] [PubMed]

44. Noroes, J.; Dreyer, G.; Santos, A.; Mendes, V.G.; Medeiros, Z.; Addiss, D. Assessment of the efficacy of diethylcarbamazine on adult *Wuchereria bancrofti* in vivo. *Trans. R. Soc. Trop. Med. Hyg.* **1997**, *91*, 78–81. [CrossRef]
45. Vanamail, P.; Ramaiah, K.D.; Pani, S.P.; Das, P.K.; Grenfell, B.T.; Bundy, D.A. Estimation of the fecund life span of *Wuchereria bancrofti* in an endemic area. *Trans. R. Soc. Trop. Med. Hyg.* **1996**, *90*, 119–121. [CrossRef]
46. WHO. WHO Recommends Triple Drug Therapy to Accelerate Global Elimination of Lymphatic Filariasis. Available online: http://www.who.int/neglected_diseases/news/WHO_recommends_triple_medicine_therapy_for_LF_elimination/en/ (accessed on 25 May 2018).
47. Lim, K.H.; Speare, R.; Thomas, G.; Graves, P. Surgical treatment of genital manifestations of lymphatic filariasis: A systematic review. *World J. Surg.* **2015**, *39*, 2885–2899. [CrossRef] [PubMed]
48. Foster, W.D. *A History of Parasitology*; E. & S. Livingstone LTD.: Edinburgh/London, UK, 1965; pp. 89–104.
49. Peard, J.G. *Race, Place, and Medicine: The Idea of the Tropics in Nineteenth-Century Brazil: The Politics of Disease*; Duke University Press: Durham, NC, USA, 1999.
50. Cobbold, T.S. On the discovery of the intermediate host of *Filaria sanguinis hominis*. *Lancet* **1878**, *1*, 69.
51. Bahiana. Heróis da Saúde na Bahia: Otto Edwar Heinrich Wucherer. Available online: http://www.bahiana.edu.br/herois/heroi.aspx?id=MQ== (accessed on 10 January 2018).
52. Bancroft, P. Discussion of a paper by E. S. Jackson. *Aust. Med. Gaz.* **1893**, *12*, 261–262.
53. Bancroft, J. Diseases of animals and plants that interfere with colonial progress. *Divin. Hall Rec.* **1879**, *1*, 1–14.
54. Sweet, W.C. Report on malaria and filaria survey of Australia and on mosquito surveys in Queensland, Western Australia and Northern Territory. In *Final Report Australian Hookworm Campaign*; Australian Hookworm Campaign: Brisbane, Australia, 1924; Part II; pp. 1–37.
55. Mackerras, I.M.; Marks, E.N. The Bancrofts: A century of scientific endeavour. *Proc. R. Soc. Qld.* **1973**, *84*, 1–34.
56. Cobbold, T.S. Discovery of the adult representative of microscopic filariae. *Lancet* **1877**, *2*, 70–71.
57. Cobbold, T.S. On filaria bancrofti. *Lancet* **1877**, *2*, 495–496. [CrossRef]
58. Cobbold, T.S. Verification of recent haematozoal discoveries in Australia and Egypt. *Br. Med. J.* **1876**, *1*, 780. [CrossRef]
59. Bourne, A.G. A note on *Filaria sanguinis hominis*: With a description of a male specimen. *Br. Med. J.* **1888**, *1*, 1050. [CrossRef] [PubMed]
60. Trewin, B.J.; Darbro, J.M.; Jansen, C.C.; Schellhorn, N.A.; Zalucki, M.P.; Hurst, T.P.; Devine, G.J. The elimination of the dengue vector, *Aedes aegypti*, from Brisbane, Australia: The role of surveillance, larval habitat removal and policy. *PLoS Negl. Trop. Dis.* **2017**, *11*, e0005848. [CrossRef] [PubMed]
61. Bancroft, T.L. Notes on filaria in Queensland. *Aust. Med. Gaz.* **1901**, *29*, 233–234.
62. Bancroft, T.L. Filarial metamorphosis in the mosquito. *Aust. Med. Gaz.* **1899**, *18*, 120.
63. Mackerras, I.M. Metamorphosis of *Filaria bancrofti* Cobbold. *Br. Med. J.* **1933**, *2*, 36. [CrossRef]
64. Manson, P. On the development of *Filaria sanguinis hominis*, and on the mosquito considered as a nurse. *J. Linn. Soc. Lond. Zool.* **1878**, *14*, 304–311. [CrossRef]
65. Bancroft, T.L.; Edin, M.B. On a proposed technique for the prevention of dengue fever and filariasis. *Aust. Med. Gaz.* **11912**, *31*, 80–81.
66. Turner, P.; Copeman, B.; Gerisi, D.; Speare, R. A comparison of the Og4C3 antigen capture ELISA, the Knott test, an IgG4 assay and clinical signs, in the diagnosis of Bancroftian filariasis. *Trop. Med. Parasitol.* **1993**, *44*, 45–48. [PubMed]
67. Burkot, T.R.; Durrheim, D.N.; Melrose, W.D.; Speare, R.; Ichimori, K. The argument for integrating vector control with multiple drug administration campaigns to ensure elimination of lymphatic filariasis. *Filaria J.* **2006**, *5*, 10. [CrossRef] [PubMed]
68. Zeldenryk, L.M.; Gray, M.; Speare, R.; Gordon, S.; Melrose, W. The emerging story of disability associated with lymphatic filariasis: A critical review. *PLoS Negl. Trop. Dis.* **2011**, *5*, e1366. [CrossRef] [PubMed]
69. Zeldenryk, L.; Gordon, S.; Gray, M.; Speare, R.; Melrose, W. Disability Measurement for Lymphatic Filariasis: A Review of Generic Tools Used within Morbidity Management Programs. *PLoS Negl. Trop. Dis.* **2012**, *6*. [CrossRef] [PubMed]
70. Durrheim, D.N.; Nelesone, T.; Speare, R.; Melrose, W. Certifying lymphatic filariasis elimination in the Pacific—The need for new tools. *Pac. Health Dialog* **2003**, *10*, 149–154. [PubMed]

71. Harrington, H.; Asugeni, J.; Jimuru, C.; Gwalaa, J.; Ribeyro, E.; Bradbury, R.; Joseph, H.; Melrose, W.; MacLaren, D.; Speare, R. A practical strategy for responding to a case of lymphatic filariasis post-elimination in Pacific islands. *Parasit. Vectors* **2013**, *6*, 218. [CrossRef] [PubMed]
72. Michael, E.; Bundy, D.A. Global mapping of lymphatic filariasis. *Parasitol. Today* **1997**, *13*, 472–476. [CrossRef]
73. JCU. James Cook University: WHO Collaborating Centres. Available online: https://research.jcu.edu.au/who-collaborating-centres (accessed on 20 January 2018).
74. Bockarie, M.J.; Tisch, D.J.; Kastens, W.; Alexander, N.D.; Dimber, Z.; Bockarie, F.; Ibam, E.; Alpers, M.P.; Kazura, J.W. Mass treatment to eliminate filariasis in Papua New Guinea. *N. Engl. J. Med.* **2002**, *347*, 1841–1848. [CrossRef] [PubMed]
75. Erickson, S.M.; Thomsen, E.K.; Keven, J.B.; Vincent, N.; Koimbu, G.; Siba, P.M.; Christensen, B.M.; Reimer, L.J. Mosquito-parasite interactions can shape filariasis transmission dynamics and impact elimination programs. *PLoS Negl. Trop. Dis.* **2013**, *7*, e2433. [CrossRef] [PubMed]
76. Tisch, D.J.; Alexander, N.D.; Kiniboro, B.; Dagoro, H.; Siba, P.M.; Bockarie, M.J.; Alpers, M.P.; Kazura, J.W. Reduction in acute filariasis morbidity during a mass drug administration trial to eliminate lymphatic filariasis in Papua New Guinea. *PLoS Negl. Trop. Dis.* **2011**, *5*, e1241. [CrossRef] [PubMed]
77. Tisch, D.J.; Bockarie, M.J.; Dimber, Z.; Kiniboro, B.; Tarongka, N.; Hazlett, F.E.; Kastens, W.; Alpers, M.P.; Kazura, J.W. Mass drug administration trial to eliminate lymphatic filariasis in Papua New Guinea: Changes in microfilaremia, filarial antigen, and Bm14 antibody after cessation. *Am. J. Trop. Med. Hyg.* **2008**, *78*, 289–293. [PubMed]
78. Weil, G.J.; Kastens, W.; Susapu, M.; Laney, S.J.; Williams, S.A.; King, C.L.; Kazura, J.W.; Bockarie, M.J. The impact of repeated rounds of mass drug administration with diethylcarbamazine plus albendazole on bancroftian filariasis in Papua New Guinea. *PLoS Negl. Trop. Dis.* **2008**, *2*, e344. [CrossRef] [PubMed]
79. WHO. Pacific Program to Eliminate Lymphatic Filariasis: Country Programs. Available online: http://www.wpro.who.int/southpacific/pacelf/countries/en/ (accessed on 25 January 2018).
80. Hotez, P.J.; Bottazzi, M.E.; Strych, U.; Chang, L.Y.; Lim, Y.A.; Goodenow, M.M.; AbuBakar, S. Neglected tropical diseases among the Association of Southeast Asian Nations (ASEAN): Overview and update. *PLoS Negl. Trop. Dis.* **2015**, *9*, e0003575. [CrossRef] [PubMed]
81. Wibawa, T.; Satoto, T.B.T. Magnitude of neglected tropical diseases in Indonesia at postmillennium Development Goals Era. *J. Trop. Med.* **2016**, *2016*, 9. [CrossRef] [PubMed]
82. Oemijati, S. Current status of filariasis in Indonesia. *Southeast Asian J. Trop. Med. Public Health* **1993**, *24* (Suppl. 2), 2–4. [PubMed]
83. Wahyono, T.Y.M.; Purwantyastuti; Supali, T. *Filariasis di Indonesia*; Buletin Jendela Epidemiologi: Jakarta, Indonesia, 2010.
84. *2015 Indonesian Health Profile*; Ministry of Health RI: Jakarta, Indonesia, 2016.
85. Krentel, A.; Damayanti, R.; Titaley, C.R.; Suharno, N.; Bradley, M.; Lynam, T. Improving coverage and compliance in mass drug administration for the elimination of LF in two 'endgame' districts in Indonesia using micronarrative surveys. *PLoS Negl. Trop. Dis.* **2016**, *10*, e0005027. [CrossRef] [PubMed]
86. Krentel, A.; Fischer, P.; Manoempil, P.; Supali, T.; Servais, G.; Ruckert, P. Using knowledge, attitudes and practice (KAP) surveys on lymphatic filariasis to prepare a health promotion campaign for mass drug administration in Alor District, Indonesia. *Trop. Med. Int. Health* **2006**, *11*, 1731–1740. [CrossRef] [PubMed]
87. Martins, N.; McMinn, P.; de Jesus Gomes, M.S.; Freitas, L.T.; Counahan, M.; Freitas, C. *Timor-Leste National Parasite Survey: Report and Recommendations*; Ministerio da Saude: Dili, Timor-Leste, 2012.
88. Frances, S.P.; Baade, L.M.; Kubofcik, J.; Nutman, T.B.; Melrose, W.D.; McCarthy, J.S.; Nissen, M.D. Seroconversion to filarial antigens in Australian defence force personnel in Timor-Leste. *Am. J. Trop. Med. Hyg.* **2008**, *78*, 560–563. [PubMed]
89. Lau, C.L.; Won, K.Y.; Becker, L.; Soares Magalhaes, R.J.; Fuimaono, S.; Melrose, W.; Lammie, P.J.; Graves, P.M. Seroprevalence and spatial epidemiology of lymphatic filariasis in American Samoa after successful mass drug administration. *PLoS Negl. Trop. Dis.* **2014**, *8*, e3297. [CrossRef] [PubMed]
90. Lau, C.L.; Sheridan, S.; Ryan, S.; Roineau, M.; Andreosso, A.; Fuimaono, S.; Tufa, J.; Graves, P.M. Detecting and confirming residual hotspots of lymphatic filariasis transmission in American Samoa 8 years after stopping mass drug administration. *PLoS Negl. Trop. Dis.* **2017**, *11*, e0005914. [CrossRef] [PubMed]
91. Monchy, D.; Barny, S.; Rougier, Y.; Baudet, J.M.; Gentile, B. Survey of lymphatic filariasis on Ouvea Island in New Caledonia. *Med. Trop.* **1999**, *59*, 146–150.

92. Daures, M.; Champagnat, J.; Pfannstiel, A.; Ringuenoire, F.; Grangeon, J.P.; Musso, D. Filariasis serosurvey, New Caledonia, South Pacific, 2013. *Parasit. Vectors* **2015**, *8*, 102. [CrossRef] [PubMed]
93. Pretrick, M.; Melrose, W.; Chaine, J.P.; Canyon, D.; Carron, J.; Graves, P.M.; Bradbury, R.S. Identification and control of an isolated, but intense focus of lymphatic filariasis on Satawal Island, Federated States of Micronesia, in 2003. *Trop. Med. Health* **2017**, *45*, 17. [CrossRef] [PubMed]
94. WHO. *Weekly Epidemiological Record*; WHO: Geneva, Switzerland, 2010; pp. 365–372.
95. Fraser, M.; Taleo, G.; Taleo, F.; Yaviong, J.; Amos, M.; Babu, M.; Kalkoa, M. Evaluation of the program to eliminate lymphatic filariasis in Vanuatu following two years of mass drug administration implementation: Results and methodologic approach. *Am. J. Trop. Med. Hyg.* **2005**, *73*, 753–758. [PubMed]
96. Allen, T.; Taleo, F.; Graves, P.M.; Wood, P.; Taleo, G.; Baker, M.C.; Bradley, M.; Ichimori, K. Impact of the Lymphatic Filariasis Control Program towards elimination of filariasis in Vanuatu, 1997–2006. *Trop. Med. Health* **2017**, *45*, 8. [CrossRef] [PubMed]
97. Taleo, F.; Taleo, G.; Graves, P.M.; Wood, P.; Kim, S.H.; Ozaki, M.; Joseph, H.; Chu, B.; Pavluck, A.; Yajima, A.; et al. Surveillance efforts after mass drug administration to validate elimination of lymphatic filariasis as a public health problem in Vanuatu. *Trop. Med. Health* **2017**, *45*, 18. [CrossRef] [PubMed]
98. WHO. *Cambodia, Cook Islands, Niue and Vanuatu Eliminate Lymphatic Filariasis as a Public Health Problem*; WHO: Geneva, Switzerland, 2016.
99. Australian Bureau of Statistics. Migration, Australia, 2015–16. Available online: http://www.abs.gov.au/ausstats/abs@.nsf/mf/3412.0 (accessed on 4 July 2017).
100. Lowichik, A.; Lowrie, R.C., Jr. Uptake and development of *Wuchereria bancrofti* in *Aedes aegypti* and Haitian *Culex quinquefasciatus* that were fed on a monkey with low-density microfilaremia. *Trop. Med. Parasitol.* **1988**, *39*, 227–229. [PubMed]
101. Queensland Government. Dengue Outbreaks. Available online: https://www.health.qld.gov.au/clinical-practice/guidelines-procedures/diseases-infection/diseases/mosquito-borne/dengue/dengue-outbreaks (accessed on 28 January 2018).
102. Queensland Government. *Queensland Dengue Management Plan 2015–2020*; State of Queensland (Queensland Health): Brisbane, Australia, 2015.
103. Queensland Government. Mosquito Control. Available online: https://www.qld.gov.au/health/conditions/all/prevention/mosquito-borne/control/breeding-sites (accessed on 28 January 2018).
104. Ciota, A.; Kramer, L. Vector-virus interactions and transmission dynamics of West Nile virus. *Viruses* **2013**, *5*, 3021–3047. [CrossRef] [PubMed]
105. Kovendan, K.; Murugan, K.; Vincent, S.; Kamalakannan, S. Larvicidal efficacy of *Jatropha curcas* and bacterial insecticide, *Bacillus thuringiensis*, against lymphatic filarial vector, *Culex quinquefasciatus* Say (Diptera: culicidae). *Parasitol. Res.* **2011**, *109*, 1251–1257. [CrossRef] [PubMed]
106. Muzari, M.O.; Devine, G.; Davis, J.; Crunkhorn, B.; van den Hurk, A.; Whelan, P.; Russell, R.; Walker, J.; Horne, P.; Ehlers, G.; et al. Holding back the tiger: Successful control program protects Australia from *Aedes albopictus* expansion. *PLoS Negl. Trop. Dis.* **2017**, *11*, e0005286. [CrossRef] [PubMed]
107. Proestos, Y.; Christophides, G.K.; Erguler, K.; Tanarhte, M.; Waldock, J.; Lelieveld, J. Present and future projections of habitat suitability of the Asian tiger mosquito, a vector of viral pathogens, from global climate simulation. *Philos. Trans. R. Soc. Lond. B Biol. Sci.* **2015**, *370*. [CrossRef]
108. Southgate, B.A. Intensity and efficiency of transmission and the development of microfilaraemia and disease: Their relationship in lymphatic filariasis. *J. Trop. Med. Hyg.* **1992**, *95*, 1–12. [PubMed]
109. Subramanian, S.; Krishnamoorthy, K.; Ramaiah, K.D.; Habbema, J.D.; Das, P.K.; Plaisier, A.P. The relationship between microfilarial load in the human host and uptake and development of *Wuchereria bancrofti* microfilariae by *Culex quinquefasciatus*: A study under natural conditions. *Parasitology* **1998**, *116 Pt 3*, 243–255. [CrossRef] [PubMed]
110. Bryan, J.H.; McMahon, P.; Barnes, A. Factors affecting transmission of *Wuchereria bancrofti* by anopheline mosquitoes. 3. Uptake and damage to ingested microfilariae by *Anopheles gambiae*, *An. arabiensis*, *An. merus* and *An. funestus* in east Africa. *Trans. R. Soc. Trop. Med. Hyg.* **1990**, *84*, 265–268. [CrossRef]
111. Bryan, J.H.; Southgate, B.A. Factors affecting transmission of *Wuchereria bancrofti* by anopheline mosquitoes. 1. Uptake of microfilariae. *Trans. R. Soc. Trop. Med. Hyg.* **1988**, *82*, 128–137. [CrossRef]

112. Bryan, J.H.; Southgate, B.A. Factors affecting transmission of *Wuchereria bancrofti* by anopheline mosquitoes. 2. Damage to ingested microfilariae by mosquito foregut armatures and development of filarial larvae in mosquitoes. *Trans. R. Soc. Trop. Med. Hyg.* **1988**, *82*, 138–145. [CrossRef]

113. Southgate, B.A.; Bryan, J.H. Factors affecting transmission of *Wuchereria bancrofti* by anopheline mosquitoes. 4. Facilitation, limitation, proportionality and their epidemiological significance. *Trans. R. Soc. Trop. Med. Hyg.* **1992**, *86*, 523–530. [CrossRef]

114. Boakye, D.A.; Wilson, M.D.; Appawu, M.A.; Gyapong, J. Vector competence, for *Wuchereria bancrofti*, of the *Anopheles* populations in the Bongo district of Ghana. *Ann. Trop. Med. Parasitol.* **2004**, *98*, 501–508. [CrossRef] [PubMed]

115. Manson, P. *The Filaria Sanguinis Hominis and Certain Forms of Parasitic Disease in India, China and Warm Countries*; H. K. Lewis: London, UK, 1883.

116. Shriram, A.N.; Ramaiah, K.D.; Krishnamoorthy, K.; Sehgal, S.C. Diurnal pattern of human-biting activity and transmission of subperiodic *Wuchereria bancrofti* (Filariidea: Dipetalonematidae) by *Ochlerotatus niveus* (Diptera: Culicidae) on the Andaman and Nicobar islands of India. *Am. J. Trop. Med. Hyg.* **2005**, *72*, 273–277. [PubMed]

117. Samarawickrema, W.A.; Kimura, E.; Spears, G.F.; Penaia, L.; Sone, F.; Paulson, G.S.; Cummings, R.F. Distribution of vectors, transmission indices and microfilaria rates of subperiodic *Wuchereria bancrofti* in relation to village ecotypes in Samoa. *Trans. R. Soc. Trop. Med. Hyg.* **1987**, *81*, 129–135. [CrossRef]

118. Russell, R.C.; Webb, C.E.; Davies, N. *Aedes aegypti* (L.) and *Aedes polynesiensis* Marks (Diptera: Culicidae) in Moorea, French Polynesia: A Study of adult population structures and pathogen (*Wuchereria bancrofti* and *Dirofilaria immitis*) infection rates to indicate regional and seasonal epidemiological risk for dengue and filariasis. *J. Med. Entomol.* **2005**, *42*, 1045–1056. [CrossRef] [PubMed]

119. Ariani, C.V.; Juneja, P.; Smith, S.; Tinsley, M.C.; Jiggins, F.M. Vector competence of *Aedes aegypti* mosquitoes for filarial nematodes is affected by age and nutrient limitation. *Exp. Gerontol.* **2015**, *61*, 47–53. [CrossRef] [PubMed]

120. Beebe, N.W.; Cooper, R.D.; Mottram, P.; Sweeney, A.W. Australia's dengue risk driven by human adaptation to climate change. *PLoS Negl. Trop. Dis.* **2009**, *3*, e429. [CrossRef] [PubMed]

121. Richard, V.; Paoaafaite, T.; Cao-Lormeau, V.M. Vector competence of *Aedes aegypti* and *Aedes polynesiensis* populations from French Polynesia for chikungunya virus. *PLoS Negl. Trop. Dis.* **2016**, *10*, e0004694. [CrossRef] [PubMed]

122. Gilotra, S.K.; Shah, K.V. Laboratory studies on transmission of chikungunya virus by mosquitoes. *Am. J. Epidemiol.* **1967**, *86*, 379–385. [CrossRef] [PubMed]

123. Gubler, D.J. Transmission of Ross River virus by *Aedes polynesiensis* and *Aedes aegypti*. *Am. J. Trop. Med. Hyg.* **1981**, *30*, 1303–1306. [CrossRef] [PubMed]

124. Rollins, A. TB Superbug Makes Landfall in Australia. Available online: https://ama.com.au/ausmed/tb-superbug-makes-landfall-australia (accessed on 29 March 2018).

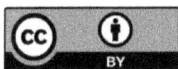

Tropical Medicine and
Infectious Disease

MDPI

Review

An Overview of Brucellosis in Cattle and Humans, and its Serological and Molecular Diagnosis in Control Strategies

Muhammad Zahoor Khan [1] and Muhammad Zahoor [2,*]

[1] Key Laboratory of Agricultural Animal Genetics and Breeding, National Engineering Laboratory for Animal Breeding, College of Animal Science and Technology, China Agricultural University, Beijing 100193, China; zahoorkhattak91@yahoo.com
[2] Department of Molecular Medicine, Institute of Basic Medical Sciences, University of Oslo, Sognsvannsveien, 90372 Oslo, Norway
* Correspondence: muhammad.zahoor@medisin.uio.no; Tel.: +47-97-17-8583

Received: 28 April 2018; Accepted: 9 June 2018; Published: 14 June 2018

Abstract: Brucellosis is one of the most common contagious and communicable zoonotic diseases with high rates of morbidity and lifetime sterility. There has been a momentous increase over the recent years in intra/interspecific infection rates, due to poor management and limited resources, especially in developing countries. Abortion in the last trimester is a predominant sign, followed by reduced milk yield and high temperature in cattle, while in humans it is characterized by undulant fever, general malaise, and arthritis. While the clinical picture of brucellosis in humans and cattle is not clear and often misleading with the classical serological diagnosis, efforts have been made to overcome the limitations of current serological assays through the development of PCR-based diagnosis. Due to its complex nature, brucellosis remains a serious threat to public health and livestock in developing countries. In this review, we summarized the recent literature, significant advancements, and challenges in the treatment and vaccination against brucellosis, with a special focus on developing countries.

Keywords: brucellosis; cattle; human; serological and molecular methods

1. Introduction

Brucellosis is thought to have been identified in the late Roman era, named because of its resemblance to the organism *Brucellae* (later called *Brucella*) from carbonized cheese. Brucellosis has been associated with military campaigns, predominantly in the Mediterranean region. The disease was first expounded by Sir David Bruce, Hughes, and Zammit while working in Malta; hence the name 'Malta fever' is occasionally used for typical fever conditions caused by *Brucella* and its two most common species *B. abortus* and *B. melitensis*. *B. abortus* was first reported as a causative agent of premature delivery in cattle and intermittent fever in humans [1,2]. Brucellosis stands first in the list of zoonotic bacterial diseases, and 500,000 cases are reported annually in disease-endemic regions [3–7].

Although brucellosis is a widespread livestock infection in the Middle East and North Africa, it has not been studied in detail, except for rough figures about the epidemiology of the infection in these regions [8]. The bacteria infect reproductive tissues, lymph nodes, and the spleen, and therefore cause inflammation, edema, and necrosis. In pregnant animals it causes placental lesions and increases the risks of abortion [9,10]. Brucellosis gains public health importance when the bacteria are transmitted to human via unpasteurized milk, meat, and animal byproducts, from infected animals [11]. Proper diagnosis is one of the key obstacles for the complete eradication of brucellosis. Although several serological tests such as the Rose Bengal tube test, serum agglutination test, and enzyme-linked immunosorbent assay (ELISA) are used for disease diagnosis in cattle; however, these are often found to be misleading [12]. In recent years, PCR-based validation along with serological tests are widely used to ensure proper diagnoses [13]. Apart from the risk to public health, it also raises financial concerns to livestock stakeholders or latent product consumers. Figure 1 is a graphical summarization of brucellosis infection [14,15].

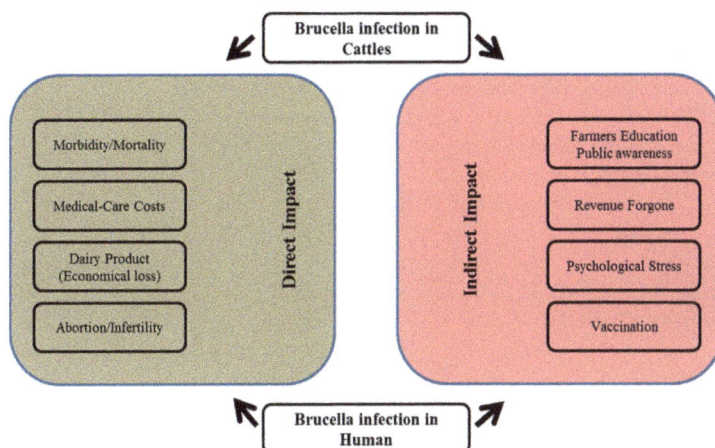

Figure 1. Summarizing the impact of *Brucella* infection in humans as well in cattle.

1.1. Brucella: The Causative Agent of Brucellosis

Brucellosis is caused by *Brucella*, a Gram-negative, aerobic, and facultative intracellular coccobacillus [16]. Based on taxonomic distribution, *Brucella* is classified as α-proteobacteria, which is further divided into six species, each including several biovars. The species *B. melitensis* biovars 1–3 have been reported in sheep and goats, and *B. abortus* biovars 1–6 and 9 in cattle. Similarly, the *B. suis* biovars 1–3 are known to infect pigs, while *B. suis* biovar 4 and 5 are more common for infection in reindeer and small rodents. Among other common species, *B. canis is* found in dogs, *B. ovis* in sheep, and *B. neotomae* in desert wood rats. Recently, *B. pinnipedialis* (in seals) and *B. ceti* (in whales and dolphins) are newly reported species, infecting marine animals [17].

The genome structure of *Brucella* is composed of two chromosomes, without plasmids, making it unique in Bacteriaceae. The recent introduction of genome sequence projects and genome information of *B. melitensis* (Gene Bank NC003317) and (NC003318), *B. suis* (Gene Bank NC002969), and *B. abortus* has opened up further gates towards the understanding of the disease pathogenicity and its mode of virulence [18,19]. Classification is usually based on the distinction between pathogenicity and host partiality [20]. *B. abortus* and *B. melitensis* are the key bovine brucellosis bacteria, while *B. abortus*, *B. melitensis*, *B. suis*, and *B. canis* are known for their infectivity in humans. Studies have also reported *B. melitensis* infection in sheep and goats [21,22].

1.2. Brucellosis Transmission

The infection of *Brucella* species is commonly mediated by direct contact with the placenta, fetus, fetal fluids, and vaginal discharges or byproducts (e.g., milk, meat, and cheese) from infected animals [23,24]. This explains why the typical route of infection is either direct ingestion or via mucous membranes, broken skin, and in rare cases intact skin [25,26]. Professional health workers are frequent victims of *Brucella* infection, especially in regions of prevalent disease, and it is documented that nearly 12% of laboratory workers in Spain get brucellosis during fieldwork [27,28]. In addition, in utero transmission, person-to-person transmission, and transmission associated with tissue transplantation have been observed in rare cases [29–31]. Aerial bacteria also remain a severe threat of infection, either by inhaling organisms or through the conjunctiva. Brucellosis also spreads via vertical transmission, by infecting new-born calves and lambs in the uterus [32].

1.3. Global Public Health Concerns

Brucellosis has been reported in 86 different countries worldwide and is a serious threat not only to livestock but also to human health globally. Despite its brutal impact on economic loss, it is also associated with high morbidity, both for humans and animals in developing countries [25,33]. North African and Near East countries are listed at the top for infection and cross-infection of brucellosis [34,35]. *Brucella melitensis* and *B. abortus* persistence has been confirmed in most Middle Eastern countries, but African and Asian continents are not spared either [36,37]. *Brucella abortus* and *B. suis* infection is widespread throughout Central America [38]. In Europe, human brucellosis is thought to be associated with travellers and immigrants from the Middle East or the private import of dairy products from endemic areas [37,39–41].

Brucella infection is widespread in several South Asian/Asian countries including Pakistan, India, China, and Sri Lanka, in humans as well as in animals [42–45]. In 1950, *Brucella* was for the first time reported in animals in Malaysia, and the government undertook an eradication strategy for bovine, ovine, and caprine brucellosis (National Surveillance Program for Animal Brucellosis) since 1978 [46]. Additionally, a series of studies documented the seropositive cases of brucellosis in humans mainly in veterinary professionals and farmers that had close contact with animals. The prevalence of brucellosis is more common in males (90%) ranging from 20–45 years old in Malaysia [47]. This showed that *Brucella* infection is highly zoonotic, as males are commonly involved in the handling of livestock and their products in Malaysia. Brucellosis occurrence fluctuates extensively, not only between countries but also within a country.

Though we lack solid evidence, a report suggests that in Iraq and Egypt occupation and socioeconomic status are associated with the rate of *Brucella* infection [35,48]. This possibly explains the high brucellosis incidence in low- and middle-income countries. To further endorse this, it was not surprising that brucellosis is more common in specific communities even in developed countries, such as Turkish immigrants in Germany or Hispanics in the USA—communities with poor socioeconomic status [49,50]. The studies above are enough to assume that though brucellosis is common in underdeveloped/developing countries or even in communities with poor socioeconomic status, in developed countries due to its infectious nature, the risk circle of *Brucella* infection might potentially extend to safe havens in the near future [51,52].

Dissecting the occupational hazard of brucellosis, the disease is commonly found in shepherds, people working in the dairy or meat industry, veterinarians, and laboratory professionals. Males are more prone to infection compared to females, being more likely to adopt such occupations. However, in rural areas where women handle livestock, the incidence rate is elevated in females [53,54]. Brucellosis prevalence is common in people of the age group 13–40 years; in northern Saudi Arabia, it decreases in the older aged group [55]. However, vulnerability gets worse in aged groups, and can even lead to destructive localized brucellosis of the spine in cases of acute localized brucellosis [56]. Children are rarely susceptible to brucellosis, except in the regions that lack the proper pasteurization of milk [57]. This leads us to conclude that brucellosis does not associate with gender and age, but rather occupation and exposure to bacterial infection.

1.4. Clinical Picture of Brucellosis in Cattle

Brucellosis is a widespread reproductive disease, commonly causing abortion, death of young ones, stillbirth, retained placenta or birth of weak calves, delayed calving, male infertility, and marked reduction in milk yield [37,58–60]. It infects almost all domestic species except cats, which are naturally resistant to *Brucella* infection [59]. In bulls, the disease is characterized by fever, vesiculitis, orchitis, and epididymitis. In severe cases, it can also be the reason for testicular abscesses, metritis or orchitis that can lead to lifetime infertility. In animals, brucellosis symptoms can be varied from severe acute to sub-acute or chronic, depending upon the organ of infection and the type of animal [60]. When a pregnant animal is infected by *Brucella*, a visible swelling of the mammary gland to the navel region and bleeding from the vagina is not uncommon, even if the cow does not abort. The enlarged udder size (appearance of the 9th month of a pregnant cow) could be used as an indication for the high stage of the disease, where animals shed bacteria in urine, milk, and vaginal discharges.

1.5. Human Brucellosis

Human brucellosis is known by many different names such as Malta fever, Cyprus or Mediterranean fever, intermittent typhoid, rock fever of Gibraltar, and more commonly, undulant fever [61]. The usual incubation period of one to four weeks can be extended up to several months before complete symptoms appear. Infection among children is generally more benign than in adults, concerning the likelihood and severity of complications and response to treatment [62].

Fever is one of the most common symptoms across patients; intermittent in 60% of patients with acute and chronic brucellosis, while undulant in 40% of patients with subacute brucellosis. Fever is thought to be linked to relative bradycardia and fever of unknown origin (FUO) is a more common initial diagnosis in patients in areas of low endemicity. Nearly 80% of patients suffer from chills, and 20% of patients develop a cough and dyspnea without any active pulmonary involvement. Additionally, pleuritic chest pain may affect patients with underlying empyema [16,63,64].

Brucellosis also increases the risk of spontaneous abortion, premature delivery, miscarriage, and intrauterine infection with fetal death in humans as well, which is accompanied with malaise, fatigue, and arthritis [28,63]. Septicemias with sudden onset followed by high fever, emaciation, restlessness, undulant fever, sexual impotence, insomnia, headache, loss of appetite, and weight loss can also be seen in an infected patient [65]. The detailed symptoms of brucellosis have been documented; however, due to their protean and complex nature, clinical manifestations cannot be relied on for diagnosis [66]. In humans, brucellosis is not confined to the reproductive system, but is also known to cause neurobrucellosis with clinical manifestation of meningitis, encephalitis, stroke, radiculitis, myelitis, peripheral neuropathies, and neuropsychiatric features [67,68]. Studies have also reported sensorineural deafness, spastic paraparesis, followed by brisk tendon reflexes, bilateral ankle clonus, and extensor plantar responses [69].

2. Diagnosis of Brucellosis

2.1. Serological Tests

At the moment, no specific diagnostic test is available to identify *Brucella*. Therefore, conventional serological examination must be accompanied with more supportive analysis [59,70]. Serological methods are used for the initial screening of human brucellosis, as well as during follow-up treatment. Due to the consistent false negativity of serological tests in early days of infection, serial serological testing is usually recommended, which will not only help in proper diagnosis but also add to monitoring for response to treatment.

During the first week of illness, the changes in immunoglobulin (Ig) M isotype antibodies predominate, followed by an elevated level of IgG in the second week [71]. The titers of both subtypes continuously increase and reaches the peak within four weeks. Generally, a decline in antibody levels can be seen after antibiotic treatment, while relapse is often characterized by a second peak of anti-*Brucella* IgG and IgA, but not IgM [72]. At present, no standardized reference antigen for serological tests is available, therefore, combinations of several serological tests are recommended.

The investigative antigen of standard serological tests is usually prepared from whole-cell extract, which is majorly constituted of smooth lipopolysaccharides (S-LPS). During natural infection, the humoral immune reaction is characterized by antibody production against S-LPS, and therefore, diagnostic assays identify agglutinating and non-agglutinating antibodies. However, the diagnostic tool based on anti-LPS detection might lose its specificity due to its cross-reactivity with other clinically-relevant bacteria.

The immune-dominant epitope of the *Brucella* O-polysaccharide shows similarities with many other bacteria, such as *Yersinia enterocolitica* O:9, *Salmonella urbana* group N, *Vibrio cholerae*, *Francisella tularensis*, *Escherichia coli* O157, and *Stenotrophomonas maltophilia* [72,73]. Some *Brucella* species do not share similarities in S-LPS antigen, due to which the current conventional serological test loses its global application. Canine brucellosis, caused by *B. canis*, lacks S-LPS antigen, and thus cannot be diagnosed by standard S-LPS-based serological assays [74].

Among the serological methods currently in practice, the serum agglutination test (SAT) is commonly used for the diagnosis of *Brucella* infection in humans [72]. The updated serum tests (slide, plate, and card agglutination) have replaced the laborious and time consuming methods (i.e., Wright test) that were routinely used for clinical diagnosis of brucellosis. The Rose Bengal test (RBT) is an example of a card test used in endemic countries for the rapid diagnosis and screening of patients in emergency departments [75]. However, it is generally recommended that the RBT must be used in combination with other standard serological tests for more reliable detection and to avoid false positives. In high-risk populations, testing of diluted sera using the RBT might be a reasonable choice to reduce the need for a huge number of assenting tests [76]. The significance of diagnostic titers in follow-up sera from patients with brucellosis can be examined only within the circumstance of a well-matched clinical representation [69]. The lateral flow assay is another tool appropriate for rapid field or bedside testing in low socio-economic endemic areas, where laboratories lack modern facilities. This assay is even considered more accurate and specific than the SAT in chronic and complex cases [77].

Acomparative analysis of three tests (RBT, SAT, and Coombs' test (CT)) recommended Coombs gel test regarding specificity and sensitivity [78]. Several other serological tests are also used for diagnosis including the standard tube agglutination test (STAT), enzyme-linked immunosorbent assay (ELISA), milk ring test (MRT), and fluorescence polarization assay (FPA) [79]. Among them the SAT remained the most popular and used test for routine diagnostic practice worldwide [49]. Immunoglobulins including immunoglobulin M (IgM), IgG, and IgA measurement by ELISA reflect the better image of clinical disease manifestation. Compared to the SAT, ELISA yields higher sensitivity and specificity, therefore it is widely used in the diagnosis of chronic cases of brucellosis to detect incomplete antibodies [80,81].

Complement fixation test (CFT) is an option developed for the detection of IgG, but mostly used as a confirmatory test because of its cross-reactivity with *B. abortus* S19 vaccinated cattle [82]. The classical CT helps in the detection of incomplete, non-agglutinating or blocking antibodies, and is considered a suitable test to detect slight changes in anti-*Brucella* antibody titers during relapse and chronic courses [73].

Despite the fact that several serological assays are available in clinics, none of them meet the standard criteria for a convincing diagnosis. None of the assays are recommended to be used alone in endemic areas, and a verification test is often required [83].

Due to the lack of specificity and sensitivity of serological tests and culture techniques, different molecular methods have been optimized both for the diagnosis of bovine and human brucellosis [84].

2.2. Molecular Diagnosis

Polymerase chain reaction (PCR)-based diagnosis has been adopted in recent decades and is rapidly replacing conventional assays for diagnosis in clinical laboratories. In the same fashion, PCR-based detection of *Brucella* has also emerged as a novel and much more efficient diagnostic tool. Moreover, it not only detects but also accurately distinguishes between acute, subacute, and chronic infection. The pioneering approach using PCR for *Brucella* diagnosis was reported in early 1990s [85]. Blood is an easy source of DNA for the diagnosis of *Brucella* infection. In addition, various other clinical specimens including serum, urine, and cerebrospinal, synovial or pleural fluid and pus can also be used for *Brucella* detection [86,87]. In recent years, serum is the preferred source of DNA in molecular diagnostic assays, due to its anticoagulant and hemoglobin-free nature.

The detection of *Brucella* DNA in patients is considered a challenging task because of the lower number of bacteria in infected tissue and the inhibitory effects taking place from surrounding substances [88]. The standard methods used for sample preparation must include a step that reduces matrix inhibitory influences and deliberate bacterial DNA. Additionally, the residual PCR inhibition by complex matrices can also be overcome through the use of proper internal amplification control [89]. The QIAamp™ DNA Mini Kit (Qiagen Inc., Valencia, CA, USA) and the UltraClean™ DNA Blood Spin Kit (MO BIO Laboratories Inc., Carlsbad, CA, USA) are commercially-available kits, ready to be used for *Brucella* DNA extraction from serum, blood, and other tissue samples [90]. The circulating macrophages engulf and processes bacteria and negatively affect the PCR-based detection. However, the modern PCR method has the ability to detect even the non-viable or phagocytosed microorganisms [91]. *Brucella* DNA has also been successfully detected in milk samples from an infected animal using PCR-based assay [92].

Various gene and loci have been identified as potential targets for PCR-based amplification [50,93]. For example, *IS711* insertion element is a potential target that can be used for the detection of traceable bacteria as its multiple copies are found in the *Brucella* chromosomes [94]. Moreover, 16S rRNA also serves as a potential target, not only for *Brucella* but also related microorganisms [95]. The species-specific real-time PCR and conventional Bruce-ladder PCR assays are also considered to be key tools, used for confirmation and delineation of *Brucella* species [96]. For the diagnosis of human brucellosis, multilocus variable number tandem repeat analysis 16 loci panel (MLVA-16) is considered to be an authentic target [97].

Summarizing the facts, molecular diagnostics have the edge over conventional methods as they are robust and versatile, and due to the non-infectious nature of DNA, therefore safer for laboratory personnel. PCR-based detection is also more reliable and specific when compared to the serum plate agglutination test (SPAT) [98,99]. However, for a PCR-based assay, a specialized machine like a conventional thermocycler or real-time PCR is required along with skilled personnel. Moreover, specific primers for each *Brucella* species will be required.

3. Treatment of Brucellosis

Though the complex nature of brucellosis makes it harder to treat, long-term treatment with an antibiotic is thought to be beneficial. In most cases, antibiotics in combination are found to be more effective against the infection; however, the state of the disease still does not lose its importance [100,101]. Several conventional antibiotics including tetracycline, trimethoprim-sulfamethoxazole, aminoglycosides, rifampicin, quinolones, chloramphenicol, doxycycline, and streptomycin are commonly used in clinics [102,103]. In several cases, the application of antibiotics in a specific order has given best results. Likewise, a case reported that treatment with doxycycline for six months, followed by streptomycin for three weeks was found very effective against brucellosis in human [104]. Another study reported that the alkaloid columbamine in combination with jatrorrhizine were more effective against brucellosis caused by *B. abortus* compared to a combination of streptomycin and rifampicin [105]. The World Health Organization recommends that acute brucellosis cases be treated with oral doxycycline and rifampicin (600 mg for six weeks) [106]. However, rifampicin monotherapy is in common practice for treating brucellosis in pregnant women, and a combined therapy of sulphamethoxazole and trimethoprim is recommended for children [107]. In underdeveloped countries, treatment of cattle is not a common practice; however, the infected animals are isolated, culled or slaughtered to prevent the spreading of infection to other herd and at substantial veterinary costs.

In China, a case of subdural empyema complicated by intracerebral abscess due to *Brucella* infection was effectively treated with antibiotic therapy (ceftriaxone, doxycycline, rifapentine) [108]. In line with this, several reports suggested the combination therapy of doxycycline and rifampicin for six weeks is enough to eradicate *Brucella* infection, as well as associated complications [46,109–111]. This combination of doxycycline and rifampicin has also been proven experimentally [112]. As a result of continued efforts by the scientific community to develop an effective therapeutics, *Caryopteris mongolica* Bunge (Lamiaceae) has been tested in combination with doxycycline [113,114]. Despite the fact that several therapeutics are in practice which makes the disease manageable, an effective therapeutic is required for the complete treatment of brucellosis.

4. Vaccination against Brucellosis

To overcome the widespread intra- and inter-species infection of brucellosis, potent vaccination would be the best strategy [115]. Currently, several vaccines including S19, RB51, *B. melitensis* Rev.1, lysate, live vectored vaccine, mucosal vaccine subunit, and DNA vaccines are available for brucellosis [116–118]. In cattle, *B. abortus* strain 19 and RB 51 are the most commonly practiced vaccines [119,120]. S19 is used to vaccinate young female calves (3 to 12 months); however, it is not recommended for pregnant cattle, as it results in abortion [121]. S19 was found more effective in developing long-term immunity, when compared with RB51, in young calves [116,122,123]. However, RB51 does not interfere with serological diagnosis [124,125].

S19 and RB51 are live attenuated vaccines derived from *B. abortus* [126]. A cocktail lysate of S19 and RB51 was also tested as an immune-therapy to treat the bracelet infected cattle [114]. DNA vaccines have also been tested and show promising results when compared with S19 and RB51; however, several boosters were required to achieve the desired immunity [127,128]. In China, the S2 vaccine is widely in practice; however, it triggers an innate immune response and causes increased inflammation [129]. In conclusion, no effective and relatively safe vaccine is available that provides long-term protection against brucellosis.

5. Control Strategies for Prevention of Brucellosis

An effective approach should be adopted to eradicate and prevent brucellosis in cattle and humans. Diagnosing, curing/eradicating, and prevention are the golden rules often recommended by experts [130,131]. The slaughtering and proper disposal of seropositive animals to decrease the incidence of infection in healthy animals and effective vaccination and hygienic practices would reduce the disease spreading in/from endemic regions [132]. Vaccination is an effective strategy to prevent the spread of brucellosis and is in practice worldwide. However, there is demand for the development of new vaccines that are safer and more effective [9].

To cover the zoonotic aspects of brucellosis, proper education of field farmers, field workers, and the local community in endemic regions is required. The effective pasteurization of milk and other products and disinfection of meat is of key importance before consumption. The regular sterilization of labwares and laboratory tools would also result in a decrease in infection of clinical laboratory personnel [133].

Apart from local efforts, an effective global policy is required for the complete eradication of brucellosis. Proper veterinary legislation must be implemented and policies regarding animal health need to be encouraged. Modern updated knowledge on brucellosis should be delivered to farmers, veterinary professionals, and health educators, especially for rural populations, which will help to prevail over the dispersal of *Brucella* infection [134,135].

6. Conclusions

Brucellosis is not only a threat to livestock but also a global public health issue. Unfortunately, we lack not only a proper treatment but also a reliable diagnosis. Adequate and timely diagnosis of brucellosis is necessary to control and treat the disease in the best way. Different serological and molecular methods are used for the screening of the disease. However, each test has some drawbacks in one way or another. So here we suggest that due to the zoonotic importance of the *Brucella* infection, it is necessary to handle the disease in a proper way and a combination of particular tests should be used to screen for brucellosis in both humans and animals. The different cited studies regarding brucellosis in humans and cattle revealed that the combination of both the molecular and serological methods must be practiced for accurate diagnosis. If the infected animals are in chronic infected condition, they should be culled to prevent the disease spreading. The formal education and necessary training of farmers, especially those living in rural areas, would also help to get control over the disease. With rising interest of the scientific community in brucellosis, a significant improvement in diagnosis and treatment is expected. We are also in need of a broad-spectrum vaccine against *Brucella* for complete eradication of the disease worldwide.

Author Contributions: M.Z.K. and M.Z. wrote this review paper; moreover, M.Z. designed, supervised, and revised the manuscript.

Conflicts of Interest: The authors declare no conflict of interest.

References

1. Cutler, S.J.; Whatmore, A.M.; Commander, N.J. Brucellosis—New aspects of an old disease. *J. Appl. Microbiol.* **2005**, *98*, 1270–1281. [CrossRef] [PubMed]
2. Christopher, S.; Umapathy, B.; Ravikumar, K. Brucellosis: Review on the recent trends in pathogenicity and laboratory diagnosis. *J. Lab. Physicians* **2010**, *2*, 55–60. [CrossRef] [PubMed]
3. Johansen, M.V.; Welburn, S.C.; Dorny, P.; Brattig, W.N. Control of neglected zoonotic diseases. *Acta Trop.* **2017**, *165*, 1–2. [CrossRef] [PubMed]
4. Olsen, S.C.; Palmer, M.V. Advancement of knowledge of *Brucella* over the past 50 years. *Vet. Pathol.* **2014**, *51*, 1076–1089. [CrossRef] [PubMed]
5. Byndloss, M.X.; Tsolis, R.M. *Brucella* spp. Virulence factors and immunity. *Annu. Rev. Anim. Biosci.* **2016**, *4*, 111–127. [CrossRef] [PubMed]
6. Von Bargen, K.; Gorvel, J.P.; Salcedo, S.P. Internal affairs: Investigating the *Brucella* intracellular lifestyle. *FEMS Microbiol. Rev.* **2012**, *36*, 533–562. [CrossRef] [PubMed]
7. Pappas, G.; Papadimitriou, P.; Akritidis, N.; Christou, L.; Tsianos, V.E. The new global map of human brucellosis. *Lancet Infect. Dis.* **2006**, *6*, 91–99. [CrossRef]
8. Foster, J.T.; Walker, M.F.; Rannals, D.B.; Hussain, H.M.; Drees, P.K.; Tiller, V.R.; Hoffmaster, R.A.; Al-Rawahi, A.; Keim, P.; Saqib, M. African lineage *Brucella melitensis* isolates from Omani livestock. *Front. Microbiol.* **2017**, *8*, 2702. [CrossRef] [PubMed]
9. Wernery, U. Camelid brucellosis: A review. *Rev. Sci. Tech.* **2014**, *33*, 839–857. [CrossRef] [PubMed]
10. Narnaware, S.D.; Dahiya, S.S.; Kumar, S.; Tuteja, C.F.; Nath, K.; Patil, V.N. Pathological and diagnostic investigations of abortions and neonatal mortality associated with natural infection of *Brucella abortus* in dromedary camels. *Comp. Clin. Pathol.* **2017**, *26*, 79–85. [CrossRef]
11. Garcell, H.G.; Garcia, G.E.; Pueyo, V.P.; Martin, R.I.; Arias, V.A.; Alfonso Serrano, N.R. Outbreaks of brucellosis related to the consumption of unpasteurized camel milk. *J. Infect. Public Health* **2016**, *9*, 523–527. [CrossRef] [PubMed]
12. Gwida, M.M.; El-Gohary, H.A.; Melzer, F.; Khan, I.; Rosler, U.; Neubauer, H. Brucellosis in camels. *Res. Vet. Sci.* **2012**, *92*, 351–355. [CrossRef] [PubMed]
13. Gwida, M.M.; El-Gohary, H.A.; Melzer, F.; Tomaso, H.; Wernery, U.; Wernery, R.; Elschner, C.M.; Eickhoff, M.; Schoner, D.; Khan, I.; et al. Comparison of diagnostic tests for the detection of *Brucella* spp. in camel sera. *BMC Res. Notes* **2011**, *4*, 525. [CrossRef] [PubMed]
14. Rushton, J.; Thornton, P.K.; Otte, M.J. Methods of economic impact assessment. *Rev. Sci. Tech.* **1999**, *18*, 315–342. [CrossRef] [PubMed]
15. Jo, C. Cost-of-illness studies: Concepts, scopes, and methods. *Clin. Mol. Hepatol.* **2014**, *20*, 327–337. [CrossRef] [PubMed]
16. Pappas, G.; Bosilkovski, M.; Akritidis, N.; Tsianos, V.E. Brucellosis. *N. Engl. J. Med.* **2005**, *352*, 2325–2336. [CrossRef] [PubMed]
17. Foster, G.; Osterman, S.B.; Godfroid, J.; Jacques, I.; Cloeckaert, A. *Brucella ceti* sp. nov. and *Brucella pinnipedialis* sp. nov. for *Brucella* strains with cetaceans and seals as their preferred hosts. *Int. J. Syst. Evol. Microbiol.* **2007**, *57*, 2688–2693. [CrossRef] [PubMed]

18. DelVecchio, V.G.; Kapatral, V.; Redkar, R.J.; Patra, G.; Mujer, C.; Los, T.; Ivanova, N.; Anderson, I.; Bhattacharyya, A.; Lykidis, A.; et al. The genome sequence of the facultative intracellular pathogen *Brucella melitensis. Proc. Natl. Acad. Sci. USA* **2002**, *99*, 443–448. [CrossRef] [PubMed]

19. Sanchez, D.O.; Zandomeni, O.R.; Cravero, S.; Verdun, E.R.; Pierrou, E.; Faccio, P.; Diaz, G.; Lanzavecchia, S.; Aguero, F.; Frasch, C.A.; Andersson, G.S.; et al. Gene discovery through genomic sequencing of *Brucella abortus. Infect. Immun.* **2001**, *69*, 865–868. [CrossRef] [PubMed]

20. Moreno, E.; Cloeckaert, A.; Moriyon, I. *Brucella* evolution and taxonomy. *Vet. Microbiol.* **2002**, *90*, 209–227. [CrossRef]

21. Niza, M.M.R.E.; Félix, N.; Vilela, C.L.; Peleteiro, M.C.; Ferreira, A.J.A. Cutaneous and ocular adverse reactions in a dog following meloxicam administration. *Vet. Dermatol.* **2007**, *18*, 45–49. [CrossRef] [PubMed]

22. Liu, F.; Li, M.J.; Zeng, L.F.; Zong, Y.; Leng, X.; Shi, K.; Diao, C.N.; Li, D.; Li, Y.B.; Zhao, Q.; Du, R. Prevalence and risk factors of brucellosis, chlamydiosis, and bluetongue among Sika deer in Jilin Province in China. *Vector Borne Zoonotic Dis.* **2018**, *18*, 226–230. [CrossRef] [PubMed]

23. Godfroid, J.; Cloeckaert, A.; Liautard, P.J.; Kohler, S.; Fretin, D.; Walravens, K.; Garin-Bastuji, B.; Letesson, J.J. From the discovery of the Malta fever's agent to the discovery of a marine mammal reservoir, brucellosis has continuously been a re-emerging zoonosis. *Vet. Res.* **2005**, *36*, 313–326. [CrossRef] [PubMed]

24. Ferrero, M.C.; Hielpos, S.M.; Carvalho, B.N.; Barrionuevo, P.; Corsetti, P.P.; Giambartolomei, H.G.; Oliveira, C.S.; Baldi, C.P. Key role of toll-like receptor 2 in the inflammatory response and major histocompatibility complex class ii downregulation in *Brucella abortus*-infected alveolar macrophages. *Infect. Immun.* **2014**, *82*, 626–639. [CrossRef] [PubMed]

25. Tadesse, G. Brucellosis seropositivity in animals and humans in Ethiopia: A meta-analysis. *PLoS Negl. Trop. Dis.* **2016**, *10*, e0005006. [CrossRef] [PubMed]

26. Poester, F.P.; Samartino, L.E.; Santos, R.L. Pathogenesis and pathobiology of brucellosis in livestock. *Rev. Sci. Tech.* **2013**, *32*, 105–115. [CrossRef] [PubMed]

27. Bouza, E.; Sanchez-Carrillo, C.; Hernangomez, S.; Gonzalez, J.M. Laboratory-acquired brucellosis: A Spanish national survey. *J. Hosp. Infect.* **2005**, *61*, 80–83. [CrossRef] [PubMed]

28. Kose, S.; Serin Senger, S.; Akkoclu, G.; Kuzucu, L.; Ulu, Y.; Ersan, G.; Oguz, F. Clinical manifestations, complications, and treatment of brucellosis: Evaluation of 72 cases. *Turk. J. Med. Sci.* **2014**, *44*, 220–223. [CrossRef] [PubMed]

29. Giannacopoulos, I.; Eliopoulou, M.I.; Ziambaras, T.; Papanastasiou, D.A. Transplacentally transmitted congenital brucellosis due to *Brucella abortus. J. Infect.* **2002**, *45*, 209–210. [CrossRef] [PubMed]

30. Kotton, C.N. Zoonoses in solid-organ and hematopoietic stem cell transplant recipients. *Clin. Infect. Dis.* **2007**, *44*, 857–866. [CrossRef] [PubMed]

31. Tuon, F.F.; Gondolfo, R.B.; Cerchiari, N. Human-to-human transmission of *Brucella*—A systematic review. *Trop. Med. Int. Health* **2017**, *22*, 539–546. [CrossRef] [PubMed]

32. Rossetti, C.A.; Arenas-Gamboa, A.M.; Maurizio, E. Caprine brucellosis: A historically neglected disease with significant impact on public health. *PLoS Negl. Trop. Dis.* **2017**, *11*, e0005692. [CrossRef] [PubMed]

33. Colmenero, J.D.; Reguera, M.J.; Martos, F.; Sanchez-De-Mora, D.; Delgado, M.; Causse, M.; Martin-Farfan, A.; Juarez, C. Complications associated with *Brucella melitensis* infection: A study of 530 cases. *Medicine* **1996**, *75*, 195–211. [CrossRef] [PubMed]

34. Aggad, H.; Boukraa, L. Prevalence of bovine and human brucellosis in western Algeria: Comparison of screening tests. *East Mediterr. Health J.* **2006**, *12*, 119–128. [PubMed]

35. Jennings, G.J.; Hajjeh, A.R.; Girgis, Y.F.; Fadeel, A.M.; Maksoud, A.M.; Wasfy, O.M.; El-Sayed, N.; Srikantiah, P.; Luby, P.S.; Earhart, K.; et al. Brucellosis as a cause of acute febrile illness in Egypt. *Trans. R. Soc. Trop. Med. Hyg.* **2007**, *101*, 707–713. [CrossRef] [PubMed]

36. Musallam, I.I.; Abo-Shehada, N.M.; Hegazy, M.Y.; Holt, R.H.; Guitian, J.F. Systematic review of brucellosis in the Middle East: Disease frequency in ruminants and humans and risk factors for human infection. *Epidemiol. Infect.* **2016**, *144*, 671–685. [CrossRef] [PubMed]

37. Garofolo, G.; Fasanella, A.; Di Giannatale, E.; Platone, I.; Sacchini, L.; Persiani, T.; Boskani, T.; Rizzardi, K.; Wahab, T. Cases of human brucellosis in Sweden linked to Middle East and Africa. *BMC Res. Notes* **2016**, *9*, 277. [CrossRef] [PubMed]

38. McDermott, J.; Grace, D.; Zinsstag, J. Economics of brucellosis impact and control in low-income countries. *Rev. Sci. Tech.* **2013**, *32*, 249–261. [CrossRef] [PubMed]

39. Moreno, E. Brucellosis in Central America. *Vet. Microbiol.* **2002**, *90*, 31–38. [CrossRef]
40. Hanot Mambres, D.; Boarbi, S.; Michel, P.; Bouker, N.; Escobar-Calle, L.; Desqueper, D.; Fancello, T.; Van Esbroeck, M.; Godfroid, J.; Fretin, D. Imported human brucellosis in Belgium: Bio- and molecular typing of bacterial isolates, 1996–2015. *PLoS ONE* **2017**, *12*, e0174756. [CrossRef] [PubMed]
41. Georgi, E.; Walter, C.M.; Pfalzgraf, T.M.; Northoff, H.B.; Holdt, M.L.; Scholz, C.H.; Zoeller, L.; Zange, S.; Antwerpen, H.M. Whole genome sequencing of *Brucella melitensis* isolated from 57 patients in Germany reveals high diversity in strains from Middle East. *PLoS ONE* **2017**, *12*, e0175425. [CrossRef] [PubMed]
42. Norman, F.F.; Monge-Maillo, B.; Chamorro-Tojeiro, S.; Perez-Molina, A.J.; Lopez-Velez, R. Imported brucellosis: A case series and literature review. *Travel Med. Infect. Dis.* **2016**, *14*, 182–199. [CrossRef] [PubMed]
43. Neha, A.K.; Kumar, A.; Ahmed, I. Comparative efficacy of serological diagnostic methods and evaluation of polymerase chain reaction for diagnosis of bovine brucellosis. *Iran. J. Vet. Res.* **2017**, *18*, 279–281. [PubMed]
44. Tiwari, S.; Kumar, A.; Thavaselvam, D.; Mangalgi, S.; Rathod, V.; Prakash, A.; Barua, A.; Arora, S.; Sathyaseelan, K. Development and comparative evaluation of a plate enzyme-linked immunosorbent assay based on recombinant outer membrane antigens Omp28 and Omp31 for diagnosis of human brucellosis. *Clin. Vaccine Immunol.* **2013**, *20*, 1217–1222. [CrossRef] [PubMed]
45. Chen, Q.; Lai, S.; Yin, W.; Zhou, H.; Li, Y.; Mu, D.; Li, Z.; Yu, H.; Yang, W. Epidemic characteristics, high-risk townships and space-time clusters of human brucellosis in Shanxi Province of China, 2005–2014. *BMC Infect. Dis.* **2016**, *16*, 760. [CrossRef] [PubMed]
46. Hartady, T.; Saad, Z.M.; Bejo, K.S.; Salisi, S.M. Clinical human brucellosis in Malaysia: A case report. *Asian Pac. J. Trop. Dis.* **2014**, *4*, 150–153. [CrossRef]
47. Tay, B.Y.; Ahmad, N.; Hashim, R.; Mohamed Zahidi, A.J.; Thong, L.K.; Koh, P.X.; Mohd Noor, A. Multiple-locus variable-number tandem-repeat analysis (MLVA) genotyping of human *Brucella* isolates in Malaysia. *BMC Infect. Dis.* **2015**, *15*, 220. [CrossRef] [PubMed]
48. Garba, B.; Bahaman, R.A.; Khairani-Bejo, S.; Zakaria, Z.; Mutalib, R.A. Retrospective study of leptospirosis in Malaysia. *Ecohealth* **2017**, *14*, 389–398. [CrossRef] [PubMed]
49. Yacoub, A.A.; Bakr, S.; Hameed, M.A.; Al-Thamery, A.A.; Fartoci, J.M. Seroepidemiology of selected zoonotic infections in Basra region of Iraq. *East Mediterr. Health J.* **2006**, *12*, 112–118. [PubMed]
50. Al Dahouk, S.; Neubauer, H.; Hensel, A.; Schoneberg, I.; Nockler, K.; Alpers, K.; Merzenich, H.; Stark, K.; Jansen, A. Changing epidemiology of human brucellosis, Germany, 1962–2005. *Emerg. Infect. Dis.* **2007**, *13*, 1895–1900. [CrossRef] [PubMed]
51. Doyle, T.J.; Bryan, R.T. Infectious disease morbidity in the US region bordering Mexico, 1990–1998. *J. Infect. Dis.* **2000**, *182*, 1503–1510. [CrossRef] [PubMed]
52. Leiser, O.P.; Corn, L.J.; Schmit, S.B.; Keim, S.P.; Foster, T.J. Feral swine brucellosis in the United States and prospective genomic techniques for disease epidemiology. *Vet. Microbiol.* **2013**, *166*, 1–10. [CrossRef] [PubMed]
53. Boschiroli, M.L.; Foulongne, V.; O'Callaghan, D. Brucellosis: A worldwide zoonosis. *Curr. Opin. Microbiol.* **2001**, *4*, 58–64. [CrossRef]
54. Mantur, B.G.; Biradar, S.M.; Bidri, C.R.; Mulimani, S.M.; Veerappa, P.; Kariholu, P.; Patil, B.S.; Mangalgi, S.S. Protean clinical manifestations and diagnostic challenges of human brucellosis in adults: 16 years' experience in an endemic area. *J. Med. Microbiol.* **2006**, *55*, 897–903. [CrossRef] [PubMed]
55. Makita, K.; Fevre, M.E.; Waiswa, C.; Kaboyo, W.; De Clare Bronsvoort, M.B.; Eisler, C.M.; Welburn, C.S. Human brucellosis in urban and peri-urban areas of Kampala, Uganda. *Ann. N. Y. Acad. Sci.* **2008**, *1149*, 309–311. [CrossRef] [PubMed]
56. Fallatah, S.M.; Oduloju, J.S.; Al-Dusari, N.S.; Fakunle, M.Y. Human brucellosis in *Northern* Saudi Arabia. *Saudi Med. J.* **2005**, *26*, 1562–1566. [PubMed]
57. Alp, E.; Doganay, M. Current therapeutic strategy in spinal brucellosis. *Int. J. Infect. Dis.* **2008**, *12*, 573–577. [CrossRef] [PubMed]
58. Celebi, G.; Külah, C.; Kiliç, S.; Üstündağ, G. Asymptomatic *Brucella* bacteraemia and isolation of *Brucella melitensis* biovar 3 from human breast milk. *Scand. J. Infect. Dis.* **2007**, *39*, 205–208. [CrossRef] [PubMed]
59. Arif, S.; Thomson, C.P.; Hernandez-Jover, M.; McGill, M.D.; Warriach, M.H.; Heller, J. Knowledge, attitudes and practices (KAP) relating to brucellosis in smallholder dairy farmers in two provinces in Pakistan. *PLoS ONE* **2017**, *12*, e0173365. [CrossRef] [PubMed]

60. Currò, V.; Marineo, S.; Vicari, D.; Galuppo, L.; Galluzzo, P.; Nifosì, D.; Pugliese, M.; Migliazzo, A.; Torina, A.; Caracappa, S. The isolation of *Brucella* spp. from sheep and goat farms in Sicily. *Small Rumin. Res.* **2012**, *106*, S2–S5.

61. Buzgan, T.; Karahocagil, K.M.; Irmak, H.; Baran, I.A.; Karsen, H.; Evirgen, O.; Akdeniz, H. Clinical manifestations and complications in 1028 cases of brucellosis: A retrospective evaluation and review of the literature. *Int. J. Infect. Dis.* **2010**, *14*, e469–e478. [CrossRef] [PubMed]

62. Al Dahouk, S.; Tomaso, H.; Nockler, K.; Neubauer, H.; Frangoulidis, D. Laboratory-based diagnosis of brucellosis—A review of the literature. Part II: Serological tests for brucellosis. *Clin. Lab.* **2003**, *49*, 577–589. [PubMed]

63. Mili, N.; Auckenthaler, R.; Nicod, L.P. Chronic brucella empyema. *Chest* **1993**, *103*, 620–621. [CrossRef] [PubMed]

64. Sharda, D.C.; Lubani, M. A study of brucellosis in childhood. *Clin. Pediatr.* **1986**, *25*, 492–495. [CrossRef] [PubMed]

65. Franco, M.P.; Mulder, M.; Gilman, H.R.; Smits, L.H. Human brucellosis. *Lancet Infect. Dis.* **2007**, *7*, 775–786. [CrossRef]

66. Guven, T.; Ugurlu, K.; Ergonul, O.; Celikbas, K.A.; Gok, E.S.; Comoglu, S.; Baykam, N.; Dokuzoguz, B. Neurobrucellosis: Clinical and diagnostic features. *Clin. Infect. Dis.* **2013**, *56*, 1407–1412. [CrossRef] [PubMed]

67. Gunduz, T.; Tekturk, T.P.; Yapici, Z.; Kurtuncu, M.; Somer, A.; Torun, M.S.; Eraksoy, M. Characteristics of isolated spinal cord involvement in neurobrucellosis with no corresponding MRI activity: A case report and review of the literature. *J. Neurol. Sci.* **2017**, *372*, 305–306. [CrossRef] [PubMed]

68. Dias, S.P.; Sequeira, J.; Almeida, M. Spastic paraparesis and sensorineural hearing loss: Keep brucellosis in mind. *J. Neurol. Sci.* **2018**, *385*, 144–145. [CrossRef] [PubMed]

69. Ducrotoy, M.J.; Muñoz, M.P.; Conde-Álvarez, R.; Blasco, M.J.; Moriyón, I. A systematic review of current immunological tests for the diagnosis of cattle brucellosis. *Prev. Vet. Med.* **2018**, *151*, 57–72. [CrossRef] [PubMed]

70. Al Dahouk, S.; Nockler, K. Implications of laboratory diagnosis on brucellosis therapy. *Expert Rev. Anti Infect. Ther.* **2011**, *9*, 833–845. [CrossRef] [PubMed]

71. Casanova, A.; Ariza, J.; Rubio, M.; Masuet, C.; Diaz, R. BrucellaCapt versus classical tests in the serological diagnosis and management of human brucellosis. *Clin. Vaccine Immunol.* **2009**, *16*, 844–851. [CrossRef] [PubMed]

72. Lucero, N.E.; Escobar, I.G.; Ayala, M.S.; Jacob, N. Diagnosis of human brucellosis caused by *Brucella canis*. *J. Med. Microbiol.* **2005**, *54*, 457–461. [CrossRef] [PubMed]

73. Ruiz-Mesa, J.D.; Sanchez-Gonzalez, J.; Reguera, M.J.; Martin, L.; Lopez-Palmero, S.; Colmenero, D.J. Rose Bengal test: Diagnostic yield and use for the rapid diagnosis of human brucellosis in emergency departments in endemic areas. *Clin. Microbiol. Infect.* **2005**, *11*, 221–225. [CrossRef] [PubMed]

74. Harding-Esch, E.M.; Holland, J.M.; Schemann, F.J.; Molina, S.; Sarr, I.; Andreasen, A.A.; Roberts, C.; Sillah, A.; Sarr, B.; Harding, F.E.; et al. Diagnostic accuracy of a prototype point-of-care test for ocular *Chlamydia trachomatis* under field conditions in The Gambia and Senegal. *PLoS Negl. Trop. Dis.* **2011**, *5*, e1234. [CrossRef] [PubMed]

75. Zeytinoglu, A.; Turhan, A.; Altuglu, I.; Bilgic, A.; Abdoel, H.T.; Smits, L.M. Comparison of *Brucella* immunoglobulin M and G flow assays with serum agglutination and 2-mercaptoethanol tests in the diagnosis of brucellosis. *Clin. Chem. Lab. Med.* **2006**, *44*, 180–184. [CrossRef] [PubMed]

76. Roushan, M.R.H.; Amiri, S.J.S.; Laly, A.; Mostafazadeh, A.; Bijani, A. Follow-up standard agglutination and 2-mercaptoethanol tests in 175 clinically cured cases of human brucellosis. *Int. J. Infect. Dis.* **2010**, *14*, e250–e253. [CrossRef] [PubMed]

77. Hanci, H.; Igan, H.; Uyanik, M.H. Evaluation of a new and rapid serologic test for detecting brucellosis: *Brucella* Coombs gel test. *Pak. J. Biol. Sci.* **2017**, *20*, 108–112. [CrossRef] [PubMed]

78. Memish, Z.A.; Balkhy, H.H. Brucellosis and international travel. *J. Travel Med.* **2004**, *11*, 49–55. [CrossRef] [PubMed]

79. Bastos, C.R.; Mathias, A.L.; Jusi, G.M.M.; Santos, D.F.R.; Silva, D.P.C.G.; André, R.M.; Machado, Z.R.; Bürger, P.K. Evaluation of dot-blot test for serological diagnosis of bovine brucellosis. *Braz. J. Microbiol.* **2018**. [CrossRef] [PubMed]

80. Arif, S.; Heller, J.; Hernandez-Jover, M.; McGill, M.D.; Thomson, C.P. Evaluation of three serological tests for diagnosis of bovine brucellosis in smallholder farms in Pakistan by estimating sensitivity and specificity using Bayesian latent class analysis. *Prev. Vet. Med.* **2018**, *149*, 21–28. [CrossRef] [PubMed]

81. Mohseni, K.; Mirnejad, R.; Piranfar, V.; Mirkalantari, S. A comparative evaluation of ELISA, PCR, and serum agglutination tests for diagnosis of *Brucella* using human serum. *Iran J. Pathol.* **2017**, *12*, 371–376. [PubMed]

82. Bricker, B.J. PCR as a diagnostic tool for brucellosis. *Vet. Microbiol.* **2002**, *90*, 435–446. [CrossRef]

83. Ferreira, A.C.; Cardoso, R.; Travassos Dias, I.; Mariano, I.; Belo, A.; Rolao Preto, I.; Manteigas, A.; Pina Fonseca, A.; Correa De Sa, I.M. Evaluation of a modified Rose Bengal test and an indirect enzyme-linked immunosorbent assay for the diagnosis of *Brucella melitensis* infection in sheep. *Vet. Res.* **2003**, *34*, 297–305. [CrossRef] [PubMed]

84. Queipo-Ortuno, M.I.; Colmenero, D.J.; Bermudez, P.; Bravo, J.M.; Morata, P. Rapid differential diagnosis between extrapulmonary tuberculosis and focal complications of brucellosis using a multiplex real-time PCR assay. *PLoS ONE* **2009**, *4*, e4526. [CrossRef]

85. Zerva, L.; Bourantas, K.; Mitka, S.; Kansouzidou, A.; Legakis, J.N. Serum is the preferred clinical specimen for diagnosis of human brucellosis by PCR. *J. Clin. Microbiol.* **2001**, *39*, 1661–1664. [CrossRef] [PubMed]

86. Wang, Y.; Wang, Z.; Zhang, Y.; Bai, L.; Zhao, Y.; Liu, C.; Ma, A.; Yu, H. Polymerase chain reaction-based assays for the diagnosis of human brucellosis. *Ann. Clin. Microbiol. Antimicrob.* **2014**, *13*, 31. [CrossRef] [PubMed]

87. Queipo-Ortuno, M.I.; De Dios Colmenero, J.; Macias, M.; Bravo, J.M.; Morata, P. Preparation of bacterial DNA template by boiling and effect of immunoglobulin G as an inhibitor in real-time PCR for serum samples from patients with brucellosis. *Clin. Vaccine Immunol.* **2008**, *15*, 293–296. [CrossRef] [PubMed]

88. Al Dahouk, S.; Nockler, K.; Scholz, C.H.; Pfeffer, M.; Neubauer, H.; Tomaso, H. Evaluation of genus-specific and species-specific real-time PCR assays for the identification of *Brucella* spp. *Clin. Chem. Lab. Med.* **2007**, *45*, 1464–1470. [CrossRef] [PubMed]

89. Vrioni, G.; Pappas, G.; Priavali, E.; Gartzonika, C.; Levidiotou, S. An eternal microbe: *Brucella* DNA load persists for years after clinical cure. *Clin. Infect. Dis.* **2008**, *46*, e131–e136. [CrossRef] [PubMed]

90. Bounaadja, L.; Albert, D.; Chenais, B.; Henault, S.; Zygmunt, S.M.; Poliak, S.; Garin-Bastuji, B. Real-time PCR for identification of *Brucella* spp.: A comparative study of IS711, bcsp31 and per target genes. *Vet. Microbiol.* **2009**, *137*, 156–164. [CrossRef] [PubMed]

91. Hamdy, M.E.; Amin, A.S. Detection of *Brucella* species in the milk of infected cattle, sheep, goats and camels by PCR. *Vet. J.* **2002**, *163*, 299–305. [CrossRef] [PubMed]

92. Navarro, E.; Casao, M.A.; Solera, J. Diagnosis of human brucellosis using PCR. *Expert Rev Mol. Diagn.* **2004**, *4*, 115–123. [CrossRef] [PubMed]

93. Romero, C.; Lopez-Goni, I. Improved method for purification of bacterial DNA from bovine milk for detection of *Brucella* spp. by PCR. *Appl. Environ. Microbiol.* **1999**, *65*, 3735–3737. [PubMed]

94. Gee, J.E.; De, K.B.; Levett, N.P.; Whitney, M.A.; Novak, T.R.; Popovic, T. Use of 16S rRNA gene sequencing for rapid confirmatory identification of *Brucella* isolates. *J. Clin. Microbiol.* **2004**, *42*, 3649–3654. [CrossRef] [PubMed]

95. Lopez-Goni, I.; Garcia-Yoldi, D.; Marin, M.C.; de Miguel, J.M.; Barquero-Calvo, E.; Guzman-Verri, C.; Albert, D.; Garin-Bastuji, B. New Bruce-ladder multiplex PCR assay for the biovar typing of *Brucella suis* and the discrimination of *Brucella suis* and *Brucella canis*. *Vet. Microbiol.* **2011**, *154*, 152–155. [CrossRef] [PubMed]

96. Jiang, H.; Fan, M.; Chen, J.; Mi, J.; Yu, R.; Zhao, H.; Piao, D.; Ke, C.; Deng, X.; Tian, G.; et al. MLVA genotyping of Chinese human *Brucella melitensis* biovar 1, 2 and 3 isolates. *BMC Microbiol.* **2011**, *11*, 256. [CrossRef] [PubMed]

97. Navarro, E.; Segura, C.J.; Castano, J.M.; Solera, J. Use of real-time quantitative polymerase chain reaction to monitor the evolution of *Brucella melitensis* DNA load during therapy and post-therapy follow-up in patients with brucellosis. *Clin. Infect. Dis.* **2006**, *42*, 1266–1273. [CrossRef] [PubMed]

98. Castano, M.J.; Solera, J. Chronic brucellosis and persistence of *Brucella melitensis* DNA. *J. Clin. Microbiol.* **2009**, *47*, 2084–2089. [CrossRef] [PubMed]

99. Fosgate, G.T.; Adesiyun, A.A.; Hird, W.D.; Johnson, O.W.; Hietala, K.S.; Schurig, G.G.; Ryan, J. Comparison of serologic tests for detection of *Brucella* infections in cattle and water buffalo (*Bubalus bubalis*). *Am. J. Vet. Res.* **2002**, *63*, 1598–1605. [CrossRef] [PubMed]

100. Falagas, M.E.; Bliziotis, I.A. Quinolones for treatment of human brucellosis: Critical review of the evidence from microbiological and clinical studies. *Antimicrob. Agents Chemother.* **2006**, *50*, 22–33. [CrossRef] [PubMed]

101. Moon, M.S. Tuberculosis of spine: Current views in diagnosis and management. *Asian Spine J.* **2014**, *8*, 97–111. [CrossRef] [PubMed]

102. Saltoglu, N.; Tasova, Y.; Inal, S.A.; Seki, T.; Aksu, S.H. Efficacy of rifampicin plus doxycycline versus rifampicin plus quinolone in the treatment of brucellosis. *Saudi Med. J.* **2002**, *23*, 921–924. [PubMed]

103. Geyik, M.F.; Gur, A.; Nas, K.; Cevik, R.; Sarac, J.; Dikici, B.; Ayaz, C. Musculoskeletal involvement of brucellosis in different age groups: A study of 195 cases. *Swiss Med. Wkly.* **2002**, *132*, 98–105. [PubMed]

104. Yousefi-Nooraie, R.; Mortaz-Hejri, S.; Mehrani, M.; Sadeghipour, P. Antibiotics for treating human brucellosis. *Cochrane Database Syst. Rev.* **2012**, *10*, Cd007179. [CrossRef] [PubMed]

105. Azimi, G.; Hakakian, A.; Ghanadian, M.; Joumaa, A.; Alamian, S. Bioassay-directed isolation of quaternary benzylisoquinolines from *Berberis integerrima* with bactericidal activity against *Brucella abortus*. *Res. Pharm. Sci.* **2018**, *13*, 149–158. [PubMed]

106. Ersoy, Y.; Sonmez, E.; Tevfik, R.M.; But, D.A. Comparison of three different combination therapies in the treatment of human brucellosis. *Trop. Doct.* **2005**, *35*, 210–212. [CrossRef] [PubMed]

107. Karabay, O.; Sencan, I.; Kayas, D.; Sahin, I. Ofloxacin plus rifampicin versus doxycycline plus rifampicin in the treatment of brucellosis: A randomized clinical trial [ISRCTN11871179]. *BMC Infect. Dis.* **2004**, *4*, 18. [CrossRef] [PubMed]

108. Zhang, J.; Chen, Z.; Xie, L.; Zhao, C.; Zhao, H.; Fu, C.; Chen, G.; Hao, Z.; Wang, L.; Li, W. Treatment of a subdural empyema complicated by intracerebral abscess due to *Brucella* infection. *Braz. J. Med. Biol. Res.* **2017**, *50*, e5712. [CrossRef] [PubMed]

109. Solis Garcia del Pozo, J.; Solera, J. Systematic review and meta-analysis of randomized clinical trials in the treatment of human brucellosis. *PLoS ONE* **2012**, *7*, e32090. [CrossRef] [PubMed]

110. Meng, F.; Pan, X.; Tong, W. Rifampicin versus streptomycin for brucellosis treatment in humans: A meta-analysis of randomized controlled trials. *PLoS ONE* **2018**, *13*, e0191993. [CrossRef] [PubMed]

111. Kaya, S.; Elaldi, N.; Deveci, O.; Eskazan, E.A.; Bekcibasi, M.; Hosoglu, S. Cytopenia in adult brucellosis patients. *Indian J. Med. Res.* **2018**, *147*, 73–80. [CrossRef] [PubMed]

112. Yang, H.X.; Feng, J.J.; Zhang, X.Q.; Hao, E.R.; Yao, X.S.; Zhao, R.; Piao, R.D.; Cui, Y.B.; Jiang, H. A case report of spontaneous abortion caused by *Brucella melitensis* biovar 3. *Infect. Dis. Poverty* **2018**, *7*, 31. [CrossRef] [PubMed]

113. Tsevelmaa, N.; Narangerel, B.; Odgerel, O.; Dariimaa, D.; Batkhuu, J. Anti-*Brucella* activity of *Caryopteris mongolica* Bunge root extract against *Brucella melitensis* infection in mice. *BMC Complement. Altern. Med.* **2018**, *18*, 144.

114. Saxena, H.M.; Raj, S. A novel immunotherapy of *Brucellosis* in cows monitored non-invasively through a specific biomarker. *PLoS Negl. Trop. Dis.* **2018**, *12*, e0006393. [CrossRef] [PubMed]

115. Aznar, M.N.; Arregui, M.; Humblet, F.M.; Samartino, E.L.; Saegerman, C. Methodology for the assessment of brucellosis management practices and its vaccination campaign: Example in two Argentine districts. *BMC Vet. Res.* **2017**, *13*, 281. [CrossRef] [PubMed]

116. Dorneles, E.M.; Lima, K.G.; Teixeira-Carvalho, A.; Araujo, S.M.; Martins-Filho, A.O.; Sriranganathan, N.; Al Qublan, H.; Heinemann, B.M.; Lage, P.A. Immune response of calves vaccinated with *Brucella abortus* S19 or RB51 and revaccinated with RB51. *PLoS ONE* **2015**, *10*, e0136696. [CrossRef] [PubMed]

117. Avila-Calderon, E.D.; Lopez-Merino, A.; Sriranganathan, N.; Boyle, M.S.; Contreras-Rodriguez, A. A history of the development of *Brucella* vaccines. *Biomed. Res. Int.* **2013**, *2013*, 743509. [CrossRef] [PubMed]

118. Lalsiamthara, J.; Lee, J.H. Development and trial of vaccines against *Brucella*. *J. Vet. Sci.* **2017**, *18* (Suppl. S1), 281–290. [CrossRef] [PubMed]

119. Frolich, K.; Thiede, S.; Kozikowski, T.; Jakob, W. A review of mutual transmission of important infectious diseases between livestock and wildlife in Europe. *Ann. N. Y. Acad. Sci.* **2002**, *969*, 4–13. [CrossRef] [PubMed]

120. Martins, H.; Garin-Bastuji, B.; Lima, F.; Flor, L.; Pina Fonseca, A.; Boinas, F. Eradication of bovine brucellosis in the Azores, Portugal—Outcome of a 5-year programme (2002–2007) based on test-and-slaughter and RB51 vaccination. *Prev. Vet. Med.* **2009**, *90*, 80–89. [CrossRef] [PubMed]

121. Godfroid, J.; Scholz, C.H.; Barbier, T.; Nicolas, C.; Wattiau, P.; Fretin, D.; Whatmore, M.A.; Cloeckaert, A.; Blasco, M.J.; Moriyon, I.; et al. Brucellosis at the animal/ecosystem/human interface at the beginning of the 21st century. *Prev. Vet. Med.* **2011**, *102*, 118–131. [CrossRef] [PubMed]

122. Miranda, K.L.; Dorneles, M.E.; Pauletti, B.R.; Poester, P.F.; Lage, P.A. *Brucella abortus* S19 and RB51 vaccine immunogenicity test: Evaluation of three mice (BALB/c, Swiss and CD-1) and two challenge strains (544 and 2308). *Vaccine* **2015**, *33*, 507–511. [CrossRef] [PubMed]
123. Singh, R.; Basera, S.S.; Tewari, K.; Yadav, S.; Joshi, S.; Singh, B.; Mukherjee, F. Safety and immunogenicity of *Brucella abortus* strain RB51 vaccine in crossbred cattle calves in India. *Indian J. Exp. Biol.* **2012**, *50*, 239–242. [PubMed]
124. Barbosa, A.A.; Figueiredo, S.C.A.; Palhao, P.M.; Viana, M.H.J.; Fernandes, C.A.C. Safety of vaccination against brucellosis with the rough strain in pregnant cattle. *Trop. Anim. Health Prod.* **2017**, *49*, 1779–1781. [CrossRef] [PubMed]
125. Sanz, C.; Saez, L.; Alvarez, J.; Cortes, M.; Pereira, G.; Reyes, A.; Rubio, F.; Martin, J.; Garcia, N.; Dominguez, L.; et al. Mass vaccination as a complementary tool in the control of a severe outbreak of bovine brucellosis due to *Brucella abortus* in Extremadura, Spain. *Prev. Vet. Med.* **2010**, *97*, 119–125. [CrossRef] [PubMed]
126. Moriyon, I.; Grillo, J.M.; Monreal, D.; Gonzalez, D.; Marin, C.; Lopez-Goni, I.; Mainar-Jaime, C.R.; Moreno, E.; Blasco, M.J. Rough vaccines in animal brucellosis: Structural and genetic basis and present status. *Vet. Res.* **2004**, *35*, 1–38. [CrossRef] [PubMed]
127. Gomez, L.; Alvarez, F.; Betancur, D.; Onate, A. Brucellosis vaccines based on the open reading frames from genomic island 3 of *Brucella abortus*. *Vaccine* **2018**, *36*, 2928–2936. [CrossRef] [PubMed]
128. Yang, X.; Skyberg, A.J.; Cao, L.; Clapp, B.; Thornburg, T.; Pascual, W.D. Progress in *Brucella* vaccine development. *Front. Biol.* **2013**, *8*, 60–77. [CrossRef] [PubMed]
129. Jiang, H.; Dong, H.; Peng, X.; Feng, Y.; Zhu, L.; Niu, K.; Peng, Y.; Fan, H.; Ding, J. Transcriptome analysis of gene expression profiling of infected macrophages between *Brucella suis* 1330 and live attenuated vaccine strain S2 displays mechanistic implication for regulation of virulence. *Microb. Pathog.* **2018**, *119*, 241–247. [CrossRef] [PubMed]
130. Dorneles, E.M.; Sriranganathan, N.; Lage, A.P. Recent advances in *Brucella abortus* vaccines. *Vet. Res.* **2015**, *46*, 76. [CrossRef] [PubMed]
131. Hotez, P.J.; Savioli, L.; Fenwick, A. Neglected tropical diseases of the Middle East and North Africa: Review of their prevalence, distribution, and opportunities for control. *PLoS Negl. Trop. Dis.* **2012**, *6*, e1475. [CrossRef] [PubMed]
132. Li, T.; Tong, Z.; Huang, M.; Tang, L.; Zhang, H.; Chen, C. *Brucella melitensis* M5-90Δbp26 as a potential live vaccine that allows for the distinction between natural infection and immunization. *Can. J. Microbiol.* **2017**, *63*, 719–729. [CrossRef] [PubMed]
133. Roy, S.; McElwain, T.F.; Wan, Y. A network control theory approach to modeling and optimal control of zoonoses: Case study of brucellosis transmission in sub-Saharan Africa. *PLoS Negl. Trop. Dis.* **2011**, *5*, e1259. [CrossRef] [PubMed]
134. Donev, D. Brucellosis control and eradication in the south eastern European countries: Current status and perspective strategies. *Maced. J. Med. Sci.* **2010**, *3*, 220. [CrossRef]
135. Franc, K.A.; Krecek, C.R.; Hasler, N.B.; Arenas-Gamboa, M.A. Brucellosis remains a neglected disease in the developing world: A call for interdisciplinary action. *BMC Public Health* **2018**, *18*, 125. [CrossRef] [PubMed]

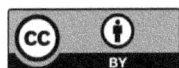

Tropical Medicine and Infectious Disease

MDPI

Case Report

Echinococcus Granulosus Infection in Two Free-Ranging Lumholtz's Tree-Kangaroo (*Dendrolagus lumholtzi*) from the Atherton Tablelands, Queensland

Amy L. Shima [1,*], Constantin C. Constantinoiu [2], Linda K. Johnson [3] and Lee F. Skerratt [1]

[1] One Health Research Group, College of Public Health, Medical and Veterinary Science (CPHMVS), James Cook University, Townsville, Queensland 4811, Australia; lee.skerratt@jcu.edu.au
[2] College of Public Health, Medical and Veterinary Science, James Cook University, Townsville, Queensland 4811, Australia; constantin.constantinoiu@jcu.edu.au
[3] University of Colorado-Denver, Aurora, CO 80045, USA; linda.k.johnson@ucdenver.edu
[*] Correspondence: dvm.shima@gmail.com; Tel.: +4-99-180-961

Received: 19 April 2018; Accepted: 1 May 2018; Published: 3 May 2018

Abstract: Infection with the larval stage of the cestode, *Echinococcus granulosus* sensu lato (s.l.), causes hydatid disease (hydatidosis) in a range of hosts, including macropods and other marsupials, cattle, and humans. Wild macropods are an important sylvatic reservoir for the life cycle of *E. granulosus* (s.l.) in Australia, and so provide a conduit for transmission of hydatid disease to domestic animals and humans. Two Lumholtz's tree-kangaroos (*Dendrolagus lumholtzi*) from the Atherton Tablelands of Far North Queensland were recently found to have hydatid cysts in both liver and lung tissues. Tree-kangaroos may travel across the ground between patches of forest but are primarily arboreal leaf-eating macropods. The finding of hydatid cysts in an arboreal folivore may indicate that the area has a high level of contamination with eggs of *E. granulosus* (s.l.). This finding may be of significance to human health as well as indicating the need for further investigation into the prevalence of hydatid disease in domestic stock, wildlife and humans living in this rapidly urbanizing region.

Keywords: echinococcus; hydatid disease; tree-kangaroo; zoonosis; public health

1. Introduction

Human echinococcosis is estimated to affect 2–3 million people worldwide with 84 to 89 new cases reported per year in Australia, yet it is a 'neglected' disease [1–4]. Human echinococcosis is caused by the cestodes *E. granulosus* (s.l.) (hydatid disease), *E. multiocularis* (alveolar hydatid disease), or *E. vogeli* and *E. oligarthus* (polycystic echinococcosis). *E. granulosus* (s.l.) is found throughout the world and canids are the definitive host. Hydatid cysts may develop in the lungs, liver, brain, or other internal organs of intermediate hosts such as humans, cattle, macropods, and other marsupials. Hydatidosis in Australia has been recognized since the 1860s. Transmission of *E. granulosus* (s.l.) in Australia has been facilitated by the presence of definitive hosts (dingoes and dogs) and naïve susceptible intermediate hosts such as macropods. Environmental conditions in eastern Australia, particularly in coastal areas and along the Great Dividing Range, with >25 mm/month rainfall for 6 months of the year, are favorable for transmission of the parasite [4].

The role of macropods as a sylvatic reservoir of the parasite has been well documented [5–7]. Jenkins [7] noted that hydatid cysts most commonly occur in the lungs of kangaroo and wallaby hosts with cysts in the liver occasionally seen in the eastern grey kangaroo, *Macropus giganteus*. Localization of cysts in pulmonary tissues of macropods such as rock wallabies likely compromises lung function and reduces fright and flight responses, making them susceptible to predation [8,9]. Banks [6] found that *E. granulosus* eggs in faeces deposited by dingoes tend to be concentrated on the verges of dense scrub where wallabies congregate, rather than in open woodland or savannah, and therefore increase the likelihood of transmission among hosts.

In this report, we describe hydatidosis in Lumholtz's tree-kangaroos for the first time. Tree-kangaroos are an iconic representative of biodiversity in the Wet Tropics World Heritage Area of Australia and their predominantly arboreal existence makes infection with a parasite present on the ground unusual. Lumholtz's tree-kangaroo is one of Australia's largest arboreal marsupials [10], coming to ground primarily to move between patches of rainforest trees or while dispersing from the maternal home range (see Supplemental Figure S1). Due to fragmentation of habitat on the Atherton Tablelands, tree-kangaroos commonly travel between patches of forest and, as such may come into contact with dingo or wild dog faeces deposited at the interface between remnant forest and grasslands. As the eggs of *E. granulosus* can survive for many months in the environment and will be dispersed over large areas by wind, rain, and insects, animals will be exposed to infective eggs as they travel across the ground [3,11]. Lumholtz's tree-kangaroo were among the 29 native prey species identified by Vernes and Dennis [12] consumed by dingoes on the Atherton Tablelands. Hence, participation in the life cycle of *E. granulosus* by Lumholtz's tree-kangaroos and dingoes is possible.

Injured and dead Lumholtz's tree-kangaroo were collected from various locations on the Atherton Tablelands as part of a mortality study conducted between August 2012 and December 2017. These were collected through a concerted campaign utilizing the local wildlife care network, media, and social media. The public was requested to notify the senior author (ALS) by telephone of injured or dead tree-kangaroos. Upon being notified of a dead or injured tree-kangaroo, the senior author visited the site, confirmed host species identity, recorded site coordinates, and performed a post-mortem examination on the carcass to determine the cause of death. Tissue samples were collected for histopathology. Presence of *E. granulosus* was confirmed by histological identification of protoscolices in the 'hydatid sand' collected from cysts and brood capsules. Molecular diagnostics would have been useful to confirm the identity of the strain of *Echinococcus* but were not carried out due to a lack of resources.

2. Cases

2.1. Case #1: 4.6 Kg Female Lumholtz's Tree-Kangaroo (Case 16-532)

A 4.6 kg female Lumholtz's tree-kangaroo was killed by a dog on a cattle property on the Atherton Tablelands, QLD. The dog responsible for killing this tree-kangaroo was on a regular program of deworming, which included praziquantel. The tree-kangaroo carcass was intact and had not been fed upon. Based on lack of enlarged teats, active ovarian tissue and dentition, the tree-kangaroo was estimated to be a nulliparous female approximately 3 years old.

On post-mortem examination, extensive bite wounds were found over the tail, head, and caudal abdomen. On opening the abdomen, large cystic structures were found occupying approximately a quarter of the liver mass (Figure 1).

Examination of the thoracic cavity revealed multiple cystic structures occupying approximately half of the total lung volume (Figure 2).

Multiple active (and fertile) *E. granulosus* hydatid cysts and cysts in various stages of degeneration were found on histopathology. Histopathologic examination of lungs revealed a well-formed, thickly encapsulated granuloma, the center of which contained a thick laminated hyaline membrane, surrounded by a thin rim of neutrophils, macrophages, and lymphocytes, consistent with a hydatid cyst. The liver showed a section of cyst wall containing numerous (up to ten) protoscolices within brood capsules (Figure 3).

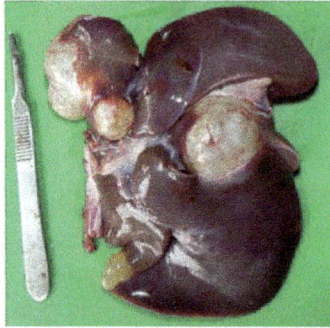

Figure 1. Liver with hydatid cysts. Photo: A. Shima.

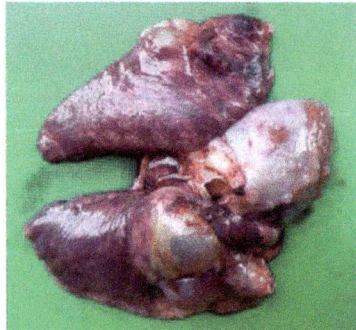

Figure 2. Lungs with hydatid cysts and heart. Photo: A. Shima.

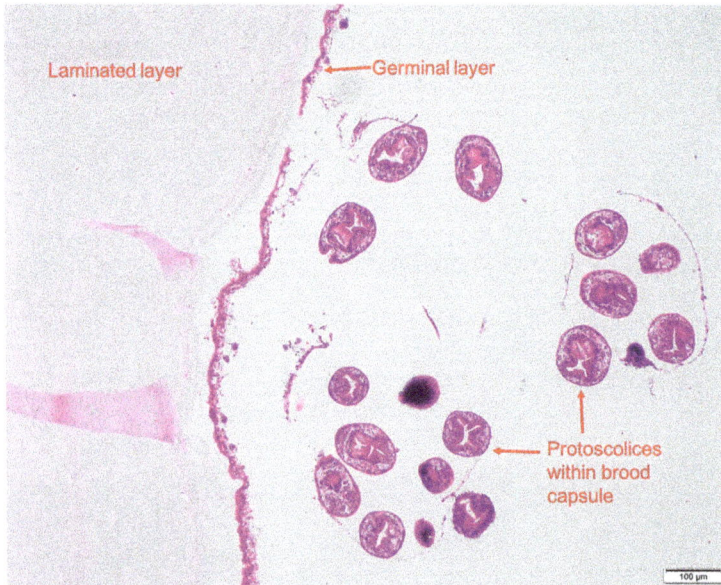

Figure 3. Protoscolices within cyst. Photo: C. Constantinoiu.

2.2. Case #2

The second case of *E. granulosus* in a Lumholtz's tree-kangaroo was an 8.5 kg adult male. Based on weight, pelage coloration and dental wear, the animal was estimated to be greater than six years old. The animal had been found in an emaciated, obtundate state on the side of a road. Clinical assessment showed 3–5% dehydration (based on skin turgor); a phthisical left globe with irregular surface to the cornea and an opaque right eye with what appeared to be a mature cataract. There was an area of moist, erosive dermatitis extending from the right inguinal region along the caudomedial aspect of the right rear limb with a 30 × 60 mm granulomatous lesion at the cranial aspect of the limb. A presumption of vehicular trauma was made, and the animal was euthanized due to age, condition, and poor prognosis.

On gross post-mortem examination, multiple hydatid cysts were found in the liver and lungs. Some had degenerate cysts which lacked a germinal membrane, others had viable protoscolices. The cyst membranes were unusually thick. They were surrounded by a fibroblastic response with giant cells, indicating chronic inflammation. Calcarous bodies were noted in the laminated layers and the germinal layers were thick (Figure 4). The lungs showed evidence of bacterial pneumonia as well as an eosinophilic response to the cysts. Multiple presumptive sarcocysts, previously reported in Lumholtz's tree-kangaroo by Speare [13], were seen in the tongue (Figure 5).

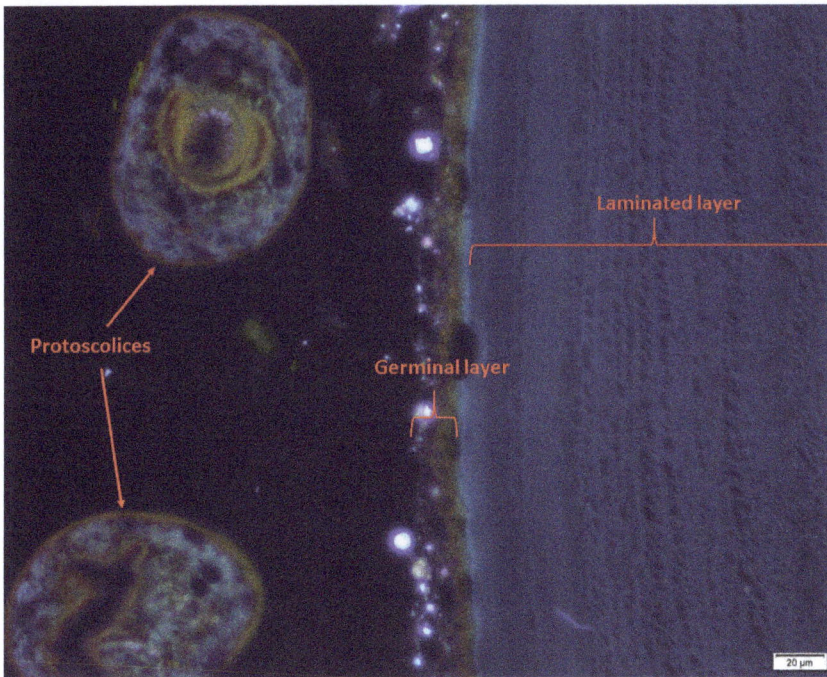

Figure 4. Showing protoscolices, germinal layer and laminated layer' photo credit: C. Constantinouiu.

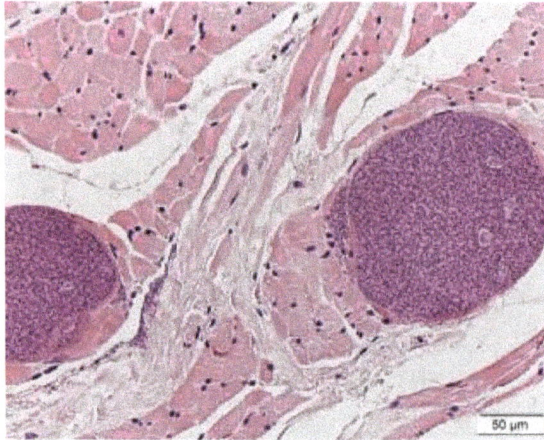

Figure 5. Section of tongue containing presumptive sarcocysts. Photo: L. Johnson.

3. Discussion and Results

Historically, *E. granulosus* (s.l.) was considered a serious and potentially fatal health threat in Australia [14]. Significant control measures were instituted, particularly in Tasmania, where the disease was subsequently eradicated. *E. granulosus* (s.l.) G1 is the only strain of echinococcus identified in Australia [15]. PCR on the samples from these two cases would have been useful to determine the strain of *E. granulosus* (s.l.); however, due to resource constraints, this was not done. The inability to eliminate the disease on the mainland has been due to the presence of a wildlife reservoir, lack of political interest and funding for disease eradication, and lack of requirements for reporting the disease in livestock and humans [16]. Hydatid disease has been demonstrated to cause depression in growth rates of some species of livestock [17]. Infection with hydatid cysts in cattle represents a significant economic loss to the beef industry in Queensland north of the Tropic of Capricorn [17]. There is no surveillance program in abattoirs for monitoring hydatidosis in livestock. Since 2008, human echinococcosis has been a non-notifiable disease in Queensland [18], yet hydatidosis is still a potentially-significant human health risk in Australia, with approximately 80–100 human cases diagnosed each year [4,19]. In humans, cystic echinococcosis can have a long period of asymptomatic incubation before the cysts grow large enough to cause one or more of the following: a fracture, abdominal pain, hepatomegaly or, if the cysts burst, anaphylaxis [20,21].

The Atherton Tablelands is an agricultural area of increasing human population, growing from 26,320 in 1976 to 44,350 in 2007, with considerable interface between forest and scrub, pasture for mainly cattle, farmland and residential areas [22,23]. Finding tree-kangaroos, a species that does not spend much of its time on the ground, infected with hydatid cysts may indicate that the abundance of dogs (either dingoes, feral or domestic dogs) infected with *E. granulosus* (s.l.) on the Atherton Tablelands is relatively high and increasing and therefore, an under-estimated zoonotic risk. There is considerable beef and dairy production as well as a growing human population, especially in semi-rural town areas in the region. *E. granulosus* may have relatively high transmission rates on the Atherton Tablelands as eggs would remain viable in the environment for a year under favorable conditions (shady, cool, damp) [4]. *E. granulosus* eggs in canid faeces are immediately infective to humans and coprophagous flies can be an important conduit for spreading infection by feeding on dingo/wild dog faeces and then moving onto human food [11,16]. Encroachment of dingoes into urban areas as well as the increasing use of domestic dogs for pig-hunting may be increasing the risk of transmission of *E. granulosus* to humans in urban and rural residential regions [6,16,24,25].

This study reports detection of *E. granulosus* cysts through post-mortem examination of Lumholtz's tree-kangaroos as part of a wildlife health surveillance PhD project. Macropods, including tree-kangaroos, are commonly identified by wildlife carers as having 'pneumonia'; they may actually have compromised lung function due to hydatid cysts or other infectious diseases (e.g., toxoplasmosis) [26–28]. Macropods entering the wildlife care network may not be examined by a veterinarian and few receive post-mortem examination, so quantifying the disease in sylvatic hosts is extremely difficult especially as attempts to develop serologic tests to diagnose hydatidosis in live animals have been unsuccessful [5,29]. Nevertheless, a one health surveillance program tailored to the Atherton Tablelands for hydatid disease via post-mortem examinations of wildlife, surveying for *Echinococcus* coproantigens in dog faeces and surveillance of livers and lungs of cattle at abattoirs may be useful in determining the prevalence and risk of transmission of *E. granulosus* (s.l.) in the region. This would enable practical measures to be undertaken to reduce the risk of human infection and the incidence of the disease in wildlife and domestic stock.

Supplementary Materials: The following are available online at http://www.mdpi.com/2414-6366/3/2/47/s1, Figure S1: Male Lumholtz's tree-kangaroo. Photo by J. Hopkinson.

Author Contributions: A.L.S. drafted the case report. L.F.S. supervised the report and, along with L.K.J. and C.C.C. reviewed and made substantive revisions. L.K.J. and C.C.C. evaluated and commented on the histopathology. All authors have read and approved of the final manuscript.

Acknowledgments: In memory of Rick Speare; the first person to identify hydatid cysts in a Lumholtz's tree-kangaroo but who never managed to get around to publishing his finding. This was not through lack of effort but rather due to a kaleidoscope of competing interests. With thanks to Ian Beveridge; Dave Spratt; Ms Karen Reeks; and Allan Kessel. Financial support was provided from the Holsworth Wildlife Research Endowment, Skyrail Rainforest Foundation, Wet Tropics Management Authority, M.A. Ingram Trust, and an Australian Postgraduate Award.

Conflicts of Interest: The authors declare they have no conflicts of interest to report.

References

1. Atkinson, J.A.M.; Gray, D.J.; Clements, A.C.A.; Barnes, T.S.; McManus, D.P.; Yang, Y.R. Environmental changes impacting *Echinococcus* transmission: Research to support predictive surveillance and control. *Glob. Chang. Biol.* **2013**, *19*, 677–688. [CrossRef] [PubMed]

2. Bristow, B.N.; Lee, S.; Shafir, S.; Sorvillo, F. Human echinococcosis mortality in the United States, 1990-2007. *PLoS Negl. Trop. Dis.* **2012**, *6*, e1524. [CrossRef] [PubMed]

3. Torgerson, P.R.; Macpherson, C.N.L. The socioeconomic burden of parasitic zoonoses: Global trends. *Vet. Parasitol.* **2011**, *182*, 79–95. [CrossRef] [PubMed]

4. Jenkins, D.J.; Macpherson, C.N.L. Transmission ecology of *Echinococcus* in wildlife in Australia and Africa. *Parasitology* **2003**, *127*, S63–S72. [CrossRef] [PubMed]

5. Barnes, T.S.; Deplazes, P.; Gottstein, B.; Jenkins, D.J.; Mathis, A.; Siles-Lucas, M.; Torgerson, P.R.; Ziadinov, I.; Heath, D.D. Challenges for diagnosis and control of cystic hydatid disease. *Acta Trop.* **2012**, *123*, 1–7. [CrossRef] [PubMed]

6. Banks, D.J.D.; Copeman, D.B.; Skerratt, L.F. *Echinococcus granulosus* in northern Queensland: 2. Ecological determinants of infection in beef cattle. *Aust. Vet. J.* **2006**, *84*, 308–311. [CrossRef] [PubMed]

7. Jenkins, D.J.; Morris, B. *Echinococcus granulosus* in wildlife in and around the Kosciuszko National Park, south-eastern Australia. *Aust. Vet. J.* **2003**, *81*, 81–85. [CrossRef] [PubMed]

8. Barnes, T.S.; Hinds, L.A.; Jenkins, D.J.; Bielefeldt-Ohmann, H.; Lightowlers, M.W.; Coleman, G.T. Comparative pathology of pulmonary hydatid cysts in macropods and sheep. *J. Comp. Pathol.* **2011**, *144*, 113–122. [CrossRef] [PubMed]

9. Barnes, T.S.; Goldizen, A.W.; Morton, J.M.; Coleman, G.T. Cystic echinococcosis in a wild population of the brush-tailed rock-wallaby (*Petrogale penicillata*), a threatened macropodid. *Parasitology* **2008**, *135*, 715–723. [CrossRef] [PubMed]

10. Newell, G.R. Australia's tree-kangaroos: Current issues in their conservation. *Biol. Conserv.* **1999**, *87*, 1–12. [CrossRef]

11. Lawson, J.R.; Gemmell, M.A. Transmission of taeniid tapeworm eggs via blowflies to intermediate hosts. *Parasitology* **1990**, *100*, 143–146. [CrossRef] [PubMed]

12. Vernes, K.; Dennis, A.; Winter, J. Mammalian diet and broad hunting strategy of the dingo (*Canis familiaris dingo*) in the wet tropical rain forests of northeastern Australia. *Biotropica* **2001**, *33*, 339–345. [CrossRef]

13. Speare, R.; Donovan, J.A.; Thomas, A.D.; Speare, P.J. Diseases of free-ranging Macropodoidea. In *Kangaroos, Wallabies and Rat-Kangaroos*; Grigg, G., Jarman, P., Hume, I., Eds.; Surrey Beatty & Sons Pty Limited: Norton, Australia, 1989; Volume 2, pp. 705–734.

14. Gemmell, M.A. Australasian contributions to an understanding of the epidemiology and control of hydatid disease caused by *Echinococcus granulosus*—Past, present and future. *Int. J. Parasitol.* **1990**, *20*, 431–456. [CrossRef]

15. Eckert, J.; World Health Organization. *WHO/OIE Manual on Echinococcosis in Humans and Animals: A Public Health Problem of Global Concern*; World Organisation for Animal Health (Office International des Epizooties): Paris, France, 2001.

16. Jenkins, D.J.; Allen, L.; Goullet, M. Encroachment of *Echinococcus granulosus* into urban areas in eastern Queensland, Australia. *Aust. Vet. J.* **2008**, *86*, 294–300. [CrossRef] [PubMed]

17. Banks, D.J.D.; Copeman, D.B.; Skerratt, L.F.; Molina, E.C. *Echinococcus granulosus* in northern Queensland: 1. Prevalence in cattle. *Aust. Vet. J.* **2006**, *84*, 303–307. [CrossRef] [PubMed]

18. Queensland Government. Health Conditions: Category: Infections and Parasites: Hydatid Disease. Available online: http://conditions.health.qld.gov.au/HealthCondition/condition/14/165/81/Hydatid-Disease (accessed on 30 April 2018).

19. Carmena, D.; Cardona, G.A. Echinococcosis in wild carnivorous species: Epidemiology, genotypic diversity, and implications for veterinary public health. *Vet. Parasitol.* **2014**, *202*, 69–94. [CrossRef] [PubMed]

20. Mandal, S.; Deb Mandal, M. Human cystic echinococcosis: Epidemiologic, zoonotic, clinical, diagnostic and therapeutic aspects. *Asian Pac. J. Trop. Med.* **2012**, *5*, 253–260. [CrossRef]

21. WHO. WHO *Echinococcus* Fact Sheet. Available online: http://www.who.int/mediacentre/factsheets/fs377/en/ (accessed on 3 April 2018).

22. QGPIFU. Far North Queensland Region: A Demographic Profile. Available online: http://www.dilgp.qld.gov.au/resources/plan/far-north-queensland/background/demographic-report-final.pdf (accessed on 3 April 2018).

23. QGSD. Far North Queensland Region. Available online: http://www.statedevelopment.qld.gov.au/resources/factsheet/regional/far-north-queensland-region-fact-sheet.pdf (accessed on 3 April 2018).

24. Jenkins, D.J.; McKinlay, A.; Duolong, H.E.; Bradshaw, H.; Craig, P.S. Detection of *Echinococcus granulosus* coproantigens in faeces from naturally infected rural domestic dogs in south eastern Australia. *Aust. Vet. J.* **2006**, *84*, 12–16. [CrossRef] [PubMed]

25. Jenkins, D.J.; Lievaart, J.J.; Boufana, B.; Lett, W.S.; Bradshaw, H.; Armua-Fernandez, M.T. *Echinococcus granulosus* and other intestinal helminths: Current status of prevalence and management in rural dogs of eastern Australia. *Aust. Vet. J.* **2014**, *92*, 292–298. [CrossRef] [PubMed]

26. Jackson, S.M.E.C. *Australian Mammals: Biology and Captive Management*; CSIRO Publishing: Melbourne, Australia, 2003.

27. Staker, L. *The Complete Guide to the Care of Macropods*; Lynda A. Staker: Armidale, Australia, 2006.

28. Vogelnest, L.; Woods, R. *Medicine of Australian Mammals*; CSIRO Publishing: Melbourne, Australia, 2008.

29. Barnes, T.S.; Li, J.; Coleman, G.T.; McManus, D.P. Development and evaluation of immunoblot-based serodiagnostic tests for hydatid infection in macropodids. *J. Wildl. Dis.* **2008**, *44*, 1036–1040. [CrossRef] [PubMed]

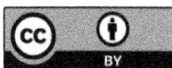

Tropical Medicine and Infectious Disease

MDPI

Article

Scabies in Resource-Poor Communities in Nasarawa State, Nigeria: Epidemiology, Clinical Features and Factors Associated with Infestation

Uade Samuel Ugbomoiko [1,*], Samuel Adeola Oyedeji [1], Olarewaju Abdulkareem Babamale [1] and Jorg Heukelbach [2,3]

[1]   Parasitology Unit, Department of Zoology, University of Ilorin, PMB 1515 Ilorin, Nigeria;
      oyedejisamed@gmail.com (S.A.O.); olas4nice2004@yahoo.co.uk (O.A.B.)
[2]   Department of Community Health, School of Medicine, Federal University of Ceará,
      Fortaleza CE 60430-140, Brazil; heukelbach@web.de
[3]   College of Public Health, Medical and Veterinary Sciences, Division of Tropical Health and Medicine,
      James Cook University, Townsville 4811, Australia
*   Correspondence: samugbomoiko@yahoo.com; Tel.: +234-8033585881

Received: 24 April 2018; Accepted: 29 May 2018; Published: 4 June 2018

Abstract: Epidemiology and clinical features of scabies remain largely unknown in Nigeria's rural communities. To fill this gap, we performed a cross-sectional study in three rural communities in north central Nigeria. A total of 500 individuals were included and examined for scabies infestation; a questionnaire was applied to collect socio-demographic and behavioral data. Scabies was diagnosed in 325 (65.0%) participants. Excoriations (68.6%), vesicles (61.8%), and papules (58.8%) were common skin lesions. Itching was the most common symptom (77.5%); 64% complained of sleep disturbances. Lymphadenopathy was identified in 48.3%. Lesions were most commonly encountered on the abdomen (35.5%), inguinal area (19.1%), and interdigital spaces (14.2%). Poverty-related variables, such as illiteracy (OR: 7.15; 95% CI: 3.71–13.95), low household income (7.25; 1.19–88.59), absence of a solid floor inside house (12.17; 2.83–52.34), and overcrowding (1.98; 1.08–2.81) were significantly associated with infestation. Individual behavior, such as sharing of beds/pillows (2.11; 1.42–3.14) and sharing of clothes (2.51; 1.57–3.99), was also highly significantly associated with scabies. Regular bathing habits (0.37; 0.24–0.56) and regular use of bathing soap (0.36; 0.21–0.53) were protective factors. Scabies is extremely common in the communities under study and is associated with considerable morbidity. The disease is intrinsically linked with extreme poverty.

Keywords: scabies; epidemiology; parasitic skin disease; cross-sectional study; Nigeria

---

1. Introduction

Scabies is a common contagious parasitic skin disease and a public health problem, mainly in tropical and subtropical countries [1,2]. Hundreds of millions of people suffer from infestation in impoverished urban and rural communities worldwide [3–6]. Outbreaks of scabies in closed groups have been reported particularly from high income countries, but the disease is more common in resource-poor communities in low and middle income countries in tropical climate zones [7–9]. High prevalence and re-infestations in endemic settings are correlated with armed conflicts, homelessness, crowding, and communal use of clothes, beds, and pillows [10,11]. Between 18% and 70% of people are reported to be affected in resource-limited communities in India, on south Pacific islands, and in Australian Aboriginal communities [1,8,12], with severe morbidity being common, such as abscess formation, lymphadenopathy, and post-streptococcal glomerulonephritis [8,13–15]. Control and prevention strategies by chemotherapy require considerable public health services and home resources, since treatment is often cumbersome and stressful [2,16].

The prevalence of scabies disease remains largely unknown in Nigeria, in the face of many other health problems considered of more severe morbidity [17–19]. Only a limited number of hospital-based studies have described scabies and other skin diseases [20–24]. However, the upsurge in communal clashes and terrorist insurgence have increased the number of refugees and infectious diseases in all cardinal zones of the country, which poses vulnerable communities at higher risk for scabies infestation. To provide information on the epidemiology of scabies in Nigeria, a cross-sectional community-based study of scabies infestation was conducted in impoverished rural communities in north central Nigeria.

2. Materials and Methods

2.1. Study Area

The study was conducted in three indigenous communities in the Lafia Local Government Area (LGA) of Nasarawa State (north central Nigeria). State health workers had communicated endemicity of scabies from these communities. The areas (latitude 8°32′ N; longitude 8°18′ E) are largely settlements with an estimated population of 3300 inhabitants (National Population Commission, 2007). The climate condition in the state is tropical with a mean daily temperature of 40 °C and relative humidity of 90% during the dry season (November–April).

In the area there have been several violent communal disturbances, with consequently many families being displaced and living under inappropriate housing conditions. Most houses are built with clay or palm products, and there is no electricity, nor a structured community waste disposal system. The inhabitants are predominantly Muslims. The people are largely illiterate subsistence farmers of food crops and cattle herders, with 84% of the households on a monthly per capital income of <N18,000 (equivalent to US$50 at the time of study), the national minimum wage. Human and animal waste is littered around compounds and is widely dispersed during heavy rains. Rivers and streams serve as the major source of water supply. Roads are caliche-topped. Public schools and health centers in the areas are deplorable and poorly staffed. School-aged children (locally called 'Almagiri') are compelled to solicit for food and finance for their daily existence.

2.2. Study Design

For the purpose of this study, the three communities under study were considered as one study area. Prior to the study, a complete household census conducted in the study area identified 390 households (about 3300 individuals), which were listed and subsequently numbered. Using the Epi Info Software package (version 6.04d), we estimated that a population of 344 individuals was sufficient for the prevalence study with 80% power and 95% confidence level. Considering a safety margin (due to expected high non-participation) and a cluster effect (household sampling), a total of 209 households comprising 1050 individuals were selected using a random number generator (Epi Info version 6.04d, Centers for Disease Control and Prevention, Atlanta, GA, USA).

The study was conducted during the dry season (data collection November 2016–April 2017). All members in the selected households were eligible for the study except for individuals who declined participation and those who had not spent at least five days per week in the previous two months in the study area. Those who consented were registered and interviewed to obtain information on their biodata (name, sex, age, and educational background), socioeconomic information, and environmental and behavioral variables, using pre-tested structured questionnaires.

Thereafter, the entire skin surface including the genital areas of each participant was carefully examined clinically for scabies infestation. Children aged <10 years were examined in the presence of their parents or caregivers. In the absence of any household members, the houses were revisited three times.

2.3. Case Definition and Skin Examination

Within the realm of this study, scabies was defined on the basis of a symptomatic description proposed and used by our group previously [9,10,13]—namely, presence of at least two of the following requirements: 1. one or more typical lesions for longer than 2 weeks; 2. pruritus that intensified at night; 3. at least one more family member with similar lesions. Typical skin lesions included papules, vesicular rash, and nodules.

For description of topographical distribution of lesions and parts of the affected skin surfaces, the entire body surface was vertically divided into left and right sides. Each side was subdivided into interdigital spaces, hand, wrist, arm, elbow, axilla, leg, foot, abdomen, thorax, mamilla/perimammillar area, back, buttock, genital/inguinal area, and head (scalp/neck/face) [6]. Primary lesions were distinguished as macular, papules, crusted papules (if a tiny hemorrhage crusts), vesicles, and nodules [3,6,8,25]. Excoriations on skin and bacterial superinfection were noted when pustules, abscess, or suppuration were observed. Lymph nodes were palpated to confirm lymphadenopathy while the intensity of itching was assessed semi-quantitatively and graded as absent, light, moderate, and heavy, using visual ordinal scales. To guarantee privacy of participants, all individuals were examined in a well-lighted room provided in the households. Examinations were performed by one male investigator (SAO) extensively trained in diagnosis of scabies, and assisted by a female senior nursing officer of the Dermatology unit of Nasarawa Central Hospital.

2.4. Statistical Analysis

Data were double-entered into a database and crosschecked for entry errors, using SPSS version 16.0 for Windows (SPSS Inc., Chicago, IL, USA). Chi-squared statistics was applied to determine the significance of differences of relative frequencies between groups. Age groups were defined as follows: ≤10 years, 11–15 years, 16–20 years, ≥21 years. Bivariate analysis and multivariate logistic regression models were applied to identify independently associated variables measured on the prevalence of scabies in the communities. Variables were checked for collinearity before inclusion in the multivariate model.

2.5. Ethical Considerations

The study protocol for this study was approval by the Ethical Review Committee of the University of Ilorin, Nigeria and the Primary Health Care Unit of the Lafia Local Government Area of Nasarawa State. Prior to the study, informed consent was obtained from adult participants and from the parents or legal guardians of minors after detailed explanation of the study protocol. In accordance with the ethical review committee requirements, patient information was made confidential.

3. Results

3.1. Characteristics of Study Population

The target population consisted of 1050 individuals (546 males and 504 females) belonging to 144 households. Seventy-eight individuals failed inclusion criteria, and 38 moved to neighbouring communities during the study. Of the remaining 934 individuals, the data records of 65 were incomplete (interview data or clinical examination). A total of 369 females declined participation for religious and cultural reasons.

Consequently, the study population consisted of 500 individuals, comprising more males ($n = 429$) than females ($n = 71$). The age of individuals ranged from 1 to 34 years (median = 14 years), and the household size ranged from 2 to 14 persons (median = 6).

The characteristics of the study population are presented in Table 1. The study population was primarily illiterate, with an illiteracy rate of almost 90%. Males and age group >21 years were disproportionately highly represented in the study population.

Table 1. Characteristics of study population (*n* = 500).

Variable	N (%)
Sex	
Male	429 (85.8)
Female	71 (14.2)
Age group (years)	
≤10	104 (20.8)
11–15	232 (46.4)
16–20	117 (23.4)
≥21	47 (9.4)
Community	
Lafia Municipal	175 (35.0)
Lafia East	160 (32.0)
Lafia North	165 (33.0)
Education	
Illiterate	440 (88.0)
Primary	48 (9.6)
Post primary	12 (2.4)
Presence of scabies-typical lesions	
Yes	325 (65.0)
No	175 (35.0)
Type of lesions	
Papules	191 (58.8)
Crusted papules	105 (32.3)
Vesicles	201 (61.8)
Macules	160 (49.2)
Pustules	132 (40.6)
Excoriations	223 (68.6)

3.2. Scabies Prevalence and Clinical Features

A total of 325 (65.0%) participants were diagnosed with scabies. Excoriations, vesicles, and papules were the most common skin lesions (Table 1). There were no cases of crusted scabies. The prevalence of scabies stratified by socio-demographic and cultural factors is presented in Table 2. Age groups <15 years showed highest prevalences (accounting for 76.3% of all infected cases), and infestation was significantly more common in females (74.6%) than in males (60.6%).

Signs and symptoms associated with scabies are presented in Table 3. Itching was the most common symptom (77.5%), with 56% presenting severe itching; 52% complained of itching-related sleep disturbance. Lymphadenopathy was identified in about half of the infected cases, commonly in the inguinal and cervical regions.

The topographic distribution of lesions is shown in Table 3. Lesions were most commonly encountered on the abdomen (35.4%), inguinal area (19.1%), and interdigital spaces (14.5%).

3.3. Factors Associated with Infestation

Table 2 presents the bivariate analysis of factors associated with scabies infestation. Prevalence in <16-year-olds was significantly higher than in older age groups. Poverty-related variables such as illiteracy, low household income, inadequate housing, unemployment, and overcrowding were significantly associated with scabies. Sharing of beds/pillows and sharing of clothes were also highly significantly associated with infestation. Regular bathing habits and regular use of bathing soap were protective factors. In multivariate logistic regression analysis, poverty-related variables remained independent factors significantly associated with infestation (Table 4).

Table 2. Prevalence of scabies and bivariate analysis of socio-demographic and behavioral factors associated with infestation.

Variable	n	% (95% CI)	OR (95% CI)	p Value
Age group				
≤10	63/104	60.6 (50.5–69.9)	2.16 (1.00–4.56)	0.013
11–15	185/232	79.7 (73.9–84.6)	2.90 (1.34–3.19)	0.016
16–20	58/117	49.6 (40.3–59.0)	1.97 (0.17–2.28)	0.585
≥21	19/47	40.4 (26.7–55.7)	Ref.	
Sex				
Male	272/429	63.4 (58.6–67.9)	0.52 (0.04–0.72)	0.015
Female	53/71	74.6 (62.7–83.9)	Ref.	
Illiteracy				
Yes	310/440	70.5 (65.9–74.6)	7.15 (3.71–13.95)	<0.001
No	15/60	25.0 (15.1–38.1)	Ref.	
Occupation				
Unemployed	304/445	68.3 (63.7–72.6)	3.83 (1.65–8.89)	<0.001
Farming	12/30	40.0 (23.2–59.2)	1.19 (0.40–3.55)	0.764
Wage earner	9/25	36.0 (18.7–57.4)	Ref.	
Monthly income (NGN)				
≤18,000	312/424	73.6 (69.1–77.7)	7.25 (1.19–88.59)	0.011
>18,000	13/76	17.1 (9.7–27.8)	Ref.	
No. of persons/room/bed				
<4	90/179	50.3 (42.8–57.8)	Ref.	
>4	235/321	73.2 (67.9–79.9)	1.98 (1.08–2.81)	0.004
House structure				
Bricks	100/168	59.5 (51.7–66.9)	Ref.	
Adobe	215/321	66.9 (61.5–72.0)	1.15 (0.18–1.28)	0.071
Palm product	10/11	90.9 (57.1–99.5)	2.20 (1.26–2.61)	0.031
Type of floor				
Sandy	29/31	93.5 (79.2–98.9)	12.17 (2.83–52.34)	0.001
Clay	184/263	70.0 (63.9–75.4)	1.96 (1.34–2.86)	0.001
Cemented	112/283	39.6 (33.9–45.6)	Ref.	
Shared beds and pillows				
Yes	247/352	70.2 (65.0–74.8)	2.11 (1.42–3.14)	<0.001
No	78/148	52.7 (44.4–60.9)	Ref.	
Sharing of clothes				
Yes	105/135	77.8 (69.7–84.3)	2.51 (1.57–3.99)	<0.001
No	220/367	59.9 (54.7–64.9)	Ref.	
Bathing habits				
Regular	193/333	58.0 (52.4–63.3)	0.37 (0.24–0.56)	<0.001
Irregular	132/167	79.0 (72.3–84.5)	Ref.	
Use of bathing soap				
Regular	204/350	58.3 52.9–63.5)	0.36 (0.21–0.53)	<0.001
Irregular	121/150	80.7 (73.2–86.5)	Ref.	

Table 3. Clinical features and topographical location of scabies infestation (*n* = 325).

Variable	N (%)
Itching	252 (77.5)
Light	45 (17.9)
Moderate	65 (25.8)
Severe	142 (56.3)
Sleeping disturbance	208 (64.0)
Due to itching	109 (52.4)
Due to pain	32 (15.4)
Others	67 (32.2)
Lymphadenopathy	157 (48.3)
Cervical	35 (22.3)
Axillar	22 (14.0)
Inguinal	100 (64.1)
Infected skin	222 (68.3)
Suppuration	119 (36.6)
No complaints	67 (20.6)
Topographical location of lesions	
Abdomen	115 (35.4)
Inguinal/thigh	62 (19.1)
Wrist	41 (12.6)
Interdigital	46 (14.5)
Legs	23 (7.1)
Elbow	9 (2.8)
Buttock	27 (8.3)
Arms	12 (3.7)
Hands	45 (13.8)
Feet	2 (0.6)
Thorax	1 (0.3)

Table 4. Multivariate analysis of factors independently associated with scabies.

Variable	Adjusted Odd Ratio	95% CI	*p* Value
Household income <1 minimum wage	3.23	1.94–3.85	0.026
Sharing of bed and pillow	3.03	2.53–3.21	0.015
Female sex	2.72	1.56–3.52	0.062
Poor housing conditions (no brick house)	2.61	1.94–3.06	<0.001
Unemployment	2.23	1.15–2.59	0.001
Sharing of clothes	2.11	1.88–2.53	0.041
Illiteracy	1.67	1.01–1.93	0.002
Irregular bathing with soap	1.96	0.97–2.13	0.011
Age ≥15 years	0.92	0.42–1.05	0.062

4. Discussion

Our study represents the first systematic community-based study on scabies conducted in Nigeria, revealing an extremely high prevalence and morbidity of scabies. The disease was associated with poverty-related variables even within the communities under study, which can be characterized as extremely resource-poor, with precarious living conditions. The high prevalence recorded in the present study indicates the under-recognition of the disease in resource-poor communities, and difficult access to the health system. The prevalence of 65% is comparable to studies in specific and high-risk populations worldwide. For example, prevalences were similar or even higher in a Bangladeshi Islamic religious school (61%) [26], displacement camps in Sierra Leone 67%) [27], Thailand orphanages (87%) [28], a Korean leprosarium (87%) [29], and in a rural village in Papua New Guinea (80%) [30].

Other studies from Nigeria reported lower prevalences of 5% to 57% [20–22]. Other African countries (Cameroon—18% [31], Malawi—36% [32]), as well as Cambodia (4.3%) [33], Brazil (9–10%) [9,10,34], and Fiji (24%) [2] also reported lower prevalences, as compared to our study.

The endemicity of scabies and the associated burden have been attributed to a wide range of intervening factors previously, including socio-economic factors, overcrowding, and behavioral and environmental variables [1,10,13,35]. Consistent with these reports, our findings confirmed poor housing conditions and behavior such as sharing of beddings and pillows—which may serve as fomites—as important risk factors. Overcrowding in the study area was worsened by internal migration of refugees from neighboring communities due to recent communal clashes and terrorist insurgencies. In fact, crowding is a known risk factor for scabies, and has been reported previously in several studies from endemic areas in Egypt [36], Sierra Leone [27], Mali [33], Brazil [10], India [26], and Thailand [28]. Similarly, other proxies for poverty such as unemployment, low income, communal use of clothing, and illiteracy were significantly associated. Multivariate analysis indicated the importance of hygiene habits as independent protective factors.

Another major outcome of this study is the uneven distribution of scabies and its morbidity. Our data show that scabies in the female study population was significantly higher, as compared to males. However, considering the high non-participation rate in females, this figure must be taken with care. There was also a considerable variation in prevalence with age. Children of school age were more frequently infested than the older age groups. This is in agreement with other studies from endemic areas [9,37], indicative of the high frequency of interaction and poor hygiene that enhances transmission amongst these highly mobile age groups. In our study area, these age groups are mostly schoolchildren of private Islamic schools that are sent out by school owners to roam around the streets as so-called Almajiri (beggars) and beg for food and money (OAB, personal observation). The observed occurrence of scabies in the middle and older age groups >21 years may be attributed to sustained contact with infested children, especially in the female population.

We also observed that the topographical distribution of the morbidity-associated features of scabies varied in the population. More than 14% of the infested had more than one type of lesion in various topographic sites, commonly on the abdomen, inguinal/thigh, interdigital space, hands, and wrists, confirming previous reports [3,6,9]. In our study area, a climate-determined behavior in which people, particularly male children, expose greater parts of the body and maintain prolonged close physical contact facilitates transmission of scabies mite. This partly explained why lesions commonly occurred on the abdomen, hands, and wrists in this study.

Our data further show that the prevalence of both itching and excoriation in the affected population was high (77.5% and 68.3%, respectively). Scabies-related itching is a host allergic immune response to mite products [38]. Usually, in resource-limited settings, secondary bacterial infection is common due to poor hygiene conditions and overcrowding [39]. Intense itching and scratching result in skin breaks and facilitates secondary bacterial infection among the affected population [9,13,32,37,40]. Lymphadenopathy has also been well correlated to secondarily-infected scabies lesions in individuals [9,34]. In the current study, high proportions of lymphadenopathy and itching were reported in the affected population. Similar conditions are, however, not uncommon with other parasitic skin disease, such as tungiasis and cutaneous larva migrans [17,41]. Severe itching has also been reported to induce sleep disturbances in scabies-affected individuals. Although other diseases may induce sleep disturbance, the observation that sleep was more often disturbed at a time that coincides with the peak activities of the sarcoptic mites indicates the involvement of this mite. Sixty-four percent of the population with scabies reported sleep disturbance. This is comparable to 77% of cases reported previously from Brazilian communities [6].

Scabies is increasingly recognised as a common parasitic skin disease in Nigerian children [20–22], particularly in poor rural communities where important infrastructural facilities including health care services are unavailable or inadequate. With the current socioeconomic and lifestyle patterns of people where living conditions are precarious—e.g., families sharing clothing and bed space—scabies will be continuously endemic, with high prevalences.

The cost of and access to healthcare services is prohibitive and difficult for many individuals at risk living in the study area and elsewhere in Nigeria in similar settings. Thus, traditional medication, which often complicates disease conditions, is an alternative choice of care by many affected people. Alleviating the scourge of potentially preventable and treatable diseases such as scabies is fundamental in public health service. In Nigeria, and indeed many other African countries, identification and treatment of cases appears to be the only management option in the face of paucity of reliable epidemiological data for control programs. The effectiveness of oral ivermectin in the treatment of scabies and other parasitic diseases such as pediculosis, lymphatic filariasis, onchocerciasis, and intestinal helminthiasis has been widely reported from endemic areas in Africa, South America, and Pacific Islands [1,3,8,13,39]. In endemic communities, control programs by oral ivermectin chemotherapy could be integrated into other existing parasite control programs with strong advocacy on health education, training of health personnel, and surveillance.

Our study is subject to several limitations, and internal and external validity of data may have suffered from the extremely difficult field conditions under which this study took place. Given the considerable difference in participation rates between males and females, and under-representation of adults, prevalence data may have suffered from participation bias. Many female non-participants declined due to cultural and religious beliefs. During field work in the community, we sought to discern other reasons for the striking gender-driven non-participation, but could confirm repeatedly during interviews with community members that the major reasons for non-participation in females in fact were of socio-cultural origin, and not related to symptomatic scabies infestation status (SAO, personal communication). Diagnosis of scabies was based on clinical features; microscopic examination of skin scrapings, videodermatoscopy, and bacteriological testing to validate the presence of mite and bacterial infection in lesions, could not be conducted in this extremely difficult field setting. In some cases diagnosis may have been inaccurate; for example, untreated onchodermatitis (due to onchocerciasis) may have been misclassified as scabies. We aimed to reduce possible diagnostic error by systematic training and supervision of field investigators, and by meticulously adapting to the diagnostic approach as proposed by Heukelbach & Feldmeier [13]. Despite the limitations mentioned, we believe that this population-based study from typical impoverished communities in Nigeria may reflect the situation in similar communities throughout the country.

5. Conclusions

Scabies is extremely common in the rural Nigerian communities under study, and associated with considerable morbidity. We have confirmed that even in the least developed and precarious communities, poverty-related variables are important risk factors for infestation and that hygiene habits may still have a protective effect, even in settings with extremely high transmission pressure. Communal clashes and disturbances related to displacement, overcrowding, and unemployment may further increase prevalence and scabies-related morbidity. Given the risk of sequelae related to chronic infestation and bacterial superinfection, an urgent response from the health care sector is mandatory. Intervention measures may be integrated into existing helminth control programs based on oral ivermectin mass treatment.

Author Contributions: U.S.U. and J.H. conceived and designed the experiments; S.A.O. performed data collection; O.A.B., U.S.U. and J.H. analyzed the data and interpreted results; U.S.U. and J.H. wrote the paper. All authors contributed substantially to the work reported.

Acknowledgments: The study was performed without any sources of funding. The authors wish to thank the communities for participation. This paper is dedicated to the memory of Rick Speare. J.H. is a class 1 research fellow at the Brazilian National Council for Scientific Development (CNPq).

Conflicts of Interest: The authors declare no conflict of interest. There were no funding sponsors.

References

1. Hay, R.; Steer, A.; Engelman, D.; Walton, S. Scabies in the developing world—Its prevalence, complications, and management. *Clin. Microbiol. Infect.* **2012**, *18*, 313–323. [CrossRef] [PubMed]
2. Romani, L.; Koroivueta, J.; Steer, A.C.; Kama, M.; Kaldor, J.M.; Wand, H.; Hamid, M.; Whitfeld, M.J. Scabies and impetigo prevalence and risk factors in Fiji: A national survey. *PLoS Negl. Trop. Dis.* **2015**, *9*, e0003452. [CrossRef] [PubMed]
3. Chosidow, O. Scabies. *N. Engl. J. Med.* **2006**, *354*, 1718–1727. [CrossRef] [PubMed]
4. Murray, C.J.; Vos, T.; Lozano, R.; Naghavi, M.; Flaxman, A.D.; Michaud, C.; Ezzati, M.; Shibuya, K.; Salomon, J.A.; Abdalla, S. Disability-adjusted life years (DALYs) for 291 diseases and injuries in 21 regions, 1990–2010: A systematic analysis for the Global Burden of Disease Study 2010. *Lancet* **2012**, *380*, 2197–2223. [CrossRef]
5. Karimkhani, C.; Colombara, D.V.; Drucker, A.M.; Norton, S.A.; Hay, R.; Engelman, D.; Steer, A.; Whitfeld, M.; Naghavi, M.; Dellavalle, R.P. The global burden of scabies: A cross-sectional analysis from the Global Burden of Disease Study 2015. *Lancet Infect. Dis.* **2017**, *17*, 1247–1254. [CrossRef]
6. Jackson, A.; Heukelbach, J.; Júnior, C.; de Barros, E.; Feldmeier, H. Clinical features and associated morbidity of scabies in a rural community in Alagoas, Brazil. *Trop. Med. Int. Health* **2007**, *12*, 493–502. [CrossRef] [PubMed]
7. Andersen, B.; Haugen, H.; Rasch, M.; Haugen, A.H.; Tageson, A. Outbreak of scabies in Norwegian nursing homes and home care patients: Control and prevention. *J. Hosp. Infect.* **2000**, *45*, 160–164. [CrossRef] [PubMed]
8. Heukelbach, J.; Mazigo, H.D.; Ugbomoiko, U.S. Impact of scabies in resource-poor communities. *Curr. Opin. Infect. Dis.* **2013**, *26*, 127–132. [CrossRef] [PubMed]
9. Heukelbach, J.; Wilcke, T.; Winter, B.; Feldmeier, H. Epidemiology and morbidity of scabies and pediculosis capitis in resource-poor communities in Brazil. *Br. J. Dermatol.* **2005**, *153*, 150–156. [CrossRef] [PubMed]
10. Feldmeier, H.; Jackson, A.; Ariza, L.; Calheiros, C.M.L.; de Lima Soares, V.; Oliveira, F.A.; Hengge, U.R.; Heukelbach, J. The epidemiology of scabies in an impoverished community in rural Brazil: Presence and severity of disease are associated with poor living conditions and illiteracy. *J. Am. Acad. Dermatol.* **2009**, *60*, 436–443. [CrossRef] [PubMed]
11. Wang, C.-H.; Lee, S.-C.; Huang, S.-S.; Kao, Y.-C.; See, L.-C.; Yang, S.-H. Risk factors for scabies in Taiwan. *J. Microbiol. Immunol. Infect.* **2012**, *45*, 276–280. [CrossRef] [PubMed]
12. Fuller, L.C. Epidemiology of scabies. *Curr. Opin. Infect. Dis.* **2013**, *26*, 123–126. [CrossRef] [PubMed]
13. Heukelbach, J.; Feldmeier, H. Scabies. *Lancet* **2006**, *367*, 1767–1774. [CrossRef]
14. Engelman, D.; Kiang, K.; Chosidow, O.; McCarthy, J.; Fuller, C.; Lammie, P.; Hay, R.; Steer, A.; on behalf of the members of the International Alliance for the Control of Scabies (IACS). Toward the global control of human scabies: Introducing the International Alliance for the Control of Scabies. *PLoS Negl. Trop. Dis.* **2013**, *7*, e2167. [CrossRef] [PubMed]
15. Hengge, U.R.; Currie, B.J.; Jäger, G.; Lupi, O.; Schwartz, R.A. Scabies: A ubiquitous neglected skin disease. *Lancet Infect. Dis.* **2006**, *6*, 769–779. [CrossRef]
16. Yeoh, D.K.; Anderson, A.; Cleland, G.; Bowen, A.C. Are scabies and impetigo 'normalised'? A cross-sectional comparative study of hospitalised children in northern Australia assessing clinical recognition and treatment of skin infections. *PLoS Negl. Trop. Dis.* **2017**, *11*, e0005726. [CrossRef] [PubMed]
17. Ugbomoiko, U.S.; Ofoezie, I.E.; Heukelbach, J. Tungiasis: High prevalence, parasite load, and morbidity in a rural community in Lagos State, Nigeria. *Int. J. Dermatol.* **2007**, *46*, 475–481. [CrossRef] [PubMed]
18. McLean, F.E. The elimination of scabies: A task for our generation. *Int. J. Dermatol.* **2013**, *52*, 1215–1223. [CrossRef] [PubMed]
19. Feldmeier, H.; Heukelbach, J.; Ugbomoiko, U.S.; Sentongo, E.; Mbabazi, P.; von Samson-Himmelstjerna, G.; Krantz, I. Tungiasis—A neglected disease with many challenges for global public health. *PLoS Negl. Trop. Dis.* **2014**, *8*, e3133. [CrossRef] [PubMed]
20. Nnoruka, E. Skin diseases in south-east Nigeria: A current perspective. *Int. J. Dermatol.* **2005**, *44*, 29–33. [CrossRef] [PubMed]
21. Onayemi, O.; Isezuo, S.A.; Njoku, C.H. Prevalence of different skin conditions in an outpatients' setting in north-western Nigeria. *Int. J. Dermatol.* **2005**, *44*, 7–11. [CrossRef] [PubMed]

22. Yahya, H. Change in pattern of skin disease in Kaduna, north-central Nigeria. *Int. J. Dermatol.* **2007**, *46*, 936–943. [CrossRef] [PubMed]
23. Okafor, O.; Akinbami, F.; Orimadegun, A.; Okafor, C.; Ogunbiyi, A. Prevalence of dermatological lesions in hospitalized children at the University College Hospital, Ibadan, Nigeria. *Niger. J. Clin. Pract.* **2011**, *14*, 287–292. [CrossRef] [PubMed]
24. Ukonu, B.; Eze, E. Pattern of skin diseases at university of Benin teaching hospital, Benin city, Edo State, South-South Nigeria: A 12 month prospective study. *Glob. J. Health Sci.* **2012**, *4*, 148. [CrossRef] [PubMed]
25. McCarthy, J.; Kemp, D.; Walton, S.; Currie, B. Scabies: More than just an irritation. *Postgrad. Med. J.* **2004**, *80*, 382–387. [CrossRef] [PubMed]
26. Oztiirkcan, S.; Ozcelik, S.; Saygi, G.; Ozcelik, S. Spread of scabies and pediculus humanus among the children at Sivas orphanage. *Indian Pediatr.* **1994**, *31*, 210–213.
27. Terry, B.; Kanjah, F.; Sahr, F.; Kortequee, S.; Dukulay, I.; Gbakima, A. *Sarcoptes scabiei* infestation among children in a displacement camp in Sierra Leone. *Public Health* **2001**, *115*, 208–211. [CrossRef]
28. Pruksachatkunakorn, C.; Wongthanee, A.; Kasiwat, V. Scabies in Thai orphanages. *Pediatr. Int.* **2003**, *45*, 719–723. [CrossRef]
29. Park, H.; Lee, C.; Park, S.; Kwon, H.; Kweon, S.-S. Scabies among elderly Korean patients with histories of leprosy. *Am. J. Trop. Med. Hyg.* **2016**, *95*, 75–76. [CrossRef] [PubMed]
30. Bockarie, M.; Alexander, N.; Kazura, J.; Bockarie, F.; Griffin, L.; Alpers, M. Treatment with ivermectin reduces the high prevalence of scabies in a village in Papua New Guinea. *Acta Trop.* **2000**, *75*, 127–130. [CrossRef]
31. Kouotou, E.A.; Nansseu, J.R.N.; Kouawa, M.K.; Bissek, A.-C.Z.-K. Prevalence and drivers of human scabies among children and adolescents living and studying in Cameroonian boarding schools. *Parasites Vectors* **2016**, *9*, 400. [CrossRef] [PubMed]
32. Kristensen, J.K. Scabies and pyoderma in Lilongwe, Malawi. *Int. J. Dermatol.* **1991**, *30*, 699–702. [CrossRef] [PubMed]
33. Landwehr, D.; Keita, S.M.; Pönnighaus, J.M.; Tounkara, C. Epidemiologic aspects of scabies in Mali, Malawi, and Cambodia. *Int. J. Dermatol.* **1998**, *37*, 588–590. [CrossRef] [PubMed]
34. Jackson, A.; Heukelbach, J.; Feldmeier, H. Transmission of scabies in a rural community. *Braz. J. Infect. Dis.* **2007**, *11*, 386–387. [CrossRef] [PubMed]
35. Feldmeier, H.; Heukelbach, J. Epidermal parasitic skin diseases: A neglected category of poverty-associated plagues. *Bull. World Health Organ.* **2009**, *87*, 152–159. [CrossRef] [PubMed]
36. Hegab, D.S.; Kato, A.M.; Kabbash, I.A.; Dabish, G.M. Scabies among primary schoolchildren in Egypt: Sociomedical environmental study in Kafr El-Sheikh administrative area. *Clin. Cosmet. Investig. Dermatol.* **2015**, *8*, 105. [CrossRef] [PubMed]
37. Steer, A.C.; Jenney, A.W.; Kado, J.; Batzloff, M.R.; La Vincente, S.; Waqatakirewa, L.; Mulholland, E.K.; Carapetis, J.R. High burden of impetigo and scabies in a tropical country. *PLoS Negl. Trop. Dis.* **2009**, *3*, e467. [CrossRef] [PubMed]
38. Worth, C.; Heukelbach, J.; Fengler, G.; Walter, B.; Liesenfeld, O.; Hengge, U.; Feldmeier, H. Acute morbidity associated with scabies and other ectoparasitoses rapidly improves after treatment with ivermectin. *Pediatr. Dermatol.* **2012**, *29*, 430–436. [CrossRef] [PubMed]
39. World Health Organization; Department of Child, Adolescent Health, WHO; UNICEF. *Handbook IMCI: Integrated Management of Childhood Illness*; WHO: Geneva, Switzerland, 2005.
40. Feldmeier, H.; Singh Chhatwal, G.; Guerra, H. Pyoderma, group A streptococci and parasitic skin diseases—A dangerous relationship. *Trop. Med. Int. Health* **2005**, *10*, 713–716. [CrossRef] [PubMed]
41. Heukelbach, J.; Wilcke, T.; Meier, A.; Moura, R.C.S.; Feldmeier, H. A longitudinal study on cutaneous larva migrans in an impoverished Brazilian township. *Travel Med. Infect. Dis.* **2003**, *1*, 213–218. [CrossRef] [PubMed]

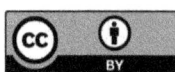

Tropical Medicine and Infectious Disease

MDPI

Article

Cross-Cultural, Aboriginal Language, Discovery Education for Health Literacy and Informed Consent in a Remote Aboriginal Community in the Northern Territory, Australia

Jennifer M. Shield [1,2,*], Thérèse M. Kearns [3], Joanne Garŋgulkpuy [4], Lisa Walpulay [3,4], Roslyn Gundjirryirr [3,4], Leanne Bundhala [3,4,†], Veronica Djarpanbuluwuy [3,4], Ross M. Andrews [3] and Jenni Judd [5,6]

[1] ARDS Aboriginal Corporation, Winnellie, NT 0821, Australia
[2] Department of Pharmacy and Applied Science, La Trobe University, Bendigo, VIC 3552, Australia
[3] Menzies School of Health Research, Charles Darwin University, Darwin, NT 0811, Australia;
     therese.kearns@menzies.edu.au (T.M.K.); walpulay@gmail.com (L.W.);
     roslyn.dhurrkay@menzies.edu.au (R.G.); djarpanbuluwuy@gmail.com (V.D.);
     ross.andrews@menzies.edu.au (R.M.A.)
[4] Yalu' Marŋgithinyaraw, Galiwin'ku, NT 0822, Australia; yaluoffice@gmail.com
[5] School of Health, Medical and Applied Sciences, Central Queensland University, Bundaberg,
     QLD 4670, Australia; j.judd@cqu.edu.au
[6] College of Medicine and Dentistry, Anton Breinl Research Centre for Health Systems Strengthening,
     James Cook University, Townsville, QLD 4811, Australia
*   Correspondence: j.shield@latrobe.edu.au; Tel.: +61-455-138-444
†   The author has passed away.

Received: 10 December 2017; Accepted: 20 January 2018; Published: 29 January 2018

Abstract: Background: Education for health literacy of Australian Aboriginal people living remotely is challenging as their languages and worldviews are quite different from English language and Western worldviews. Becoming health literate depends on receiving comprehensible information in a culturally acceptable manner. Methods: The study objective was to facilitate oral health literacy through community education about scabies and strongyloidiasis, including their transmission and control, preceding an ivermectin mass drug administration (MDA) for these diseases. A discovery education approach where health concepts are connected to cultural knowledge in the local language was used. Aboriginal and non-Aboriginal educators worked collaboratively to produce an in-depth flip-chart of the relevant stories in the local language and to share them with clan elders and 27% of the population. Results: The community health education was well received. Feedback indicated that the stories were being discussed in the community and that the mode of transmission of strongyloidiasis was understood. Two-thirds of the population participated in the MDA. This study documents the principles and practice of a method of making important Western health knowledge comprehensible to Aboriginal people. This method would be applicable wherever language and culture of the people differ from language and culture of health professionals.

Keywords: cross-cultural health education; health education; Aboriginal language; worldview; health literacy; discovery education; informed consent; scabies; strongyloidiasis

1. Introduction

Australian Aboriginal peoples, especially those who live in remote communities, experience a higher burden of disease, more than three times that of the Australian national average [1]. Most lack the knowledge about how to be healthy when living a Western lifestyle [2].

One of the factors contributing to the high burden of disease is limited health literacy [3,4]. People with low health literacy have a higher risk of poorer health outcomes [4,5]. The Australian Commission on Safety and Quality in Health Care [6] defines individual health literacy as 'the skills, knowledge, motivation and capacity of a person to access, understand, appraise and apply information to make effective decisions about health and health care and take appropriate action', and this definition is modified from Sørenson's [7] model of health literacy. This definition fits Nutbeam's concept of 'critical health literacy' [8] and assumes good literacy skills. However, Nutbeam, referring to the work of Freire [9], indicated that outcomes similar to critical health literacy could be achieved by those with low or no skills in reading and writing through interpersonal forms of communication and community-based health education [8]. Similarly, Baker [10] divides health literacy into health-related print literacy and health related oral literacy, the ability to orally communicate about health. In the context of Aboriginal people living remotely, health related oral literacy is achievable.

Both language and culture (including worldview) act as barriers for Aboriginal people in achieving health literacy in the Western cultural context, especially for those living remotely [11]. Worldview, the way people construct meaning and understand the world around them [12], is closely related to language and culture. Aboriginal languages, cultures, and worldviews are very different from the English language and Australian non-Aboriginal culture and worldview [12,13]. Aboriginal worldviews supported them adequately when living a traditional lifestyle. The difficulty arises because the traditional roles of doctor and midwife have been taken over by non-Aboriginal health professionals with a different worldview [14], so people need the necessary cross-cultural understanding to do well when in need of medical assistance [14,15].

Essential general knowledge about germs, blood circulation, immunity, and the cellular composition of the body, foundational for Western understanding about health, is not part of the general knowledge of Aboriginal people living remotely [11,14]. One group of Aboriginal people recognised that the reason that they were unable to understand information in the English language was because of missing information that they called 'the secret English' [13]. 'The secret English' was in fact general knowledge for their English-speaking informants but not for them. Some Aboriginal people even believe that key information about their sickness is deliberately hidden [15]. So when informing people about their health, relevant foundational knowledge, as well as the specific information, is needed for understanding to occur.

An essential ingredient for effective communication and health literacy is the provision of comprehensible information [4,6]. For Aboriginal and Torres Strait people to achieve health literacy, 'it is necessary for information to build on Indigenous understandings and perspectives' [6]. Aboriginal people have cultural knowledge such as the organs of the body and the behaviour and life cycles of food animals and plants that can be used as starting points to connect new health information to what they already know [14].

Aboriginal people can become health literate about a particular topic by engaging in community education when the knowledge is shared in their language, is connected to their cultural knowledge, is directed to the whole community, and is shared in a culturally sensitive manner [11,12,14,16]. For new information to become part of the cultural knowledge of an individual, it is essential that the information is accepted by the cultural group as a whole, so that it can be maintained, updated, and passed on to the next generation. This can be achieved when the majority of adults in the cultural group hear, understand, and discuss the new information [14].

This style of education, first documented in 2000 [14] and later called discovery education [16], is also known as story methodology [17]. It was developed to help Yolŋu Aboriginal people of north-east Arnhem Land understand law, economics, and health. Discovery health education uses a collaboration between non-Aboriginal and Aboriginal health educators to find connections between the health information and existing cultural general knowledge and to develop a cross-cultural story in the local language that is shared with the community.

In this study, community health education was undertaken in a remote community using a discovery education approach that focussed on the diseases scabies (caused by mites, *Sarcoptes scabei*) and strongyloidiasis (caused by roundworms, *Strongyloides stercoralis)* and the effect of treatment. The education was part of the preparation for a research project examining the effect of ivermectin mass drug administration (MDA) on the two diseases [18,19], so that potential participants could give informed consent and learn how to prevent the diseases. The education aimed to facilitate the development of health literacy in these two diseases so that in the future, the participants would be able to connect further information about infectious diseases to the foundational knowledge obtained from this education process.

2. Materials and Methods

2.1. Population

The health education took place in Galiwin'ku, a remote Aboriginal community with a population of approximately 2000, located 550 km east of Darwin, Northern Territory (NT), Australia. This project received ethical approval from the Human Research Ethics Committee of the NT Department of Health and Menzies School of Health Research (EC00153—project 09/34).

2.2. Study Objective and Evaluation

The study objective was to facilitate the development of oral health literacy through community education about the nature of scabies and strongyloidiasis, how these diseases are transmitted, and how to prevent and treat these diseases.

Expected outcomes of the education were:

- an informative cross-cultural flipchart in Djambarrpuyŋu language about scabies and strongyloidiasis, how they are transmitted, and how to prevent and treat these diseases, developed in collaboration with non-Aboriginal and Aboriginal educators;
- non-Aboriginal and Aboriginal educators conducting the education together in a conversational style;
- discussion of the educational stories by the people amongst themselves;
- feedback from community members indicating that aspects of the story are understood;
- a large number of people participating in the ivermectin MDA project.

2.3. Consultation with Clan Elders

Community-based workers facilitated informal discussions with the community elders, who gave their approval for the project.

2.4. Community Health Education Principles

The community health education followed the principles of discovery education (Table 1). Discovery education uses a culturally acceptable process and employs a collaborative approach between non-Aboriginal health educator/s and Aboriginal educator/s. The non-Aboriginal educators provide the information and have some knowledge of the language and culture, and the Aboriginal professionals know some English and have an in-depth knowledge of their language, culture, and worldview. Educational stories are developed by connecting health concepts to cultural knowledge in the local language.

Table 1. Principles of Discovery Education (Modified from Trudgen [14] (pp. 202–210).

Principle	Explanation
The educator/s are credible in the eyes of the people	Traditional Yolŋu knowledge is owned by particular clans and clan elders and only they have the authority to share it. Knowledge of modern diseases is considered by Yolŋu to be 'owned' by non-Aboriginal health professionals because Yolŋu people consider that these diseases are of European origin.
The educator/s follow 'culturally correct' steps for providing the information	The new information is presented first to the clan elders for their approval, and then shared with the whole cultural group, particularly the adults.
The information is provided in the local language	The majority of remote-living people have only a superficial knowledge of English. They can draw on sophisticated concepts in their own language to help them understand relevant health information.
The information is built on culturally accepted knowledge and truths	This involves searching for key terms and stories in the local language, and using ways, such as analogy, of connecting the new knowledge with cultural general knowledge.
The educators use a dialogue style [9]	The educator and learner are learning from each other. This enables the educator to clarify information that is not clear and to provide answers to what the learners want to know.
The information is rigorous and in-depth	Comprehensible information that can survive intellectual debate is accepted. If it is 'simplified' or superficial, it is rejected.

2.5. Development of Educational Materials

A flip-chart, information sheet, and consent form were prepared in Djambarrpuyŋu language, the local *lingua franca*, and in English. These flip-charts contained details about scabies mites, *Strongyloides* worms, and the research project. They incorporated existing educational resources [20–25] as well as components developed especially for the project. The traditional story about cycad food (*Cycas armstrongii*) was used as an analogy for the project. This story belongs to the Wangurri Clan of north-east Arnhem Land, and an elder of this clan 'an owner of the knowledge' recorded the story and gave permission to use it for the project. This story about how to collect cycad nuts, leach out the poison in running water and prepare a safe, delicious, and nutritious food, is well-known to Yolŋu people. This story was compared with eliminating scabies and *Strongyloides* from the community by washing hands, wearing shoes, stopping taps from leaking to keep the ground dry, keeping the house clean, washing clothes and airing bedding in the sun, showering, using the toilet and keeping it clean, giving faecal and/or blood samples for testing for *Strongyloides*, and taking the medicine to eliminate scabies and *Strongyloides* from the body.

The stages in the life cycle of *Strongyloides* were likened to the stages in the human life cycle. The rhabdiform larvae that exit the body via the faeces were called *Strongyloides* djamarrkuli' (*Strongyloides* children). *Strongyloides* infective larvae that can invade the body are all immature females, so were called 'wirrkuḻ*Strongyloides*' or 'wirrkuḻ mewirri' (pre-pubescent female *Strongyloides* or pre-pubescent female worms). The parasitic adults were called 'ŋänḏi *Strongyloides*' (mother *Strongyloides*) because they are all female.

Similarly, the stages of the life cycle of scabies were compared with the human life cycle. The name given to scabies was 'scabies-puy dhirrkthirrk' or scabies itch. Illustrations included scanned drawings by the Aboriginal educators, photographs prepared by the team, and photographs and drawings from pre-existing educational materials in English.

The Djambarrpuyŋu text and illustrations were assembled in a power-point presentation after each flip-chart preparation session and reviewed at the beginning of the next session. When complete, an English version was prepared, and the final formatting of both flip-charts was done by a graphic designer. The final files were printed, laminated and assembled into a flipchart (Figure 1) and are available at the following web addresses: https://www.menzies.edu.au/icms_docs/162089_Mites_and_worms_flipchart_English_version.pdf; https://www.menzies.edu.au/icms_docs/162094_Mites_and_worms_flipchart_Yolngu_version.pdf.

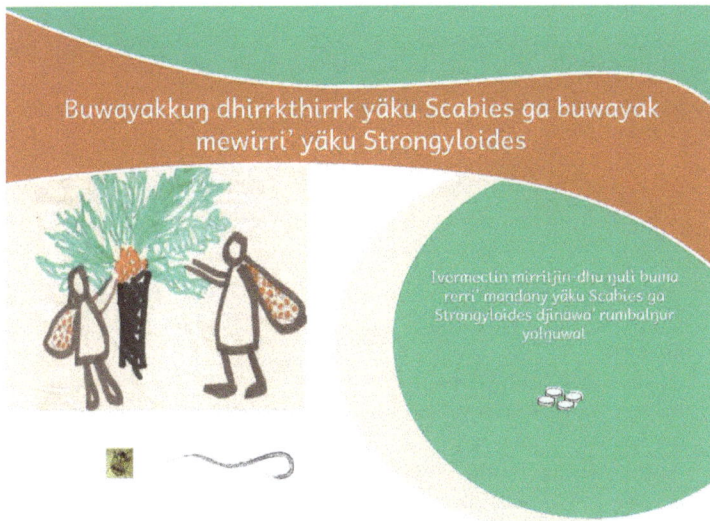

Figure 1. Title page of the flipchart. The title translates as 'Eliminating scabies mites and invisible *Strongyloides* worms'. The subtitle: 'Ivermectin medicine kills both diseases in people's bodies'. The title page includes symbols of the main components of the story: the overall analogy (the cycad story), a scabies mite, an adult female *Strongyloides* worm, and the ivermectin tablets.

2.6. Presentation of the Story to the Elders of the Community

The first educational session took place at an indoor meeting of the *Dhuni Forum*, a group comprising representative elders of each clan. The project was explained to them in English, and details of scabies and strongyloidiasis were explained in Djambarrpuyŋu language.

2.7. Carrying out Scabies and Strongyloidiasis Education

Scabies and *Strongyloides* health education took place over eight weeks in February–March 2010, prior to the commencement of the MDA project. Two community education teams were formed, one male and one female, so that men could talk with men and women with women, an important cultural issue for more traditional Aboriginal communities. Each team included a non-Aboriginal health educator and one or more Aboriginal educators. The teams visited households and work places as people were available, and engaged with either single sex groups, or family groups. Before each education session took place, usually the previous day, Aboriginal staff visited households to find a convenient time for the education. Most often, the education took place out-of-doors, on a veranda or under a tree.

2.8. Supplementary Materials

The flip-chart was supplemented by pictures of microscopes and microscope movie clips of a scabies mite, rhabitiform *Strongyloides* larvae, filariform *Strongyloides* larvae, and bacteria (responsible for secondary infection) [23]. The educational DVDs on scabies [21] and *Strongyloides* [22] were also used occasionally. An information sheet about the project in Djambarrpuyngu language (or occasionally in English if more appropriate) was left with each household.

3. Results

3.1. Flipchart

The front page of the flipchart is shown in Figure 1, and the topic of each page of the flipchart is listed in Table 2.

Table 2. Contents of the educational flipchart for the ivermectin mass drug administration (MDA) project.

Page	Contents
Title	Summary of the aim of the ivermectin research project and the effect of ivermectin (Figure 1)
1	Brief summary of the traditional story of preparing food from cycad nuts as an overall analogy for the project
2	Diagram illustrating what people can do to eliminate scabies and *Strongyloides*
3	The role of the microscope in making it possible to see bacteria, *Strongyloides* worms, and scabies mites
4	Good and bad bacteria and secondary infection
5	Immunity, focusing on the role of white cells
6	Immunity, focusing on the role of antibodies
7	Direct life cycle of *Strongyloides*, emphasizing the role of parasitic adults in reproduction, of larvae in transmission via the faeces, and immature female infective larvae in entering the body through the skin
8.	*Strongyloides* autoinfective cycle, implications for life-long infection, and overwhelming infection when the white cells cannot do their work; an assurance that ivermectin can kill *Strongyloides* in our body
9	Secondary infection occurs when *Strongyloides* larvae enter the body proper through the wall of the lower gut, accompanied by bacteria
10	Symptoms of strongyloidiasis
11	Life cycle of scabies mites
12	Symptoms of scabies
13	Secondary infection associated with scabies
14	Transmission of scabies, mainly by person-to-person contact
15	Ivermectin treatment program: testing for scabies and strongyloidiasis, and medication for different age groups
16	Ivermectin treatment program: taking medicine, following-up at 6 months, repeating after 1 year, following up again at 18 months, and informed consent
17	A detailed version of the cycad story
18	Acknowledgements
Back page	Summary of what people can do to eliminate scabies mites and *Strongyloides* worms from their bodies

3.2. Community Education

The stories from the flip-chart were shared with people from 111 houses, 70% of the houses in the community (n = 159 at the time of the education [18]). At 41 houses (37% of those visited) either the men's team or the women's team spoke with family groups. At another 43 houses (39%) the men's team spoke to men only, and at 27 houses (24%) the women's team spoke to women only. This is the culturally acceptable way of educating the community. In addition, two homelands (small outlying settlements), eight workplaces, and two schools were visited. The number in each age group as percent of the estimated 2011 population and sex are given in Table 3. The people who took part in the education were predominantly in the 30–49 years age group.

Most of the people were very interested in the stories and asked questions. The movie clips were particularly effective in giving people an understanding of disease-causing organisms, foundational to understanding scabies and *S. stercoralis* infection. The role of faecal material from infected people in the transmission of *S. stercoralis* also became clearer to people when they saw the movie clips. Children enjoyed watching the *Strongyloides* Story DVD.

Table 3. Age groups as percent of estimated population and sex of people who took part.

Age Group	Estimated Population [26]	Total Seen (% of pop.)	% Male
3–14 years	754	148 (20)	45
15–29 years	541	115 (21)	63
30–49 years	568	254 (45)	51
50+ years	260	62 (24)	47
Total	2123	579 (27)	51

3.3. Community Discussion of the Stories

People were fascinated by the idea of the 'wirrkul̲ mewirri' (pre-pubescent female worm), the infective filariform larva. The story of the wirrkul̲ mewirri spread through the community. On a number of occasions, teenagers passing by called out 'wirrkul̲ mewirri' to the non-Aboriginal educator, as they passed her in the street. The story also spread to the city through children who had visited the community and then told their father when they went home. Their father then wanted to know more. *Strongyloides* became known locally as 'wirrkul̲ mewirri'. People who had missed out on hearing the stories about scabies and *Strongyloides* were asking the Aboriginal educators why the education had stopped. In 2017, a person who was being shown gut bacteria in a movie clip that also included *Strongyloides* worms asked whether the worms were 'wirrkul̲ mewirri', demonstrating that the introduced term has currency seven years after it was introduced.

3.4. Feedback Indicating that the Mode of Transmission of Strongyloides Was Understood

Children were overheard telling each other to be careful where they put their feet, for fear of the wirrkul̲ mewirri. Teenagers were overheard teasing each other when not wearing footwear, and telling each other that the wirrkul̲ mewirri would get into them. One of the non-Aboriginal teachers at the school offered to do some shopping for her Aboriginal neighbours while she was away on leave. They asked her to bring thongs, footwear for all the family, to protect them from the wirrkul̲ mewirri, indicating that the mode of transmission was understood.

3.5. Participation in the Ivermectin MDA

A large proportion of the population participated in the MDA research project. In 2010, there were 1013 participants, and in 2011 an additional 360 people joined the project, a total of 1373 [18,19], approximately 65% of the 2011 estimated population [26].

4. Discussion

This study fills a gap in the literature by documenting the principles and practice of discovery education, an effective method of cross-cultural community education that uses a collaborative approach to make important information in the Australian western context comprehensible to Aboriginal Australians living remotely. In the Australian context, there is no generally accepted effective strategy to promote health literacy in Aboriginal people who retain their worldview and language. There are few studies reporting effective community health education in the literature [11,12,16,17]. This paper outlines an effective process of co-constructing narrative health education materials, and of face-to-face communication of community health information to improve knowledge, health literacy, and health outcomes of the community.

The large number of people who participated in the ivermectin MDA project in 2010, and the substantial number of additional people who participated in 2011, suggests that the community education described above was effective in informing people about scabies and strongyloidiasis and the benefits of the MDA. The process also helped them take a step towards achieving oral health literacy about the causes of scabies, strongyloidiasis, and infectious diseases and the benefits of treatment for these diseases.

The educational process followed the principles of discovery education (Table 1). The education was acceptable to people because the education teams included a non-Aboriginal educator, an 'owner of the knowledge', and even when the story was being told by an Aboriginal educator, it was recognised to be on behalf of the non-Aboriginal educator, who was available to answer questions and clarify any points not understood. The education was given in a 'culturally correct way', having been first approved by the respected clan leaders, and it was provided in Djambarrpuyŋu language, the local *lingua franca*, which is readily understood by everyone in the community. It covered foundational information, including microscopic organisms and cells of the body, and it was connected to cultural general knowledge, essential for understanding the life cycles of scabies mites and *Strongyloides* worms and how they affect the body. It connected important behaviours for preventing the transmission of scabies and strongyloidiasis with a cultural story, the preparation of cycad food. Thus, the information was built on Indigenous understandings and perspectives [6] (p. 22).

Interpersonal community health education in remote communities can be very effective because of the strong kinship network in these communities [27]. The kinship network is also the basis for social interactions. When information is given to a large number of people in the community, it becomes a topic of conversation. This gives people an opportunity to debate the information and decide whether it makes sense and is important to them. Feedback to the education team indicated that intellectual debate about the health stories was occurring in the community. It is likely that the information was able to survive intellectual debate.

The partnership between non-Aboriginal educators and Aboriginal educators was crucial to the success of the education. It enabled consultation with the clan elders, the preparation of comprehensible stories, and the sharing of the stories in a conversational style that encouraged the learners to ask questions and find out what they wanted to know. The stories were accurate and told in a way that provided a basis for understanding important health principles, especially the causes of infectious diseases. This foundational understanding has the potential to help people make sense of new health information in the future.

To what extent the knowledge has been incorporated into the cultural knowledge of the group, that is, whether it has been accepted, maintained, updated and re-taught by the group, is not known at this stage. Approximately 31% of people 15 years and over were directly reached by the education teams, whereas Trudgen [14] (p. 210) suggests that peer group affirmation of the majority of the adult population is needed in order for the information to become part of the cultural knowledge of the group. However, the 2017 query about the wirrkul mewirri is a positive sign that at least some of the knowledge is retained.

Although the discovery education method involves Aboriginal and non-Aboriginal people learning from each other, it is *not* the 'two-way education' that Harris [13] (p. 129) proposed for school education. He recommended that children be educated simultaneously but separately in cultural knowledge of their own people in their Aboriginal language, and Western knowledge in English. In discovery education, connections between the Western knowledge and Aboriginal general knowledge are explored so that people can incorporate the Western knowledge into their existing cultural general knowledge.

In recent years, there has been increased awareness of the importance of principles of adult learning and education for critical consciousness in primary health care for remote-living Aboriginal people [28], but the use of the local language as an integral part of the education process is not mentioned, and the use of the discovery education principles is rare. Although Australia's *Translating and Interpreting Service* offers the most extensive telephone interpreting system in the world, this service does not include Indigenous languages [29].

Trop. Med. Infect. Dis. **2018**, 3, 15

The importance of Aboriginal languages in communicating health information cannot be overemphasised. It is necessary but not sufficient for non-Aboriginal health professionals to be trained in Aboriginal culture and in cross-cultural communication skills [15]. A knowledge of the language is also needed to facilitate health literacy in Aboriginal people living remotely. Although all NT public sector agencies are required to provide cross-cultural awareness training to all employees who interact with Aboriginal people, including health professionals [30], they do not recognise the importance of language. The NT Health Promotion Framework [31] includes language barriers as one of the factors that compound the negative effect of low socioeconomic status on health, but it does not address the need to train specialised non-Aboriginal health professionals to become proficient in an Aboriginal language.

5. Conclusions

This study provides an example of the ability of a partnership of non-Aboriginal and Aboriginal health educators using a discovery education approach to develop and share a cross-cultural health story that people understood, in an Aboriginal language. The study also provides a model for community health education to facilitate the development of health literacy in Aboriginal people living remotely.

A discovery education approach to health education would be useful in any part of the world where the language and worldview of the majority of the people are different from that of health professionals.

Acknowledgments: This work was financially supported by a grant from the Cooperative Research Centre for Aboriginal Health [CRCAH—HS 331]. We thank Rick Speare for his part in developing the Ivermectin MDA project and regret that he passed away since the study. We thank the people of Galiwin'ku who participated in the study, discussed the scabies and strongyloidiasis stories among themselves, and gave feedback to us. We thank Timothy Buthimaŋ for the cycad food story and permission to use it, Peter Brown and Lorna McDonaugh for the use of their movie clip of *Strongyloides* rhabditiform larvae, Andrew Butcher for the use of his movie clip of *Strongyloides* filariform larvae, and Yvonne Coleman for the final formatting of the *Stop Scabies and Strongyloides* flipchart. We also thank colleagues at ARDS Aboriginal Corporation, particularly David Shield, Yalu' Marŋgithinyaraw, particularly George Garambaka, Mark Markurri, and Jeffrey Djakurrŋa, and Menzies School of Health Research for their assistance. We regret that Leanne Bundhala passed away since this study took place. We thank the reviewers for their helpful comments.

Author Contributions: This paper is dedicated to the memory of Rick Speare and Leanne Bundhala, both of whom recognised the value of cross-cultural, Aboriginal language community health education and community engagement for remote-living Aboriginal people as an essential tool in the control of scabies and strongyloidiasis. Rick encouraged the work of developing educational tools using this method, and recognised the discovery education method as a means to give comprehensible information to affected people about the causative organism *Strongyloides stercoralis*. Only an informed community can prevent the transmission of this parasite, and seek appropriate treatment. Bundhala was an experienced educator in a number of education programmes about scabies in her community including to the one reported here. This paper explains the principles of this culturally appropriate style of community health education called discovery education, and presents an example showing how the method was applied in a remote community. The education enabled people to make an informed choice of whether to participate in a research project in which all participants were treated for scabies and strongyloidiasis. Jennifer M. Shield, Therese M. Kearns, and Ross M. Andrews conceived and designed the study; Jennifer M. Shield, Joanne Garŋgulkpuy, Lisa Walpulay, Roslyn Gundjirryirr, Leanne Bundhala, and Veronica Djarpanbuluwuy prepared the educational materials and carried out the education; Jennifer M. Shield, Therese M. Kearns, Ross M. Andrews and Jenni Judd wrote the paper.

Conflicts of Interest: The authors declare no conflict of interest.

References

1. Zhao, Y.; You, J.; Guthridge, S. *Burden of Disease and Injury in the Northern Territory 1999–2003*; Health Gains Planning, Department of Health and Families: Darwin, NT, Australia, 2009.
2. Devitt, J.; Hall, G.; Tsey, K. *An Introduction to the Social Determinants of Health in Relation to the Northern Territory Indigenous Population*; Occasional Papers Series, Issue No. 6; Cooperative Research Centre for Aboriginal & Tropical Health: Darwin, Australia, 2001.

3. Joint Commission on Accreditation of Healthcare Organizations. *"What Did the Doctor Say?" Improving Health Literacy to Protect Patient Safety*; HCAHO: Oakbrook Terrace, IL, USA, 2007.
4. Amery, R. Recognising the communication gap in Indigenous health care. *Med. J. Aust.* **2017**, *207*, 13–15. [CrossRef] [PubMed]
5. Fransen, M.; Harris, V.C.; Essink-Bot, M.L. Low health literacy in ethnic minority patients: Understandable language is the beginning of good healthcare. *Ned. Tijdschr. Geneeskd.* **2013**, *157*, A5581. [PubMed]
6. Australian Commission on Safety and Quality in HealthCare. *Health Literacy: Taking Action to Improve Safety and Quality*; Australian Commission on Safety and Quality in HealthCare: Sydney, NSW, Australia, 2014.
7. Sørensen, K.; Van den Brouche, S.; Fullam, J.; Doyle, G.; Pelikan, J.; Slonska, Z.; Brand, H. Health literacy and public health: A systematic review and integration of definitions and models. *BMC Public Health* **2012**, *12*, 80. [CrossRef] [PubMed]
8. Nutbeam, D. Health literacy as a public health goal: A challenge for contemporary health education and communication strategies into the 21st century. *Health Promot. Int.* **2000**, *15*, 259–267. [CrossRef]
9. Freire, P. *Pedagogy of the Oppressed*; The Continuum Publishing Company: New York, NY, USA, 1972.
10. Baker, D.W. The meaning and the measure of health literacy. *J. Intern. Med.* **2006**, *21*, 878–883. [CrossRef] [PubMed]
11. Vass, A.; Mitchell, A.; Dhurrkay, Y. Health literacy and Australian Indigenous peoples: An analysis of the role of language and worldview. *Health Promot. J. Aust.* **2011**, *22*, 33–37. [CrossRef]
12. Mapleson, J. Do you speak my language? *Chronicle* **2014**, *26*, 4–6.
13. Harris, S. *Two-Way Aboriginal Schooling. Education and Cultural Survival*; Aboriginal Studies Press: Canberra, ACT, Australia, 1990.
14. Trudgen, R.T. *Why Warriors Lie Down and Die. Djambatj Mala*; Aboriginal Resource and Development Services: Darwin, NT, Australia, 2000.
15. Lowell, A.; Maypilama, E.; Yikaniwuy, S.; Rrapa, E.; Williams, T.; Dunn, S. "Hiding the story": Indigenous consumer concerns about communication related to chronic disease in one remote region of Australia. *Int. J. Speech-Lang. Path.* **2012**, *14*, 200–208. [CrossRef] [PubMed]
16. Trudgen, R.T. (Why Warriors, Nhulunbuy, Australia); Balanda (Mainstream Aboriginal, Nhulunbuy, Australia); Yolngu (East Arnhem Land Aboriginal, Nhulunbuy, Australia). Personal communication, 2017.
17. Mitchell, A.; Patel, B. Improving health literacy in the NT: Allowing language to empower. *Chronicle* **2014**, *26*, 2–5.
18. Kearns, T.M.; Speare, R.; Cheng, A.C.; McCarthy, J.; Carapetis, J.R.; Holt, D.C.; Currie, B.J.; Page, W.; Shield, J.; Gundjirryirr, R.; et al. Impact of an ivermectin mass drug administration on scabies prevalence in a remote Australian Aboriginal community. *PLoS Negl. Trop. Dis.* **2015**, *9*, E0004151. [CrossRef] [PubMed]
19. Kearns, T.M.; Speare, R.; Cheng, A.C.; McCarthy, J.; Carapetis, J.R.; Holt, D.C.; Currie, B.J.; Page, W.; Shield, J.; Gundjirryirr, R.; et al. *Strongyloides* seroprevalence before and after an ivermectin mass drug administration in a remote Australian Aboriginal community. *PLoS Negl. Trop. Dis.* **2017**, *11*, E0005607. [CrossRef] [PubMed]
20. Page, W. *Strongyloides Story*; Flipchart in Plain English; Miwatj Health: Nhulunbuy, NT, Australia, 2001.
21. Aboriginal Resource and Development Services. *Scabiespuy Dhäwu, Scabies Story*; DVD in Djambarrpuyŋu Language with English Subtitles; Aboriginal Resource and Development Services: Darwin, NT, Australia, 2008.
22. Aboriginal Resource and Development Services. *Strongyloidespuy Dhäwu, Strongyloides Story*; DVD in Djambarrpuyŋu Language with English Subtitles; Aboriginal Resource and Development Services: Darwin, NT, Australia, 2009.
23. Aboriginal Resource and Development Services. *Foundations in Health Literacy: A Train the Trainer Resource in English*; DVD; Aboriginal Resource and Development Services: Darwin, NT, Australia, 2009.
24. Menzies School of Health Research. *Healthy Skin Story: Scabies, Skin Sores, Tinea*; Menzies School of Health Research: Darwin, NT, Australia, 2009.
25. Menzies School of Health Research. *Recognising and Treating Skin Conditions*; Menzies School of Health Research: Darwin, NT, Australia, 2009.
26. Qpzm LocalStats Australia. Galiwinku Population Summary. 2011. Available online: http://galiwinku.localstats.com.au/population/nt/northern-territory/darwin/galiwinku (accessed on 18 May 2016).
27. Christie, M. *Yolngu Languages and Culture: Gupapuyngu*; Teaching & Learning Support Division, Northern Territory University: Darwin, NT, Australia, 2002.

28. Health Promotion Strategy Unit. *The Public Health Bush Book Vol. 1. Strategies and Resources*; Department of Health: Darwin, NT, Australia, 2007.
29. Phillips, C.B. Improving health outcomes for linguistically diverse patients. *Med. J. Aust.* **2016**, *204*, 209–210. [CrossRef] [PubMed]
30. Office of the Commissioner for Public Employment. *Cross Cultural Training Framework: An Implementation Guide*; Northern Territory Government: Darwin, NT, Australia, 2013.
31. Department of Health. *Northern Territory Health Promotion Framework*; Department of Health: Darwin, NT, Australia, 2013.

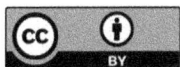

Tropical Medicine and Infectious Disease

MDPI

Review

Exotic Parasite Threats to Australia's Biosecurity—Trade, Health, and Conservation

R. C. Andrew Thompson

School of Veterinary and Life Sciences, Murdoch University, Murdoch WA 6150, Australia;
a.thompson@murdoch.edu.au

Received: 29 June 2018; Accepted: 12 July 2018; Published: 18 July 2018

Abstract: Parasites have threatened Australia's biosecurity since the early days of European settlement. Tick fever in cattle and liver fluke, along with their invertebrate hosts, and hydatid disease head the list of parasites that are still impacting livestock industries. In addition, there are many parasites that have been introduced that are of significance to public health as well as the conservation of native wildlife. As a consequence of these early arrivals, Australia has become much more aware of its vulnerability should parasites such as *Trichinella* and *Trypanosoma evansi* become established in Australia. However, recent discoveries concerning *Leishmania* and other trypanosomes have demonstrated that Australia must not become complacent and reliant on dogma when considering the potential emergence of new threats to its biosecurity. In this short review, the major parasite threats to Australia's biosecurity are summarised, some misconceptions are emphasised, and attention is given to the importance of challenging dogma in the face of a dearth of information about Australian native fauna.

Keywords: Australia; biosecurity; parasites; zoonoses; wildlife

1. Introduction

Parasites have threatened Australia's biosecurity since the early days of European settlement. Australia still suffers from some mistakes of the past when parasites were introduced during early settlement [1]. Tick fever in cattle and fascioliasis in livestock, along with their invertebrate hosts, and hydatid disease head the list of exotic parasitic diseases that are still impacting livestock industries. All three diseases were introduced as a consequence of agricultural activities. In addition, there are many introduced parasites that are of significance to public health as well as the conservation of native wildlife that were not endemic to Australia before early settlement.

These early introductions fuelled an awareness of Australia's vulnerability to exotic pests and parasites, particularly those of economic significance such as *Chrysomya bezziana* (screwworm), *Trypanosoma evansi* (surra), and *Trichinella spiralis* (trichinellosis) [1]. From a public health perspective, only *Plasmodium* seems to be a priority. Australia was declared malaria free in 1981 [2], yet Australia has a vector, *Anopheles farauti* [3]. Parasites such as *Taenia solium*, *Clonorchis sinensis*, and *Trypanosoma cruzi* are unlikely to become established in Australia, yet patients with diseases caused by these parasites migrate to Australia and there is a need for heightened awareness among clinicians about these often chronic infections [4,5].

Furthermore, recent discoveries concerning *Leishmania* and other trypanosomes (see below) have demonstrated that Australia must not become complacent and reliant on dogma when considering the potential emergence of new threats to its biosecurity.

In this review, I want to highlight the major parasite threats to Australia's biosecurity, some misconceptions, and the importance of challenging dogma in the face of a dearth of information about Australian native fauna.

2. Hydatid Disease—*Echinococcus*

Echinococcus granulosus is the causative agent of hydatid disease (or, using more recent terminology, cystic echinococcosis) in humans and livestock. It serves as perhaps the best example of a parasite that was brought into Australia in animals that were exotic to the country (principally sheep) [6] but which were essential to the development of livestock agriculture in Australia. Much has been written about the history of hydatid disease in Australia and its control [6]. Unlike the mainland, the island state of Tasmania has been able to effectively control transmission of *E. granulosus* in a dog-sheep cycle [7,8]. Although no new human cases have been reported in Tasmania, complete elimination of the parasite has proved elusive, with recent localised reports in cattle and dogs suggesting transmission may still be occurring, albeit at a low level [9]. However, this is not the case on the mainland of Australia. Tasmania had the advantage of more easily focussing a public health campaign on the dog-sheep cycle and the anthropogenic activities that sustained it, since there was no opportunity of spillover of *Echinococcus* infection to native wildlife, given the absence of the dingo [10]. On the mainland, spillover from the sheep-dog cycle has resulted in a novel cycle of transmission involving small macropods and dingoes [10]. This means that although the incidence of cystic echinococcosis has declined markedly in humans and sheep, the parasite is still maintained in a wild animal cycle and thus complete eradication of this important zoonosis will never be achieved. What was unexpected, however, has been data demonstrating the clinical impact of hydatid disease on native wildlife. Barnes and colleagues [11] investigated the growth rate and clinical presentations of hydatid cysts in macropod marsupials and demonstrated that the cysts have a major impact on respiratory capacity. Infected animals are thus potentially more susceptible to predation by wild dogs, a similar situation to the predator-prey cycle involving moose and large cervids that maintains *E. canadensis* in North America [12].

Echinococcus multilocularis is not present in Australia nor in Southeast Asia and is largely confined to the northern hemisphere [8]. This could be luck or due to the insusceptibility of native wildlife, because infected dogs are likely to have entered Australia. However, a case report of alveolar echinococcosis in a captive red-necked wallaby (*Macropus rufogriseus*) in Germany [13] demonstrates that Australia's native marsupials are likely to be susceptible to infection with the metacestode stage of *E. multilocularis*. Consequently, should an infected definitive host enter Australia, most likely a domestic dog, infection could conceivably be transmitted to free-ranging marsupials. Although quarantine restrictions should prevent an infected dog entering Australia, this depends on adequate screening, compliance with Australian quarantine regulations, and use of the most appropriate cestocidal agent. If an infected dog were to enter Australia, the post-arrival period of only 10 days in quarantine from endemic countries such as Switzerland is much less than the pre-patent period [14]. Australian authorities should guard against complacency with a parasite such as *E. multilocularis*. Within recent years, we have seen an increasing number of dogs arriving in Australia from Europe with pathogenic *Leishmania* spp. (see below) and perhaps extra vigilance may be required in post-arrival parasite checks for *E. multilocularis*.

3. Economic Threats

From an economic perspective, *Trypanosoma evansi* and *Trichinella spiralis* have always been considered major parasite threats to Australia's biosecurity [1].

Infection with *T. evansi* can lead to a disease called surra. While currently absent from Australia and Papua New Guinea, it is considered an exotic disease of concern for Australia [15–17]. The parasite has a low host specificity, and the clinical consequences of infection can be severe in a range of domestic and some wild animal species, particularly horses, camels, cattle, buffalo, cats, and dogs. In contrast, infection with *T. evansi* leads to mild or chronic disease in sheep and pigs but is often asymptomatic. Experimental evidence suggests infection with *T. evansi* is likely to lead to death in Australian macropod marsupials. *Trypanosoma evansi* has always been considered a major biosecurity risk to Australia because it is transmitted mechanically by tabanid biting flies and is endemic in a number of Southeast Asian regions in close proximity to the north of Australia [17,18]. Since pigs are highly susceptible and rarely suffer overt clinical signs, they can act as 'silent' reservoir hosts. This is a major concern given the large numbers of free-ranging feral pigs, particularly in northern Australia. Therefore, both pre- and post-border quarantine surveillance has been undertaken for many years.

Surra was diagnosed in Western Australia in a group of imported camels at Port Hedland in 1907 [19]. These animals were destroyed and there has been no further report of the disease in camels, or any other domestic or wild species of mammal, in Australia since that time. Given the widespread distribution of potential mechanical vectors of *T. evansi* in Australia and the close proximity to endemic areas, it is perhaps surprising that evidence of *T. evansi* has not been detected in Australia. Transmission of infection is related to several factors, including the size (and morphology) of the biting insect (volume of blood potentially transferred from one host to another) and insect density [15]. The latter may be particularly important in areas of northern Australia where the main potential reservoir host, feral pigs, are found. There is perhaps a need to examine vectorial density with that of feral pigs in order to re-evaluate the risk of *T. evansi* establishment in Australia.

Trichinella species have been detected worldwide in domestic and wild animals [20]. Economically, *T. spiralis* is the most important species because of its low host specificity and anthropogenic activities that perpetuate a domestic cycle involving pigs. *Trichinella spiralis* has never been reported in Australia, but *T. pseudospiralis* infection has been detected in marsupials and birds in Tasmania [21] and in a human from Tasmania [22]. Australia's domestic pig population is free from *T. pseudospiralis* and other *Trichinella* species [23]. *Trichinella papuae* has been detected in a mature boar from a Torres Strait island and has been described in pigs in New Guinea [24]. Thus, on current evidence, *Trichinella* does not appear to represent a major biosecurity risk to Australia, although continued surveillance is essential to demonstrate its absence.

4. Aboriginal Health

Early settlers brought a variety of parasites with them, including *Ancylostoma*, *Strongyloides*, *Ascaris*, *Trichuris*, *Giardia*, and *Hymenolepis/Rodentolepis* [25,26]. Following their introduction to Australia, they all became established in Aboriginal people, who probably represented a naïve host population, and were at particularly high risk of infection as community living was imposed on them. Apart from *Giardia*, these parasites are rarely seen in the general population, whereas they remain endemic in Aboriginal communities, often at high prevalence rates, particularly in children [26]. In all cases, the impact of these parasites is far more severe than in non-Aboriginal people. This is because infections are exacerbated by poor diet, are often chronic, usually involve multiple infections with several parasites, and re-infection is common. Unfortunately, the lack of ongoing surveillance in Aboriginal communities, and thus a lack of current data on the incidence of parasite infections, is a severe impediment to control.

In these situations, control has proved to be very difficult, particularly with parasites transmitted by the faecal-oral route, such as *Giardia* and *Hymenolepis/Rodentolepis*, which require improved hygiene and public health measures directed principally at children [26–28]. Similarly, although not as widespread, infections with *Ancylostoma* and *Strongyloides* have proved difficult to control once established in communities [25,29]. Control requires not just education but community-wide chemotherapy to reduce prevalence significantly and lead to eradication. Such initiatives have proved very successful for both *Ancylostoma* and *Strongyloides* in the few communities where such mass drug administrations (MDAs) have been undertaken. However, long-term success requires subsequent surveillance of the communities and the implementation of ongoing control strategies when needed. The hookworm trial was conducted over a period of six years and prevalence was reduced from 80% to 2.6% [30], but since then no follow-up prevalence surveys have been reported. The two more recent community MDAs targeting *Strongyloides* were delivered 12 months apart and resulted in a significant sustained reduction in *Strongyloides* seroprevalence over 18 months [31,32]. Recent reports of the occurrence of the zoonotic hookworm *A. ceylanicum* in Australia will further complicate control in Aboriginal communities [33,34]. The parasite has recently been reported in domestic dogs from urban area and Aboriginal communities in northern Australia and is considered an emerging public health risk [35]. Future MDAs aimed at controlling hookworm in communities must therefore take into account the role of dogs in transmission.

With global warming, parasite infections currently endemic in Aboriginal communities may become more common and more widespread within Australia. In addition, the potential for the establishment of introduced infections such as Japanese encephalitis and malaria may also increase [36].

5. Trypanosomes

Apart from surra, trypanosomes (*Trypanosoma* and *Leishmania*) have not, until recently, been considered a biosecurity issue for Australia. Although the occurrence of species of *Trypanosoma* in introduced and native wildlife has been documented since the 1950s, their impact as the causative agents of disease was not considered until recently, and attention was principally on documenting host records [16,37]. However, two recent investigations have radically changed our understanding of trypanosomes in Australia, with ramifications internationally. The first was the discovery of a novel species of *Leishmania*, *L. macropodum*, in kangaroos, which is transmitted by a new vector, a biting midge (*Forcipomyia* spp.) [38–40]. These discoveries have shattered perceived dogma calling into question the exclusivity of the *Leishmania*-phlebotomine relationship and have been followed by several reports confirming the vectorial potential of biting midges of the genus *Culicoides*, in South America and North Africa [41,42]. The biosecurity implications for Australia are that we have an indigenous *Leishmania*-competent vector in *Forcipomyia* that could transmit pathogenic zoonotic species of *Leishmania*, such as *L. infantum*, that are regularly introduced into Australia in humans and domestic dogs [43,44].

Similarly, *Trypanosoma cruzi* has received little attention in Australia, with the belief that it was restricted to South America where its known triatomid vectors are found. However, recent studies on native Australian species of *Trypanosoma* have not only revealed considerable genetic diversity, with some species closely related to *T. cruzi*, but also that some species are phenotypically similar to *T. cruzi* in their invasive nature at the cellular level, and opportunistic pathogens in some marsupial species contributing to their decline [44–46]. Little is known about the vectors of Australian trypanosomes, but the close relationship of some such as *T. noyesi* to *T. cruzi* indicates that their vectors could transmit *T. cruzi*. The vectors of Australian trypanosomes have yet to be identified, although ticks, tabanids, and biting midges may play a role [37,44,47]. Migrants from *T. cruzi*-endemic areas in South America who contracted Chagas' disease before arriving in Australia could be a source of infection to humans, dogs, or wildlife if local vectors of wildlife species of *Trypanosoma* are capable of transmitting *T. cruzi*.

Ongoing surveillance is required to monitor and address the potential biosecurity concerns of exotic trypanosomes becoming established in Australian mammals [16]. For example, in 1951, forty brush-tailed possums and a single short-beaked echidna were experimentally infected with *T. cruzi*, with the majority of animals dying between 21 and 35 days after inoculation [48]. Given the wide host range of *T. noyesi* in Australia and its genetic relationship with *T. cruzi*, it is possible that the vector of *T. noyesi* could transmit *T. cruzi* from humans (of which there were an estimated 1400–3000 human cases in Australia in 2006 [49,50]) toindigenous Australian mammals. The consequences of infection could lead to disease in naïve wildlife hosts as well as establishing a local reservoir of infection in those animals that do not succumb to infection.

In addition to the pathogenic potential of some Australian trypanosomes to native wildlife, there is increasing evidence that an exotic species of *Trypanosoma*, *T. lewisi*, introduced with rats and their fleas at the time of European settlement, or earlier, could have been responsible for reported declines of native wildlife, in a similar way that its introduction to Christmas Island has recently been found to have been responsible for the extinction of the Maclear's and bulldog rats [51]. Using ancient DNA methodology, Wyatt et al. [52] demonstrated that native trypanosomes were absent from the indigenous rodents on Christmas Island prior to the introduction of the black rat, and that after 1899 both the Maclear's and bulldog rat were infected with *T. lewisi* [16]. *Trypanosoma lewisi* was first reported in Australia by Bancroft in 1888 in an introduced *Rattus* sp. [44]. It was subsequently reported in native bush rats and water rats (*Hydromys chrysogaster*) [53]. Its origin within native wildlife is likely to have been from black and brown rats on ships arriving from Europe, or it could have been present before their arrival. Given the pathogenic potential of *T. lewisi* in naïve hosts, as demonstrated on Christmas Island, it has been suggested that *T. lewisi* may have played a role in the decline of native wildlife in Australia [37,44]. Trypanosomes have been demonstrated to vary in virulence when they encounter a new or naïve host species [37,44]. The exotic *T. lewisi* could possibly have played a role in the fauna declines identified in Australia between 1875 and 1925 [54] and since this time a more balanced host/parasite relationship has developed. Investigating the presence of *T. lewisi* in densely populated areas within Australia may assist in answering these questions [37].

Insufficient consideration has been given to the impact of introduced parasites on Australian native wildlife. Although there has been speculation in the past that *Toxoplasma* may have played a role in the decline of some native species of wildlife, recent evidence suggests that *Toxoplasma* may have been in Australia before European settlement and its ubiquity in native wildlife with little evidence of clinical disease in free-ranging wildlife attests to the evolution of a balanced host-parasite relationship [55,56]. It has always been considered that *Toxoplasma* was introduced into Australia in domestic cats and sheep at the time of European settlement [56]. Subsequently, *Toxoplasma* was linked historically to the population declines of native wildlife and has generally been believed to be pathogenic to Australia's mammalian and avian fauna [54,56]. However, there is little evidence to support these assumptions. The evidence that *Toxoplasma* is a significant cause of disease in native wildlife is largely based on the impact of infection in captive animals [56]. The dogma that *Toxoplasma* is a serious pathogen in Australian wildlife may have overshadowed the potential impact of other parasites such as *T. lewisi*.

6. Concluding Comments

Surveillance, pre- and post-border, of both parasites and their vectors, is the key to maintaining Australia's biosecurity. This has been demonstrated very well with parasites such as *Chrysomya bezziana*. Australia has also recognised which exotic parasites pose threats to Australia's biosecurity, particularly from an economic perspective. *Trichinella spiralis* and *Trypanosoma evansi* are good examples of parasites that fall into this category, although it is unfortunate that parasites of public health significance are not afforded the same attention. Furthermore, the recent discovery of both a novel species of *Leishmania* and its vector illustrates how little we know about the parasites of Australia's native fauna. As such, the dangers of local transmission of *Trypanosoma cruzi* in Australia should not be dismissed, given its emergence in the USA and involvement of native vectors. It should not be necessary to wait until a species is in danger of extinction before doing this [57], but such studies should be ongoing and the importance of doing so recognised by appropriate conservation agencies and granting agencies.

Funding: This research received no external funding.

Conflicts of Interest: The author declares no conflict of interest.

References

1. Thompson, R.C.A.; Owen, I.L.; Puana, I.; Banks, D.; Davis, T.M.E.; Reid, S.A. Parasites and iosecurity—The example of Australia. *Trends Parasitol.* **2003**, *19*, 410–416. [CrossRef]
2. World Health Organization. Synopsis of the world malaria situation in 1981. *Wkly. Epidemiol. Rec.* **1983**, *58*, 197–199.
3. Preston-Thomas, A.; Gair, R.W.; Hosking, K.A.; Devine, G.J.; Donohue, S.D. An outbreak of *Plasmodium falciparum* malaria in the Torres Strait. *Commun. Dis. Intell. Q. Rep.* **2012**, *36*, E180–E185. [PubMed]

4. Hughes, A.J.; Biggs, B.A. Parasitic worms of the central nervous system: An Australian perspective. *Intern. Med. J.* **2002**, *32*, 541–543. [CrossRef] [PubMed]
5. Thompson, R.C.A.; Conlan, J.V. Emerging issues and parasite zoonoses in the SE Asian region. *Vet. Parasitol.* **2011**, *181*, 69–73. [CrossRef] [PubMed]
6. Gemmell, M.A. Australasian contributions to an understanding of the epidemiology and control of hydatid disease caused by *Echinococcus granulosus*-past, present and future. *Int. J. Parasitol.* **1990**, *20*, 431–456. [CrossRef]
7. Thompson, R.C.A.; Jenkins, D.J. *Echinococcus* as a model system. *Int. J. Parasitol.* **2014**, *44*, 865–877. [CrossRef] [PubMed]
8. Deplazes, P.; Rinaldi, L.; Alvarez Rojas, C.A.; Torgerson, P.R.; Harandi, M.F.; Romig, T.; Antolova, D.; Schurer, J.M.; Lahmar, S.; Cringoli, G.; et al. Global distribution of cystic and alveolar echinococcosis. *Adv. Parasitol.* **2017**, *95*, 315–493. [PubMed]
9. Jenkins, D.J.; Lievaart, J.J.; Boufana, B.; Lett, W.S.; Bradshaw, H.; Armua-Fernandez, M.T. *Echinococcus granulosus* and other intestinal helminths: Current status of prevalence and management in rural dogs of eastern Australia. *Aust. Vet. J.* **2014**, *92*, 292–298. [CrossRef] [PubMed]
10. Thompson, R.C.A. Parasite zoonoses and wildlife: One health, spillover and human activity. *Int. J. Parasitol.* **2013**, *43*, 1079–1088. [CrossRef] [PubMed]
11. Barnes, T.S.; Morton, J.M.; Coleman, G.T. Clustering of hydatid infection in macropodids. *Int. J. Parasitol.* **2007**, *37*, 943–952. [CrossRef] [PubMed]
12. Schurer, J.M.; Gesy, K.M.; Elken, B.T.; Jenkins, E.J. *Echinococcus multilocularis* and *E. canadensis* in wolves from western Canada. *Parasitology* **2014**, *141*, 159–163. [CrossRef] [PubMed]
13. Peters, M.; Kilwinski, J.; Wohlsein, P.; Conraths, F.J. Alveolar echinococcosis in a captive red-necked wallaby (*Macropus rufogriseus*). *Berl. Tierartztl. Wochenschr.* **2010**, *123*, 63–69.
14. Bringing Cats and Dogs (and Other Pets) to Australia. Available online: http://www.agriculture.gov.au (accessed on 29 June 2018).
15. Desquesnes, M.; Holzmuller, P.; Lai, D.-H.; Dargantes, A.; Lun, Z.-R.; Jittaplapong, S. *Trypanosoma evansi* and surra: A review and perspectives on origin, history, distribution, taxonomy, morphology, hosts, and pathogenic effects. *BioMed Res. Int.* **2013**, *2013*, 194176. [CrossRef] [PubMed]
16. Thompson, C.K.; Godfrey, S.S.; Thompson, R.C.A. Trypanosomes of Australian mammals: A review. *Int. J. Parasitol. Parasites Wildl.* **2014**, *3*, 57–66. [CrossRef] [PubMed]
17. DAWR. Surra. 2016. Available online: http://www.agriculture.gov.au/biosecurity/australia/naqs/naqs-targetlists/surra (accessed on 29 June 2018).
18. Luckins, A. Epidemiology of surra: Unanswered questions. *J. Protozool. Res.* **1998**, *8*, 106–119.
19. Cleland, J. Trypanosomiasis in camels. *J. Agric. West. Aust.* **1907**, *15*, 517–518.
20. Pozio, E. World distribution of *Trichinella* spp. infections in animals and humans. *Vet. Parasitol.* **2007**, *149*, 3–21. [CrossRef] [PubMed]
21. Obendorf, D.; Handlinger, J.; Mason, R.; Clarke, K.; Forman, A.; Hooper, P.; Smith, S.; Holdsworth, M. *Trichinella pseudospiralis* infection in Tasmanian wildlife. *Aust. Vet. J.* **1990**, *67*, 108–110. [CrossRef] [PubMed]
22. Andrews, J.R.; Ainsworth, R.; Abernethy, D. *Trichinella pseudospiralis* in humans: Description of a case and its treatment. *Trans. R. Soc. Trop. Med. Hyg.* **1994**, *88*, 200–203. [CrossRef]
23. Wildlife Health Australia. Trichinellosis and Australian Wildlife. Available online: https://wildlifehealthaustralia.com.au/Portals/0/Documents/FactSheets/Public%20health/Trichinellosis%20and%20Australian%20Wildlife%20May%202017%20%281.2%29.pdf (accessed on 29 June 2018).
24. Cuttell, L.; Cookson, B.; Jackson, L.; Gray, C.; Traub, R. First report of a *Trichinella papuae* infection in a wild pig (*Sus scrofa*) from an Australian island in the Torres Strait region. *Vet. Parasitol.* **2012**, *185*, 343–345. [CrossRef] [PubMed]
25. Holt, D.C.; McCarthy, J.S.; Carapetis, J.R. Parasitic diseases of remote Indigenous communities in Australia. *Int. J. Parasitol.* **2010**, *40*, 1119–1126. [CrossRef] [PubMed]
26. Shield, J.; Aland, K.; Kearns, T.; Gongdjalk, G.; Holt, D.; Currie, B.; Prociv, P. Intestinal parasites of children and adults in a remote Aboriginal community of the Northern Territory, Australia, 1994–1996. *WPSAR* **2015**, *6*, 44–51. [CrossRef] [PubMed]
27. Thompson, R.C.A.; Smith, A. Zoonotic enteric protozoa. *Vet. Parasitol.* **2011**, *182*, 70–78. [CrossRef] [PubMed]

28. Thompson, R.C.A. Neglected zoonotic helminths: Hymenolepis nana, Echinococcus canadensis and Ancylostoma ceylanicum. *Clin. Microbiol. Infect.* **2015**, *21*, 426–432. [CrossRef] [PubMed]

29. Reynoldson, J.A.; Behnke, J.M.; Gracey, M.; Horton, R.J.; Spargo, R.; Hopkins, R.; Constantine, C.C.; Gilbert, F.; Stead, C.; Hobbs, R.P.; et al. Efficacy of albendazole against *Giardia* and hookworm in a remote Aboriginal community in the north of Western Australia. *Acta Trop.* **1998**, *71*, 27–44. [CrossRef]

30. Thompson, R.C.A.; Reynoldson, J.A.; Garrow, S.C.; McCarthy, J.S.; Behnke, J.M. Towards the eradication of hookworm in an isolated Australian community. *Lancet* **2001**, *357*, 9258. [CrossRef]

31. Hays, R.; Esterman, A.; McDermott, R. Control of chronic *Strongyloides stercoralis* infection in an endemic community may be possible by pharmacological means alone: Results of a three-year cohort study. *PLoS Negl. Trop. Dis.* **2017**, *11*, e0005825. [CrossRef] [PubMed]

32. Kearns, T.M.; Currie, B.J.; Cheng, A.C.; McCarthy, J.; Carapetis, J.R.; Holt, D.C.; Page, W.; Shield, J.; Gundjirryirr, R.; Mulholland, E.; et al. *Strongyloides* seroprevalence before and after an ivermectin mass drug administration in a remote Australian Aboriginal community. *PLoS Negl. Trop. Dis.* **2017**, *11*, e0005607. [CrossRef] [PubMed]

33. Palmer, C.S.; Traub, R.J.; Robertson, I.D.; Hobbs, R.P.; Elliot, A.; While, L.; Rees, R.; Thompson, R.C.A.; Hobbs, R.P.; Elliot, A.; et al. The veterinary and public health significance of hookworm in dogs and cats in Australia and the status of *Ancylostoma ceylanicum*. *Vet. Parasit.* **2007**, *145*, 304–313. [CrossRef] [PubMed]

34. Smout, F.A.; Thompson, R.C.A.; Skerrat, L.F. First report of *Ancylostoma ceylanicum* in wild canids. *Int. J. Parasitol. Parasites Wildl.* **2013**, *2*, 173–177. [CrossRef] [PubMed]

35. Smout, F.A.; Skerratt, L.F.; Butler, J.R.A.; Johnson, C.N.; Congdon, B.C.; Thompson, R.C.A. The hookworm *Ancylostoma ceylanicum*: An emerging public health risk in Australian tropical rainforests and Indigenous communities. *One Health* **2017**, *3*, 66–69. [CrossRef] [PubMed]

36. Currie, B.J.; Brewster, D.R. Childhood infections in the tropical north of Australia. *J. Paed. Child Health* **2001**, *37*, 326–330. [CrossRef]

37. Cooper, C.; Clode, P.L.; Peacock, C.; Thompson, R.C.A. Host-parasite relationships and life histories of trypanosomes in Australia. *Adv. Parasitol.* **2017**, *97*, 47–109. [PubMed]

38. Rose, K.; Curtis, J.; Baldwin, T.; Mathis, A.; Kumar, B.; Sakthianandeswaren, A.; Spurck, T.; Low Choy, J.; Handman, E. Cutaneous leishmaniasis in red kangaroos: Isolation and characterisation of the causative organisms. *Int. J. Parasitol.* **2004**, *34*, 655–664. [CrossRef] [PubMed]

39. Dougall, A.; Shilton, C.; Low Choy, J.; Alexander, B.; Walton, S. New reports of Australian cutaneous leishmaniasis in northern Australian macropods. *Epidemiol. Infect.* **2009**, *137*, 1516–1520. [CrossRef] [PubMed]

40. Dougall, A.M.; Alexander, B.; Holt, D.C.; Harris, T.; Sultan, A.H.; Bates, P.A.; Rose, K.; Walton, S.F. Evidence incriminating midges (Diptera: Ceratopogonidae) as potential vectors of *Leishmania* in Australia. *Int. J. Parasitol.* **2011**, *41*, 571–579. [CrossRef] [PubMed]

41. Slama, D.; Haouas, N.; Remadi, L.; Mezhoud, H.; Babba, H.; Chaker, E. First detection of *Leishmania infantum* (Kinetoplastida: Trypanosomatidae) in *Culicoides* spp. (Diptera: Ceratopogonidae). *Parasites Vectors* **2014**, *7*, 51. [CrossRef] [PubMed]

42. Seblova, V.; Sadlova, J.; Vojtkova, B.; Votypka, J.; Carpenter, S.; Bates, P.A.; Volf, P. The biting midge *Culicoides sonorensis* (Diptera: Ceratopogonidae) is capable of developing late stage infections of *Leishmania enriettii*. *PLoS Negl. Trop. Dis.* **2015**, *9*, e0004060. [CrossRef] [PubMed]

43. Best, M.; Ash, A.; Bergfeld, J.; Barrett, J. The diagnosis and management of a case of *Leishmania infantum* infection in a dog imported to Australia. *Vet. Parasitol.* **2014**, *202*, 292–295. [CrossRef] [PubMed]

44. Thompson, C.K.; Thompson, R.C.A. Trypanosomes of Australian mammals: Knowledge gaps regarding transmission and biosecurity. *Trends Parasitol.* **2015**, *31*, 553–562. [CrossRef] [PubMed]

45. Botero, A.; Thompson, C.K.; Peacock, C.S.; Clode, P.L.; Nicholls, P.K.; Wayne, A.F.; Lymbery, A.J.; Thompson, R.C.A. Trypanosomes genetic diversity, polyparasitism, and the population decline of the critically endangered Australian marsupial, the brush tailed bettong or woylie (*Bettongia penicillata*). *Int. J. Parasitol. Parasites Wildl.* **2013**, *2*, 77–89. [CrossRef] [PubMed]

46. Botero, A.; Clode, P.L.; Peacock, C.S.; Thompson, R.C.A. Towards a better understanding of the life cycle of *Trypanosoma copemani*. *Protist* **2016**, *167*, 82–92. [CrossRef] [PubMed]

47. Botero, A.; Keatley, S.; Peacock, C.; Thompson, R.C.A. In vitro drug susceptibility of two strains of the wildlife trypanosome, *Trypanosoma copemani*: A comparison with *Trypanosoma cruzi*. *Int. J. Parasitol. Drugs Drug Resist.* **2017**, *7*, 34–41. [CrossRef] [PubMed]

48. Backhouse, T.; Bolliger, A. Transmission of Chagas' disease to the Australian marsupial *Trichosurus vulpecula*. *Trans. R. Soc. Trop. Med. Hyg.* **1952**, *44*, 521–533. [CrossRef]

49. Gascon, J.; Bern, C.; Pinazo, M.J. Chagas' disease in Spain, the United States and other non-endemic countries. *Acta Trop.* **2010**, *115*, 22–27. [CrossRef] [PubMed]

50. Schmunis, G.A.; Yadon, Z.E. Chagas' disease: A Latin American health problem becoming a world health problem. *Acta Trop.* **2010**, *115*, 14–21. [CrossRef] [PubMed]

51. Pickering, J.; Norris, C.A. New evidence concerning the extinction of the endemic murid *Rattus macleari* from Christmas Island, Indian Ocean. *Aust. Mammal.* **1996**, *19*, 19–25.

52. Wyatt, K.B.; Campos, P.F.; Gilbert, M.T.P.; Kolokotronis, S.O.; Hynes, W.H.; DeSalle, R.; Daszak, P.; MacPhee, R.D.E.; Greenwood, A.D. Historical mammal extinction on Christmas Island (Indian Ocean) correlates with introduced infectious disease. *PLoS ONE* **2008**, *3*, 1–9. [CrossRef] [PubMed]

53. Mackerras, M.J. The haematozoa of Australian mammals. *Aust. J. Zool.* **1959**, *7*, 105–135. [CrossRef]

54. Abbott, I. Mammalian faunal collapse in Western Australia, 1875–1925: The hypothesised role of epizootic disease and a conceptual model of its origin, introduction, transmission and spread. *Aust. Zool.* **2006**, *33*, 530–561. [CrossRef]

55. Pan, S.; Thompson, R.C.A.; Grigg, M.E.; Sundar, N.; Smith, A.; Lymbery, A.J. Western Australian marsupials are multiply infected with genetically diverse strains of *Toxoplasma gondii*. *PLoS ONE* **2012**, *7*, e45147. [CrossRef] [PubMed]

56. Hillman, A.E.; Lymbery, A.J.; Thompson, R.C.A. Is *Toxoplasma gondii* a threat to the conservation of free-ranging Australian marsupial populations? *Int. J. Parasitol. Parasites Wildl.* **2016**, *5*, 17–27. [CrossRef] [PubMed]

57. Thompson, R.C.A.; Lymbery, A.J.; Godfrey, S.S. Parasites at risk—insights from an endangered marsupial. *Trends Parasitol.* **2018**, *34*, 12–22. [CrossRef] [PubMed]

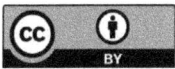

Tropical Medicine and Infectious Disease

MDPI

Article

A Survey of Intestinal Parasites of Domestic Dogs in Central Queensland

Simone Gillespie and Richard S. Bradbury *

School of Health, Medical and Applied Sciences, Central Queensland University,
North Rockhampton, QSD 4702, Australia; simone.gillespie17@hotmail.com
* Correspondence: r.bradbury@cqu.edu.au; Tel.: +1-404-718-1114

Received: 20 October 2017; Accepted: 17 November 2017; Published: 21 November 2017

Abstract: Australia has a very high rate of dog ownership, which in some circumstances may lead to exposure to zoonotic parasitic diseases from those companion animals. Domestic dog faecal samples ($n = 300$) were collected from public spaces and private property in the greater Rockhampton (Central Queensland) region and tested for intestinal helminths and protozoa by direct microscopy, two flotation methods and a modified acid-fast stain for cryptosporidia. Intestinal parasites detected included hookworms (25%), *Cystoisospora ohioensis* complex (9%), *Blastocystis hominis* (3%), *Giardia duodenalis* (3%), *Spirometra erinacei* (1%) and *Toxocara canis* (1%), *Sarcocystis* spp. (2%), *Cryptosporidium* spp. (2%) and *Cystoisospora canis* (1%). One infection each with *Trichuris vulpis*, *Dipylidium caninum* and a protozoa belonging to the *Entamoeba histolytica* complex were identified. Sheather's sucrose centrifugal flotation was more sensitive than saturated salt passive flotation, but no single test detected all cases of parasitic infection identified. The test methodologies employed are poor at recovering larva of *Strongyloides stercoralis*, *Aleurostrongylus abstrussis* and eggs of cestodes such as *Echinococcus granulosis*, so the potential presence of these parasites in Central Queensland domestic dogs cannot be excluded by this survey alone.

Keywords: dogs; canine; domestic; parasites; zoonoses; hookworm; Queensland; Australia

1. Introduction

Australia has one of the highest rates of pet ownership in the world, with 63% of households owning a pet. Dogs remain the most common companion animal, accounting for 39% of all domestic pets. It is estimated that there are 4.2 million pet dogs in Australia, correlating to 19 dogs for every 100 people [1]. The level of pet care in Australia is high, with strict legislations in place to ensure responsible pet ownership. One of the largest factors in pet ownership is parasitic infection control, which represents a major source of income for veterinarians around the country [1,2]. The close relationship between humans and their pet dogs can lead to transmission of intestinal parasitic diseases between these two species, with several parasites of dogs causing zoonotic infection in humans. Several broad surveys of domestic dog parasites have been conducted in Australia, but only one since the turn of the century. This national survey did not publish the data collected by state or climatic region [2]. No survey of all intestinal parasites of domestic dogs in an urban tropical Australia has been published until now.

Examples of zoonotic parasites reported in Australian domestic dogs that may lead to patent infection in humans following direct transmission include *Strongyloides stercoralis*, *Ancylostoma ceylanicum*, *Trichuris vulpis*, *Giardia duodenalis* and *Blastocystis hominis* [3–11]. Other parasites of domestic dogs may not reach patency in humans, but immature or larval stages have the capacity to cause significant disease in human hosts. The common dog hookworm, *Ancylostoma caninum*, may cause eosinophilic enteritis or cutaneous larva migrans in humans [3]. Visceral or ocular larva migrans disease caused by *Toxocara canis* may occur via ingestion of embryonated eggs from the environment [3].

Currently, there is limited information about the prevalence of canine gastrointestinal parasitic infections in regional and rural areas of Australia, particularly in the tropical North. The purpose of this study was to determine the prevalence and species of intestinal parasites in canines in Central Queensland, a regional and rural area within of the Tropic of Capricorn. The survey was conducted over a twelve-month period throughout the Greater Rockhampton region of Central Queensland (including Rockhampton city, Yeppoon, Cawarral, Gracemere and Emu Park areas), with a population living in both urban and rural residences. A total of 300 canine faecal samples were collected and analysed by microscopy for the presence of intestinal parasites.

2. Materials and Methods

2.1. Specimen Collection and Faecal Consistency Scoring

Specimen collection occurred once per week between January and October 2015, thereby including the end of the 2014/2015 wet season and the whole of the 2015 dry season. Fresh (based upon appearance and consistency) domestic dog (*Canis lupus familiaris*) faecal samples were collected and analysed from public spaces including parks, beaches and popular walking paths between 5 am and 9 am ($n = 174$). Residential area collections ($n = 120$) were performed with full consent and supervision from the property owner. Six samples were provided incidentally by a veterinary surgery at a time when the researchers were attending to collect ticks taken from animals for a separate study. These were all from domestic dogs held overnight for observation at the surgery. Prior to processing methods, the consistency of each sample was scored using the Purina Faecal Scoring System (Purina Faecal Scoring System for Dogs and Cats, Nestle-Purina Pet Food Co., St. Louis, MO, USA) and note of any mucous, blood, adult helminths or proglottids in the specimen was made.

2.2. Sample Processing and Direct Saline Preparation Microscopy

Gross faecal specimens were used to prepare a direct smear (12.5 mm × 25 mm in size) directly onto a glass microscope slide for later Kinyoun modified acid-fast staining. Samples were mixed with saline to form a slurry, then filtered through cotton gauze to remove larger particulate matter. A direct wet preparation was performed from this saline slurry, observing for the presence of parasitic elements and any motility of same. A portion of the slurry was then centrifuged in two 15 mL conical tubes. The centrifuged faecal deposit was corrected by removal of excess using wooden applicator sticks until the final volume of 1 mL was achieved (equivalent to 1 gram of faeces). Sheather's sucrose and salt flotation methods then performed upon sample in each of the respective conical centrifuge tubes.

2.3. Preparation of Sheather's Sucrose and Saturated Salt Solutions

Two flotation solutions were prepared in distilled water as described by Zajac et al. [12]. Briefly, Sheather's sucrose was prepared as 0.97 mol/L of sucrose (IGA, Canning Vale, Australia) in distilled water; the saturated salt solution was 6.0 mol/L NaCl (IGA, Canning Vale, Australia) in distilled water. The solutions were heated with a magnetic stirrer until completely dissolved. Mixtures were allowed to cool. 6 mL of 37% formaldehyde solution was added as a preservative to the Sheather's sucrose solution only.

The specific gravity of each batch was controlled using on a laboratory balance. An empty 15 mL plastic centrifuge tube was filled with exactly 2.0 mL of distilled water and weight checked as being 2.0 g. The same tube was then completely emptied and refilled with exactly 2.0 mL of Sheather's sucrose solution or saturated salt solution. The weights of these solutions were required to be within 2.54 ± 0.02 for Sheather's sucrose (S.G. 1.27) and 2.40 ± 0.02 for the saturated salt solution (S.G. 1.2) before use. Solutions were stored at room temperature until use.

2.4. Saturated Salt Passive Flotation Method

This method was performed as described by Zajac et al. [12]. Approximately 8 mL of saturated salt solution was added to 1 g of centrifuged faecal deposit in a 15 mL conical tube. The tube was then tightly capped and mixed vigorously to homogenise. The tube was then uncapped and placed upright in a test tube rack and topped up with the salt flotation solution to completely fill the test tube, ensuring that a slightly convex meniscus was formed. A 15 × 15 mm coverslip was placed over this meniscus, and the solution was allowed to stand for 15 min. Following this, the coverslip was carefully removed, ensuring that the drop of solution from the meniscus remained attached to the bottom of the coverslip.

2.5. Sheather's Sucrose Centrifugal Flotation Method

This method was performed as described by Zajac et al. [12], but with top-up of solution following centrifugation, despite a swing rotor centrifuge being employed. Approximately 8 mL of Sheather's sucrose solution was added to 1 g of centrifuged faecal deposit in a 15 mL conical tube. The tube was then tightly capped and mixed vigorously to homogenise. Tubes were then centrifuged at 500 g for two minutes. After centrifugation, the tubes were then uncapped and placed upright in a test tube rack, followed by topping up with Sheather's sucrose solution to completely fill the test tube, ensuring that a slightly convex meniscus was formed. A 15 mm × 15 mm coverslip was placed over this meniscus, and the solution was allowed to stand for 12 min. Following this, the coverslip was carefully removed, ensuring that the drop of solution from the meniscus remained attached to the bottom of the coverslip.

2.6. Kinyoun's Modified Acid-Fast Stain

For the staining and detection of *Cryptosporidium* oocysts, air-dried faecal smears were fixed in absolute methanol for 60 s. Slides were then flooded with Kinyoun's carbol fuchsin (Sigma-Aldrich, Darmstadt, Germany) for five minutes. Slides were briefly rinsed in 70% ethanol and then washed in tap water before de-staining with 1% acid alcohol (1 mL H_2SO_4, 99 mL ethanol) for two minutes. Slides were further washed in tap water before counterstaining with malachite green (Sigma-Aldrich, Darmstadt, Germany; 0.5 g in 100 mL distilled water) for 30 s, followed by washing in tap water and air drying.

2.7. Parasite Identification by Microscopy

The entire coverslip of the direct saline and each of the flotation preparations was placed on a microscope slide, and the entire slide was scanned at 100× and 400× magnification. The entire smears of Kinyoun's modified-acid fast-stained slides were examined at 1000× magnification, with *Cryptosporidium* oocysts identified by colour, size and distinctive morphology in the stain. Parasites were identified by size and characteristic morphology. For differentiation of the *Cystoisospora* species, *Cytoisospora canis* (size > 33 μm) was differentiated from species belonging to the *C. ohioensis* complex (size < 30 μm), based on the size of oocysts [13]. Each coverslip and Kinyoun-stained smear was examined separately by two trained morphologists (SG and RSB).

2.8. Statistical Analysis

Sample size was calculated based upon the hypergeometric distribution equation for sample size, based upon the assumption that the samples collected were random, and that no host was sampled more than once $[(1 - (1 - c)^{1/d})(N - (d/2)) + 1]$ as described by Cannon and Roe [14], where N is the population size, d is the number of infected hosts in the population, and c is the desired confidence level. The relative sensitivity and 95% confidence interval of each method employed was determined, using the combined results of each method as a reference standard. All statistical analyses were carried out in Microsoft Excel.

2.9. Ethical Approval

Ethical approval for this study was granted by the Animal Ethics Committee of Central Queensland University (approval number A15/01-325).

3. Results

3.1. Faecal Survey Results

A total of 300 canine faecal samples were collected between February and November 2015. This sample size allowed determination with 95% confidence that the prevalence of any intestinal parasite not found in our sample is at <1%, and 99% confidence that the prevalence of any parasite not recovered was <1% of the total population [14] of domestic dogs in the Greater Rockhampton region. Of these samples, 120 (40%) were positive for one or more gastrointestinal parasites; in 88 (29%) dogs, a single parasite species was identified; 27 (9%) had dual infection; and five (2%) were infected with three parasite species. Hookworm eggs were the most common parasitic element seen, being found in 24% of faecal samples analysed. Eggs of other helminths were observed only rarely; the *T. canis* or *T. vulpis* eggs detected were not larvated. The *C. ohioensis* complex was the most common protozoan parasite of domestic dogs, found in 9% of samples, while *G. duodenalis* and *B. hominis* were found in 3% of samples. Other protozoan parasites were at individual prevalences below 3% (Table 1).

3.2. Faecal Sample Consistency and Appearance

The majority (79%) of faecal specimens collected were of a healthy consistency (score 2–4); only 8% showed signs of diarrhoea (scores 5–6). No specimens collected were from dogs with watery diarrhoea (score 7). One faecal sample contained macroscopically visible mucous strands; this formed, but moist (score = 3) stool contained eggs of hookworms and cyst-like stages of *B. hominis*. Another single faecal samples had visible macroscopically visible blood; this loose and wet sample (score = 5) was found to harbour eggs of hookworm and cysts of *G. duodenalis*.

3.3. Spurious Parasites

Several samples contained mite eggs. Two samples contained eggs resembling those of *Ascaridia* spp., an ascarid intestinal helminth of birds. One sample contained eggs morphologically indistinguishable from those of *Syphacia muris*, an oxyurid intestinal helminth of rodents.

3.4. Comparison of Test Methodologies

The relative sensitivities and 95% confidence intervals for each test for hookworm were: direct saline preparation, 24% (15–35%); passive salt flotation, 83% (72–90%); and Sheather's sucrose centrifugal flotation, 91% (82–96%). For other parasite species, numbers did not reach a level at which a statistically valid test sensitivity could be achieved. No single method was ideal for the detection of *C. ohioensis* complex oocysts; in many cases, these were detected by one method and not by the other two, without any method being notably superior. There was a notable degree of variation in the sensitivity of each method employed for the detection of parasites. This was noticeable in the protozoa test results, particularly those for *C. ohioensis* complex and *B. hominis*, which were often detected in only one method, but no method seemed markedly superior in detection than another (Table 2). In four cases, *G. duodenalis* cysts were detected in the background malachite green stain of the Kinyoun *Cryptosporidium* stain and not by any other method.

Table 1. Faecal consistency and associated intestinal parasites detected in a survey of domestic dog faecal samples collected in the greater Rockhampton region of Central Queensland between February and November 2015.

	1 Hard and Dry		2 Formed but Soft		3 Formed but Moist		4 Formed and Wet		5 Semi-Formed and Wet		6 Loose and Wet		Overall Total		
	n	(%)	n	(%)	n	(%)	n	(%)	n	(%)	n	(%)	n	(%)	95% C.I.
Faecal samples	49	(16)	126	(42)	86	(29)	23	(8)	13	(4)	3	(1)	300	(100)	
Helminths													85	(28)	(23–33)
Hookworms	9	(19)	29	(23)	31	(36)	3	(13)	3	(2)	0		75	(25)	(20–30)
Spirometra erinacei	0		0		4	(5)	0		0		0		4	(1)	(0–3)
Toxocara canis	0		0		3	(3)	0		0		1	(33)	4	(1)	(0–3)
Trichuris vulpis	0		0		0		0		0		1	(33)	1	<1	(0–1)
Dipylidium caninum	0		0		1	(1)	0		0		0		1	<1	(0–1)
Protozoa													62	(21)	(16–26)
Cystoisospora ohioensis §	2	(4)	13	(10)	7	(8)	5	(22)	1		0		28	(9)	(6–13)
Blastocystis hominis	2	(4)	3	(2)	2	(2)	1	(4)	2	(15)	0		10	(3)	(1–5)
Giardia duodenalis	0		5	(4)	2	(2)	0		1	(8)	1	(33)	9	(3)	(1–5)
Sarcocystis spp.	0		5	(4)	1	(1)	0		0		0		6	(2)	(0–4)
Cryptosporidium spp.	0		2	(2)	1	(1)	1	(4)	1	(8)	0		5	(2)	(0–3)
Cystoisospora canis	1	(2)	1	(1)	1	(1)	0		0		0		3	(1)	(0–2)
Entamoeba histolytica §	0		1	(1)	0		0		0		0		1	<1	(0–2)
Parasites not seen	38	(78)	74	(59)	50	(58)	12	(52)	4	(31)	2	(67)	180	(60)	(54–66)

* Purina Faecal Scoring System for Dogs and Cats, Nestle-Purina Pet Food Co, St Louis, Mo. § These agents each represent a morphologically identical complex of species, *sensu stricto* species cannot be confirmed by morphology alone. C.I.: Confidence interval.

Table 2. Comparison of intestinal parasite detection by three test methodologies used in a survey of 300 domestic dog faecal samples collected in the greater Rockhampton region of Central Queensland between February and November 2015.

Results	Parasite Detected by Test Methodology			Comparison of Parasite Detection by Each Test Methodology			
	Saline Prep n (% of Total *)	Salt Float n (% of Total *)	Sheather's n (% of Total *)	Detected in Saline, but Not Salt Float	Detected in Saline, but Not Sheather's	Detected in Salt Float, but Not Sheather's	Detected in Sheather's, but Not Salt Float
Parasites Detected	**46** (**31**)	**93** (**63**)	**105** (**71**)	**22**	**16**	**24**	**39**
Helminths	**22** (26)	**70** (82)	**73** (86)	**5**	**1**	**10**	**15**
Hookworms	18 (24)	62 (83)	68 (91)	4	0	7	15
Spirometra erinacei	3 (75)	4 (100)	3 (75)	0	0	1	0
Toxocara canis	1 (25)	2 (50)	1 (25)	1	1	1	0
Trichuris vulpis	0 (0)	1 (100)	1 (100)	0	0	0	0
Dipylidium caninum	0 (0)	1 (100)	0 (0)	0	0	1	0
Protozoa	**24** (39)	**23** (37)	**32** (52)	**17**	**15**	**14**	**24**
Cytoisospora ohioensis §	15 (54)	7 (25)	17 (61)	13	11	7	17
Blastocystis hominis	2 (20)	5 (50)	6 (60)	0	2	3	4
Giardia duodenalis †	3 (33)	5 (56)	3 (33)	0	0	2	0
Sarcocystis spp.	0 (0)	6 (100)	4 (67)	0	0	2	2
Cytoisospora canis	3 (100)	0 (0)	1 (20)	3	2	0	0
Entamoeba histolytica §	1 (100)	0 (0)	1 (100)	1	0	0	1
No parasites identified	**254** (**141**)	**212** (**118**)	**195** (**108**)	**54**	**62**	**30**	**14**

* Total determined by a combined reference standard of all methods employed. § These agents each represent a morphologically identical complex of species, *Sensu stricto* species cannot be confirmed by morphology alone. † Four *Giardia duodenalis* were detected in background stain of Kinyoun acid fast-stained smears only. Saline: direct saline preparation method; Salt float: saturated salt passive flotation method; Sheather's: Sheather's sucrose centrifugal flotation method.

4. Discussion

There is a high prevalence of hookworm infection in domestic dogs in coastal Central Queensland. Compared to studies performed in southern temperate regions of Australia, which found hookworm prevalence ranging between 1.9% and 6.7% [2], the Greater Rockhampton region hookworm prevalence is unusually high. However, this reported prevalence is compatible with that found in comparable tropical and warm temperate regions, both in Australia and overseas [2,15–17]. Indeed, compared to previous studies of hookworm prevalence in Queensland, such as the 76.3% prevalence in domestic dogs found in 1973 [16] and more recent studies finding up to 100% prevalence in wild and domestic dogs in remote communities [5,18], the prevalence reported here is relatively moderate. The species of hookworms infecting dogs has an important impact on their risk and potential severity as zoonotic pathogens of humans. It is known that *A. caninum*, *A. braziliense* and *A. ceylanicum* may infect dogs in Queensland [18,19]. *A. ceylanicum* is of particular concern due to its demonstrated capacity to cause patent infections in humans in Australia [20]. *A. caninum* may also cause significant disease, with many cases of eosinophilic enteritis caused by this organism having previously been reported in Queensland [21]. Cutaneous larva migrans is a documented zoonoses occurring in Central Queensland [22], acquired by exposure of unprotected skin to the filariform larvae of *A. braziliense* and possibly also *A. caninum*. Without further molecular analysis to determine species, the degree and type of zoonotic disease risks presented by the high hookworm prevalence in domestic dogs in Rockhampton is unclear.

There was a low prevalence of *T. canis* and *T. vulpis* infection. The fact that the eggs seen were morulated, rather than embryonated, demonstrates that these were true infections, rather than egg passage following coprophagy. A risk of visceral or ocular migrans exists from *T. canis* and rarely, infections with *T. vulpis* in humans have been documented [7–9]. Given the low prevalence of these two helminths in Central Queensland dogs, the risk of such human infections is low in this region. However, to further minimise risk, it is advisable that specific hygiene practices are followed by dog owners. Attention to the removal and safe disposal of domestic dog faeces, to avoid contamination of the immediate environment with viable eggs, hand washing to reduce the risk of faecal-oral exposure to eggs and regular deworming of domestic dogs, are all suggested as activities reducing the risk of *Toxocara* larva migrans [3], and will be effective in reducing the risk of zoonotic infections from domestic dogs more generally.

Although *G. duodenalis* was the most prevalent intestinal parasite of dogs in some studies in southern, temperate regions of Australia [2], its prevalence in the dogs we tested was only 3%. This also represents a lower percentage prevalence than those previously reported Australian studies, which have been between 7.7% and 30.7% [2]. *G. duodenalis* may infect both humans and dogs; this species has several genetic assemblages (A–G) that are quite host specific [23]. Only two assemblages, A and B, have been found to infect humans in Australia [20,24]. Studies of the genetic assemblages of *Giardia* in Australian dogs have found that almost all were assemblages C or D, with the single assemblage A infection, considered to be a possible anthroponosis [24]. Therefore, the presence of *G. duodenalis* cysts and trophozoites in the faeces of companion animal dogs presents little or no zoonotic risk to the owners or others.

Cryptosporidium oocysts were found in the faeces of several dogs in this study. Based on the findings of a previous Australian study, it may reasonably be assumed that the majority of these are *Cryptosporidium canis* [24]. Although occasional reports do exist of transmission of *C. canis* from dogs to humans [25], given the high level of exposure to this agent from domestic dogs, such cases are quite rare and present only a very limited zoonotic risk. As an example, a study of 2414 human cases of cryptosporidiosis in the United Kingdom found only 0.04% attributable to *C. canis* [26].

One *E. histolytica* complex cyst was observed in the faeces of a dog in this study. *E. histolytica* infection has previously been reported from both dogs and humans [27] and may cause significant intestinal disease in both species. The *E. histolytica* complex includes five morphologically identical species of amoeba, of which only *E. histolytica* sensu stricto causes dysentery. Without PCR analysis, the exact species recovered here cannot be determined.

Cysts of *C. ohioensis* and *C. canis* were recovered from a number of dogs. Although there is no documented zoonotic risk from these coccidia, ingestion of the oocysts may lead to the formation of persistent monozoic tissue cysts in paratenic hosts. Canine *Cystoisospora* are capable of forming such cysts in human cell culture lines [28]. However, this does not necessarily reflect a capacity to form persistent cysts in the tissues of immunocompetent humans, as host immunity plays an important role in parasite biology. Regardless, the potential for such cysts to form in humans, especially in those who are severely immunocompromised or immunosuppressed, cannot be entirely excluded.

A number of specimens examined contained spurious parasites. The finding of *Ascaridia*-like and *S. muris*-like eggs in dog faeces at first seems exceptional, given that dogs are not hosts for these animals. However, such findings are not unusual, representing passage of eggs consumed with the definitive host by the dogs concerned. These dogs are simply passing eggs without any infection being established following meals of definitive host birds (chickens, turkeys, pigeons, some parrots) for the *Ascaridia* or rodents (rats and mice) for *S. muris*. These findings highlight the potential confounding effect of coprophagy on faecal examinations among dogs [29]. Similarly, mite eggs were seen in a number of the samples tested in this study. These are often seen in parasite screens of dog faeces. These eggs closely resemble those of hookworm, but may be differentiated by observing size, as most mite eggs are larger than those of hookworm (>65 μm) and also by examining the embryo, in which developing mite legs may be observed, rather than the development of a hookworm larva.

Methodological limitations were present in this study. The absence of watery samples (Purina Faecal Scoring System score = 7) may be attributed to the fact that the samples used in this study were collected from parks and yards, where such watery samples would seep into the ground and be unobtainable. This may have biased our results away from parasites that may cause watery diarrhoea, such as the *Cryptosporidium* spp. The detection of *G. duodenalis* is best performed by the use of permanently stained slides; not having employed such slides may have reduced the number of *Giardia* infections identified. The absence of larva of *S. stercoralis* and *Aleurostrongylus abstrussis* is attributable to both the flotation methodology employed and the low faecal larval output in both infections. The minimal amounts of faeces examined in the initial wet-preparation microscopy is insufficient to detect infections with these agents and the larvae do not float in saturated salt solution or Sheather's sucrose and thus would not have been seen in the microscopy. Overall parasite detection, for both helminths and protozoa, was best using the Sheather's sucrose centrifugal flotation method. Previous studies have determined slightly improved recovery with centrifugal flotation compared to passive flotation in zinc sulphate and Sheather's sucrose solutions [30,31], although neither method detected all infections when compared to necropsy [31]. Further comparison of each flotation solution used in this study by both passive and centrifugal flotation is warranted. Therefore, the absence of these in the findings of this study should not be interpreted as their absence from the Greater Rockhampton region. Other helminth infections, specifically trematode and cestode, that produce eggs of a higher specific gravity than the flotation solutions will not have been detected by this study. Our detection of cestode infections is likely a gross underestimate, based on the methodology employed. Previous work showing that Sheather's sucrose centrifugal flotation methods only detected 6.3% of *D. caninum* infections detected on necropsy [31]. Recovery of *Taenia* sp. was similarly poor at 57.3% by centrifugal flotation and 14.3% by passive flotation [31]. This is particularly important in the case of our non-detection of *Echinococcus granulosis*, an extremely pathogenic zoonotic parasite from dogs. The eggs of this species have a specific gravity too high (S.G. = 1.3−1.4) to easily float in the solutions used, and the sensitivity of the methods employed here range between only 3% and 33% for detection of this parasite [32]. Therefore, the results of this study should under no circumstances be interpreted as suggesting that there is no risk for hydatid disease from domestic dogs in Central Queensland. Sampling of dog scats in parks and other public places may have led to a bias towards collections from adult dogs, as smaller puppies are often not walked by owners for the first few months of life. Parasitic infections more prevalent in puppies might have been detected at higher prevalence, had a deliberate stratified age sampling approach been employed.

5. Conclusions

Hookworm infection of domestic dogs in the greater Rockhampton region of Central Queensland is common, but not inconsistent with previous studies in tropical urban environments. A limited zoonotic risk exists from domestic dogs in this region, but this cannot be fully determined without further molecular identification of the species recovered. Of the methods employed in this study, Sheather's sucrose centrifugal flotation is the overall most effective method for the recovery of canine intestinal parasites, but no single method detected all infections. The use of flotation and direct saline preparation methodologies means that accurate estimates of the prevalence of *S. stercoralis*, *A. abstrussis*, as well as many trematodes and cestodes, including *E. granulosis*, in Central Queensland cannot be inferred based on the results of this study alone.

Acknowledgments: The authors would like to acknowledge the assistance of Chyna Williams and Tanja Jovic in sample collection and laboratory work towards this study. We also thank Sarah Sapp, of the University of Georgia, who provided very helpful comments on the draft manuscript.

Author Contributions: R.S.B. conceived and designed the experiments; S.G. and R.S.B. performed the experiments; S.G. and R.S.B. analysed the data; R.S.B. wrote the paper; S.G. provided input into paper drafts. Richard Bradbury wrote this paper in his personal capacity and in his capacity as an adjunct academic at Central Queensland University.

Conflicts of Interest: The authors declare no conflict of interest.

Dedication: This work is dedicated to the memory of Emeritus Professor Rick Speare. As both a Vet and a Medical Doctor, Rick was always involved in parasitology, zoonotic disease and 'One Health' research such as the work presented here. We hope that he would feel this paper to be suitable contribution to this edition of *Tropical Medicine and Infectious Diseases* in honour of the great and generous man that Rick was. He is sorely missed in his passing.

References

1. Animal Health Alliance. *Pet Ownership in Australia Summary 2013*; Animal Health Alliance (Australia) Ltd.: Canberra, Australia, 2013.
2. Palmer, C.S.; Thompson, R.A.; Traub, R.J.; Rees, R.; Robertson, I.D. National study of the gastrointestinal parasites of dogs and cats in Australia. *J. Vet. Parasitol.* **2008**, *151*, 181–190. [CrossRef] [PubMed]
3. Robertson, I.D.; Thompson, R.C. Enteric parasitic zoonoses of domesticated dogs and cats. *Microbes Infect.* **2002**, *4*, 867–873. [CrossRef]
4. Jaleta, T.G.; Zhou, S.; Bemm, F.M.; Schär, F.; Khieu, V.; Muth, S.; Odermatt, P.; Lok, J.B.; Streit, A. Different but overlapping populations of *Strongyloides stercoralis* in dogs and humans—Dogs as a possible source for zoonotic strongyloidiasis. *PLoS Negl. Trop. Dis.* **2017**, *11*, e0005752. [CrossRef] [PubMed]
5. Smout, F.A.; Skerratt, L.F.; Butler, J.R.A.; Johnson, C.N.; Congdon, B.C.; Thompson, R.C.A. The hookworm *Ancylostoma ceylanicum*: An emerging public health risk in Australian tropical rainforests and Indigenous communities. *One Health* **2017**, *3*, 66–69. [CrossRef] [PubMed]
6. Smout, F.; Schrieber, L.; Speare, R.; Skerratt, L.F. More bark than bite: Comparative studies are needed to determine the importance of canine zoonoses in Aboriginal communities. A critical review of published research. *Zoonoses Public Health* **2017**, *64*, 495–504. [CrossRef] [PubMed]
7. Areekul, P.; Putaporntip, C.; Pattanawong, U.; Jongwutiwes, S. *Trichuris vulpis* and *T. trichiura* infections among schoolchildren of a rural community in northwestern Thailand: The possible role of dogs in disease transmission. *Asian Biomed.* **2010**, *4*, 49–60.
8. Dunn, J.J.; Columbus, S.T.; Aldeen, W.E.; Davis, M.; Carroll, K.C. *Trichuris vulpis* recovered from a patient with chronic diarrhea and five dogs. *J. Clin. Microbiol.* **2002**, *40*, 2703–2704. [CrossRef] [PubMed]
9. George, S.; Geldhof, P.; Albonico, M.; Ame, S.M.; Bethony, J.M.; Engels, D.; Mekonnen, Z.; Montresor, A.; Hem, S.; Tchuem-Tchuenté, L.A.; et al. The molecular speciation of soil-transmitted helminth eggs collected from schoolchildren across six endemic countries. *Trans. R. Soc. Trop. Med. Hyg.* **2016**, *110*, 657–663.
10. Gordon, C.; Kursheid, J.; Jones, M.; Gray, D.; McManus, D. Soil-transmitted helminths in Tropical Australia and Asia. *Trop. Med. Infect. Dis.* **2017**, *2*, 56. [CrossRef]

11. Roberts, T.; Stark, D.; Harkness, J.; Ellis, J. Subtype distribution of *Blastocystis* isolates from a variety of animals from New South Wales, Australia. *Vet. Parasitol.* **2013**, *196*, 85–89. [CrossRef] [PubMed]
12. Zajac, A.M.; Conboy, G.A. *Veterinary Clinical Parasitology*, 8th ed.; John Wiley & Sons: Blacksburg, VA, USA, 2012; pp. 5–8.
13. Houk, A.E.; O'connor, T.; Pena, H.F.; Gennari, S.M.; Zajac, A.M.; Lindsay, D.S. experimentally induced clinical *Cystoisospora canis* coccidiosis in dogs with prior natural patent *Cystoisospora ohioensis*–like or *C. canis* infections. *J. Parasitol.* **2013**, *99*, 892–895. [CrossRef] [PubMed]
14. Cannon, R.M.; Roe, R.T. *Livestock Disease Surveys: A Field Manual for Veterinarians*; Australian Bureau of Animal Health: Canberra, Australia, 1982.
15. Katagiri, S.; Oliveira-Sequeira, T.C. Prevalence of dog intestinal parasites and risk perception of zoonotic infection by dog owners in Sao Paulo State, Brazil. *Zoonoses Public Health* **2008**, *55*, 406–413. [CrossRef] [PubMed]
16. Setsuban, P.; Waddell, H. Hookworms in cats and dogs in Queensland. *Aust. Vet. J.* **1973**, *49*, 110. [CrossRef]
17. Palmer, C.S.; Traub, R.J.; Robertson, I.D.; Hobbs, R.P.; Elliot, A.; While, L.; Rees, R.; Thompson, R.A. The veterinary and public health significance of hookworm in dogs and cats in Australia and the status of *A. ceylanicum*. *Vet. Parasitol.* **2007**, *145*, 304–313. [CrossRef] [PubMed]
18. Smout, F.A.; Thompson, R.A.; Skerratt, L.F. First report of *Ancylostoma ceylanicum* in wild canids. *Int. J. Parasitol. Parasites Wildl.* **2013**, *2*, 173–177. [CrossRef] [PubMed]
19. Traub, R.J.; Hobbs, R.P.; Adams, P.J.; Behnke, J.M.; Harris, P.D.; Thompson, R.C. A case of mistaken identity—Reappraisal of the species of canid and felid hookworms (*Ancylostoma*) present in Australia and India. *Parasitology* **2007**, *134*, 113–119. [CrossRef] [PubMed]
20. Koehler, A.V.; Bradbury, R.S.; Stevens, M.A.; Haydon, S.R.; Jex, A.R.; Gasser, R.B. Genetic characterization of selected parasites from people with histories of gastrointestinal disorders using a mutation scanning-coupled approach. *Electrophoresis* **2013**, *34*, 1720–1728. [CrossRef] [PubMed]
21. Walker, N.I.; Croese, J.; Clouston, A.D.; Loukas, A.; Prociv, P. Eosinophilic enteritis in northeastern Australia: pathology, association with *Ancylostoma caninum*, and implications. *Am. J. Surg. Pathol.* **1995**, *19*, 328–337. [CrossRef] [PubMed]
22. Lord, R.J. Cutaneous Larva Migrans in Central Queensland. Master's Thesis, Central Queensland University, North Rockhampton, Australia, 1997.
23. Monis, P.T.; Andrews, R.H.; Mayrhofer, G.; Ey, P.L. Genetic diversity within the morphological species *Giardia duodenalis* and its relationship to host origin. *Infect. Genet. Evol.* **2003**, *3*, 29–38. [CrossRef]
24. Palmer, C.S.; Traub, R.J.; Robertson, I.D.; Devlin, G.; Rees, R.; Thompson, R.A. Determining the zoonotic significance of *Giardia* and *Cryptosporidium* in Australian dogs and cats. *Vet. Parasitol.* **2008**, *154*, 142–147. [CrossRef] [PubMed]
25. Xiao, L.; Cama, V.A.; Cabrera, L.; Ortega, Y.; Pearson, J.; Gilman, R.H. Possible transmission of *Cryptosporidium canis* among children and a dog in a household. *J. Clin. Microbiol.* **2007**, *45*, 2014–2016. [CrossRef] [PubMed]
26. Leoni, F.; Amar, C.; Nichols, G.; Pedraza-Diaz, S.; McLauchlin, J. Genetic analysis of *Cryptosporidium* from 2414 humans with diarrhoea in England between 1985 and 2000. *J. Med. Microbiol.* **2006**, *55*, 703–707. [CrossRef] [PubMed]
27. Morcos, Z. *Entamoeba histolytica* in dogs. *J. Egypt. Med. Assoc.* **1936**, *19*, 63–64. [CrossRef]
28. Lindsay, D.S.; Houk, A.E.; Mitchell, S.M.; Dubey, J.P. Developmental biology of *Cystoisospora* (Apicomplexa: Sarcocystidae) monozoic tissue cysts. *J. Parasitol.* **2014**, *100*, 392–398. [CrossRef] [PubMed]
29. Nijsse, R.; Mughini-Gras, L.; Wagenaar, J.A.; Ploeger, H.W. Coprophagy in dogs interferes in the diagnosis of parasitic infections by faecal examination. *Vet. Parasitol.* **2014**, *204*, 304–309. [CrossRef] [PubMed]
30. Zajac, A.M.; Johnson, J.; King, S.E. Evaluation of the importance of centrifugation as a component of zinc sulfate fecal flotation examinations. *J. Am. Anim. Hosp. Assoc.* **2002**, *38*, 221–224. [CrossRef] [PubMed]
31. Adolph, C.; Barnett, S.; Beall, M.; Drake, J.; Elsemore, D.; Thomas, J.; Little, S. Diagnostic strategies to reveal covert infections with intestinal helminths in dogs. *Vet. Parasitol.* **2017**, *247*, 108–112. [CrossRef] [PubMed]
32. Széll, Z.; Sréter-Lancz, Z.; Sréter, T. Evaluation of faecal flotation methods followed by species-specific PCR for detection of *Echinococcus multilocularis* in the definitive hosts. *Acta Parasitol.* **2014**, *59*, 331–336. [CrossRef] [PubMed]

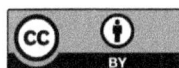

Tropical Medicine and
Infectious Disease

MDPI

Article

Hospitalizations and Deaths Associated with Diarrhea and Respiratory Diseases among Children Aged 0–5 Years in a Referral Hospital of Mauritania

Mohamed Lemine Cheikh Brahim Ahmed [1,2,3,*], Abdellahi Weddih [4], Mohammed Benhafid [2], Mohamed Abdellahi Bollahi [3,4], Mariem Sidatt [4], Khattry Makhalla [4], Ali H. Mokdad [5], Jorg Heukelbach [6,7] and Abdelkarim Filali-Maltouf [1]

[1] Department of Biology, University Mohammed V, Rabat 10010, Morocco; filalimaltouf@gmail.com
[2] Department of Virology, National Institute of Hygiene, Rabat 10010, Morocco; benhafidm@yahoo.fr
[3] Institut National de Recherche en Santé Publique (INRSP), Nouakchott 2373, Mauritania; boullahi01@gmail.com
[4] Ministry of Health and University of Nouakchott, Department of Pediatrics, Nouakchott 2373, Mauritania; aoueddih@gmail.com (A.W.); mariemsi@hotmail.fr (M.S.); drkhattry2006@yahoo.fr (K.M.)
[5] Institute for Health Metrics and Evaluation, University of Washington, Seattle, WD 98195, USA; mokdaa@uw.edu
[6] Department of Community Health, School of Medicine, Federal University of Ceará, Fortaleza CE60430-140, Brazil; heukelbach@web.de
[7] College of Public Health, Medical and Veterinary Sciences, Division of Tropical Health and Medicine, James Cook University, Townville, QLD 4810, Australia
* Correspondence: lemine1987@hotmail.fr; Tel.: +222-46-60-60-51

Received: 29 July 2018; Accepted: 11 September 2018; Published: 17 September 2018

Abstract: Diarrhea and respiratory diseases are the leading causes of morbidity and mortality among <5-year-olds worldwide, but systematic data are not available from Mauritania. We conducted a hospital-based retrospective study. Data on admissions to Mauritania's National Referral Hospital (the main pediatric referral center in the country), due to diarrhea and respiratory diseases, during 2011–2014, were analyzed. A total of 3695 children <5 years were hospitalized during this period; 665 (18.0%) due to respiratory diseases, and 829 (22.4%) due to diarrhea. Case fatality rates in the respiratory diseases and diarrhea groups were 18.0% (120/665) and 14.1% (117/829), respectively. The highest frequency of deaths due to diarrhea occurred in the age group 2–5 years (16/76; 21.0%), and due to respiratory diseases in the age group 6–12 months (32/141; 22.6%). We conclude that case fatality rates caused by respiratory diseases and diarrhea are extremely high in children hospitalized at the National Referral Hospital. These data call for intensified efforts to reduce deaths among hospitalized Mauritanian children, and also for integrated control measures to prevent and reduce the burden of both diseases. Additional studies are needed to show the effectiveness of the introduction of vaccination programs for pneumococcal diseases and rotavirus infection in the child population, which were launched in November 2013 and December 2014, respectively.

Keywords: respiratory diseases; diarrhea; hospitalizations; children; Mauritania; deaths

1. Introduction

Diarrhea and respiratory diseases are the leading causes of morbidity and mortality among children under five years of age, over the world [1,2]. Despite the decline in the burden of diarrhea and respiratory diseases since 2005, they still pose a major public health burden [3]. Both of these infectious diseases have always been in the 10 top causes of deaths among children, especially in low- and middle-income countries [4]. Globally, rotavirus and *Streptococcus pneumoniae* are the most common causes of severe diarrhea and respiratory infections in children, contributing to 28% and 18% of diarrhea cases and respiratory infections, respectively [2,5]. Given the high morbidity and mortality of diseases caused by these pathogens, the World Health Organization (WHO) recommended vaccination with rotavirus and pneumococcal conjugate vaccines (PCV13) [6,7].

Mauritania is an Arabic–African country, located between North and West Africa, on the Atlantic Ocean. It has a population of approximately 3.5 million and more than one-third of the population lives in Nouakchott territory [8]. The number of children aged 0–5 years was estimated to be 17% of the general population in 2015 [9]. In the Arabic region, including Mauritania, respiratory diseases and diarrhea account for about 50% of all post-neonatal deaths [10].

The Global Burden of Diseases study estimated that, in Mauritania, mortality from diarrhea was 10.5% (95% CI: 7.6%–14.4%) and that from respiratory disease was 12.8% (9.4%–17.1%) of the total deaths, among children <5 years [3]. From 2005 to 2016, the mortality associated with these diseases in the country decreased by 33.5% and 12.2%, respectively. In spite of this decrease, respiratory diseases are still the second leading cause of deaths [3]. Diarrhea also remains the third leading cause of deaths among children aged 0–5 years. The death rate per 100,000 was estimated at 110.3 in 1990, 85 in 2005 and 50.2 in 2016 [3].

There are no systematic baseline data available on the burden of diarrhea and respiratory diseases among children aged 0–5 years, in Mauritania. The aim of this study was to identify the proportion and case fatality rates of diarrhea and respiratory diseases in children of age 0–5 years, who have been hospitalized during 2011–2014, at the largest pediatric referral hospital in Mauritania.

2. Materials and Methods

2.1. Setting

The study was performed in Nouakchott territory, which represents 1/3 of Mauritania population, at the National Referral Hospital—the main pediatric referral hospital in Mauritania. The hospital was constructed in 1966 with more than 450 beds. It was the first and largest tertiary hospital in Mauritania and aimed to receive severely-ill patients, transferred from any health facilities throughout the country. The pediatric services at this hospital have a capacity of about 100 beds with 1000–1500 hospitalizations annually, and receive about 300–500 high-risk children, transferred annually from outside of Nouakchott, to be admitted to this hospital.

2.2. Inclusion Criteria and Variables

We conducted a retrospective study based on analyses of the registries of pediatric admissions to the hospital. All hospitalizations of children aged 0–5 years due to respiratory diseases or diarrhea, from 1 January 2011 to 31 December 2014, were included. We aimed to describe the status before effective implementation of the vaccination programs, whose significant effects were expected to start after this period. Case definitions are presented in Table 1.

Table 1. Case definitions of diarrhea and respiratory diseases used for data abstraction (ICD-10 codes).

Diarrhea	Respiratory Diseases
Non-infectious gastroenteritis (K52)	Pneumonia, bronchopneumonia, pneumonitis, acute respiratory infection (J18; J13; J15; J22)
Infectious gastroenteritis (A09)	Bronchitis, acute respiratory distress syndrome, asthma (J06; J20; J22; J80)

Data available included age, sex, admission and discharge dates, diagnosis on admission and discharge, and outcome (deceased, discharged). If the patient had a diagnosis of both diarrhea and respiratory diseases, we recorded it as both cases, but hospitalization was counted only once.

2.3. Data Analysis

Data were entered into Microsoft Office Excel 2007 spreadsheets, checked for entry-related errors and analyzed using Statistical Package for the Social Sciences (SPSS, version 22) (IBM, SPSS Inc., Chicago, IL, USA). Death and discharge rates were calculated based on the total number of hospitalizations in the corresponding diagnostic groups. Statistical significance of differences between groups was evaluated by the chi-squared test.

3. Results

3.1. General Characteristics

From 1 January 2011 to 31 December 2014, a total of 3695 children aged 0–5 years was hospitalized. Children aged 0–5 months accounted for 38%, those aged 0–11 months for 50.4%, and those aged 0–23 months for 73.4% of all hospitalized children. Most children were living in Nouakchott territory (81.9%), while those transferred from other regions accounted for 18.1%. Vaccination cards were complete and up-to-date in 55% of cases, incomplete in 35% of cases, and absent or not clear in 10%.

From these hospitalizations, 665 (18.0%) were admitted due to respiratory diseases, and 829 (22.4%) due to diarrhea (Table 2). The highest relative frequency of hospitalizations that occurred in <6-month-olds were 47.0% for respiratory diseases, and 31.9% for diarrhea. A total of 68% of all hospitalizations were treated with an antibiotic. Infectious gastroenteritis accounted for 65% of diarrheal diseases, and 78% of respiratory diseases were related to bronchopneumonia.

Table 2. Characteristics of children admitted due to diarrhea and/or respiratory diseases (*n* = 1494).

Characteristics	Diarrhea n (%)	Respiratory Diseases n (%)	Total n (%)
Sex:			
Male	347 (41.8)	296 (44.5)	643 (43)
Female	482 (58.2)	369 (55.5)	851(57)
Age:			
<6 months	264 (31.8)	312 (46.9)	576 (38.6)
6 months <1 year	258 (31.2)	141 (21.2)	399 (26.7)
1 year <2 years	231 (27.8)	109 (16.4)	340 (22.7)
2 years <5 years	76 (9.2)	103 (15.5)	179 (12)
Year of admission:			
2011	203 (24.7)	166 (24.9)	369 (24.7)
2012	207 (24.9)	165 (24.8)	372 (24.9)
2013	258 (28.2)	163 (24.5)	421 (28.2)
2014	161 (22.2)	171 (25.7)	332 (22.2)
Total	829 (55.4)	665 (44.6)	1494 (100)

There was no clear seasonal pattern of diarrhea, with the exception of a prominent peak in August 2013 (*n* = 69; Figure 1a). The frequency of cases of respiratory diseases varied, throughout the years and months, without any clear seasonal patterns (Figure 1b). The highest number of respiratory cases was observed in January 2011 (*n* = 36).

(a)

(b)

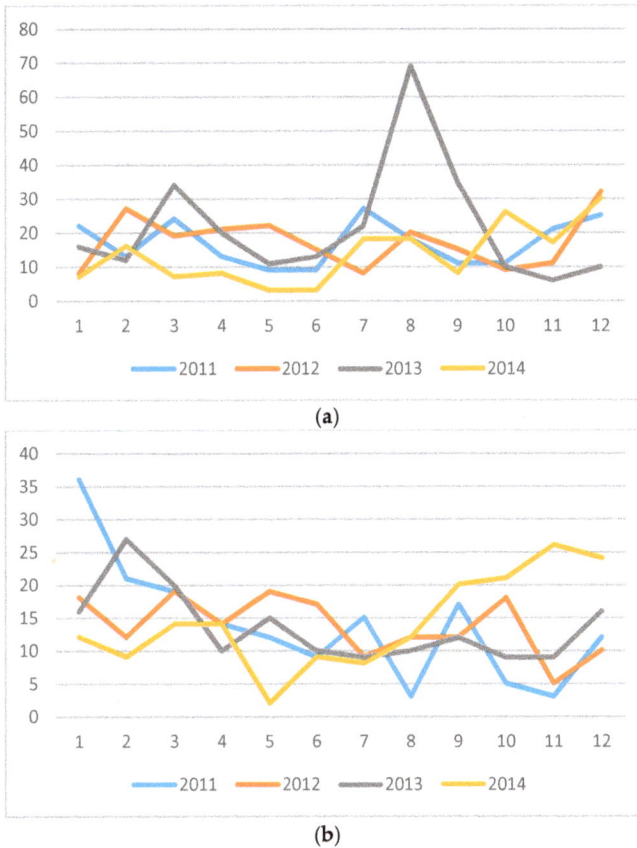

Figure 1. (**a**) Monthly variation of cases of diarrhea, stratified by year. X-axis: months of the year; y-axis: absolute number of cases. (**b**) Monthly variation of cases of respiratory diseases, stratified by year. X-axis: months of the year; y-axis: absolute number of cases.

3.2. Outcomes and Associated Factors

About 1/7 of the hospitalized children with diarrhea or respiratory diseases died (Table 3). Case fatality rates were similarly high for both groups (Table 3). The highest frequency of deaths after admission due to diarrhea occurred in the <6-month-olds (15.9%) and in the >2-year-olds (21.0%, Table 4). The case fatality rates due to respiratory disease were highest in infants, with 19.5% in <6-month-olds, and 22.6% in 6–11-month-olds. (Table 4).

Table 3. Outcome of diarrhea and respiratory diseases and the average of hospitalization periods in children <5 years of age.

Outcome	Diarrhea *n* (%)	Respiratory Diseases *n* (%)
Discharge	712 (85.9)	545 (81.9)
Death	117 (14.1)	120 (18.1)
Average length of stay in days (mean and SD)	5.28 (4.36)	5.66 (4.86)

Table 4. Case fatality rates due to diarrhea and respiratory diseases, stratified by sex, age and year of submission.

Variable	Diarrhea Deaths n (%)	p Value	Respiratory Diseases Deaths n (%)	p Value
Sex:				
Male	44/347 (12.6)		60/296 (20.2)	
Female	73/482 (15.1)	0.35	60/369 (16.2)	0.16
Age:				
<6 months	42/264 (15.9)		61/312 (19.5)	
6 months <1 year	30/258 (11.6)		32/141 (22.6)	
1 year <2 years	29/231 (12.5)		15/109 (13.7)	
2 years <5 years	16/76 (21.0)	0.74	12/103 (11.6)	0.049
Year of submission:				
2011	22/203 (10.8)		33/166 (19.8)	
2012	41/207 (19.8)		33/165 (20.0)	
2013	39/258 (15.1)		31/163 (19.0)	
2014	15/161 (9.3)	0.58	23/171 (13.4)	0.15

Table 4 presents case fatality rates due to both diarrhea and respiratory diseases, stratified by age, sex and year of submission. Case fatality rates were slightly, but not significantly, higher in females, in the diarrhea group, and slightly higher in males, in the respiratory disease group. There was a considerable decrease in case fatality rates in both groups in the year 2014, as compared to the previous years.

4. Discussion

To the best of our knowledge, this is the first systematic, hospital-based study on the burden of diarrhea and respiratory diseases among hospitalized children in Mauritania. Our study was conducted in the highest populated city in Mauritania. The data show that both diseases were important causes for hospitalization, and that they caused extremely high case-fatality rates, in the child population. These results are in line with previous studies that have shown that diarrhea and respiratory diseases contribute to a high morbidity and mortality among pediatric patients in developing countries [2,11–13].

At the time of this study, there was only one referral hospital in the country, particularly in Nouakchott city, with poor quality of care services, in addition to poor general hygiene conditions in the city. Being a referral center, the hospital receives the most complicated cases from all different regions of the country, annually. These factors may explain the extremely high case fatality rates in pediatric patients hospitalized with diarrhea and respiratory diseases. In fact, according to a study conducted in 2012, 2150 people, including 1700 children less than five years of age, die each year from diarrhea in Mauritania, and 90% of these deaths are directly attributable to the poor quality of water, sanitation, and hygiene [14]. In addition, many patients present to the health system after a relatively high time lapse since the start of symptoms, as a result of difficult access to the health system, and also a low awareness of the urgency of these conditions, in the child population.

Despite the progress made by the government in order to reduce the morbidity and case fatality of both diarrhea and respiratory diseases, such as the promotion of effective interventions and the improvement of available treatment and vaccines, the Ministry of Health of Mauritania still lists respiratory diseases and diarrhea as the first and second leading causes of death, respectively, among children aged 0–5 years [15]. The Ministry of Health of Mauritania officially introduced pneumococcal vaccine (PCV13) in November 2013 and rotavirus vaccine (Rotarix) in December 2014. As our study mostly covers the period before the effective introduction of these vaccine programs, and some time is needed until the effect can be observed on a population level, additional studies are needed to show the effect of these interventions on child health in the country. In addition, two new hospitals were inaugurated in Nouakchott, in 2013, with a possible positive effect on health outcomes.

Of the 55% of cases in which a vaccination card was available, 60% were vaccinated with PCV13 by December 2014. The decrease in the number of hospitalizations due to respiratory diseases in 2014, as compared to the previous years (as was observed in our study), might already indicate the first effect of PCV13 vaccine introduction in 2013 in Mauritania. However, it could also be expected that the most significant effects of vaccination programs will only be observed after the study period. In fact, in other countries, a significant reduction of morbidity and mortality has been reported after the introduction of vaccine programs. For example, in South Africa, pneumococcal vaccination programs contributed to a reduction of 69% of the incidence of invasive pneumococcal disease [7]. In Mexico, rotavirus vaccine contributed to a 38% reduction in diarrhea associated with hospitalization [16], and a 50% reduction in diarrhea associated with death [17].

The number of hospitalizations due to diarrheal diseases in the <6-month-olds were the highest among all age groups. In contrast, the highest frequency of hospitalization due to respiratory diseases was among children aged 6–11 months. This finding may further indicate that the introduction of rotavirus vaccine (at age of 6 and 10 weeks) and PCV13 vaccine (at age of 6, 10 and 14 weeks) will have a major impact in reducing the burden of diarrhea and respiratory diseases. Our results were supported by other findings that reported the highest number of hospitalizations was among children aged 0–11 months, in other countries [1,2,18,19]. These two age groups were also the most common age groups hospitalized for a long period, with a minimum of two days of stay at the hospital.

The majority of hospitalizations in our study were for females (57%), and diarrhea-associated deaths were also higher among them, similar to a previous study from Bangladesh [20]. On the other hand, respiratory disease-associated deaths were more common in males than females (20% vs. 16%). This finding is supported by previous studies from low, middle and high-income countries that reported the occurrence of respiratory diseases to be more frequent in males than females [21–23]. However, the differences found in our study were not statistically significant, and it is difficult to speculate on reasons for these sex differences based on the nature of the study design.

We did not observe any clear seasonal patterns for either of the diseases, as climatic conditions are similar throughout the year, with the exception of rainfall that almost exclusively occurs in July, August, and September. Singular peaks during different months throughout the years as observed in our study indicate outbreaks, such as a diarrhea outbreak during the rainy season in 2013, especially in Brakna region, with the majority of cases being transferred to the National Hospital in Nouakchott. However, the etiological agent of this outbreak was not known, and the event was only rudimentarily documented in the lay media [24].

Our study was subject to limitations. The analysis of secondary hospital data might present inconsistencies in quantity (such as missing information) and quality (such as diagnostic errors). In addition, the number of variables to be analyzed was limited. Despite these limitations, the analyzed data can be considered as consistent, as they are derived from a single source, and are based on standardized procedures, within the National Referral Hospital, which did not change throughout the study period. As the hospital was the unique referral hospital nationwide, during the study period, data may be considered representative for hospitalized children in the country. However, as this was not a population-based study, we were unable to calculate any hospitalization or incidence rates. We also could not directly conclude on the epidemiological situation of the diseases, under study, in the country. This is because access to the health system is not equal and the rural areas are especially underserved. Therefore, children may have presented at a late stage of the disease with a considerably increased risk of death, and others may have died on their long way to the hospital. As laboratory testing for diarrhea and pneumonia is not provided on a routine basis in Mauritania, and as the study was performed without any funding, information on pathogens was not available.

Difficult access to health facilities and to effective treatment remains a major hindrance to prevention and treatment of childhood diseases. The quality of healthcare services still suffers from

Trop. Med. Infect. Dis. **2018**, *3*, 103

some drawbacks, and many children are treated outside health facilities. Primary healthcare facilities are insufficient. Recent studies conducted in Nouakchott reported that less than 44% of children were taken to a healthcare facility, and only 26% of households had access to safe drinking water sources, while 70% of the population had access to improved latrines [9,14]. The situation in rural areas is even worse.

5. Conclusions

Our study demonstrated that diarrhea and respiratory diseases accounted for a high number of hospitalizations and deaths among children aged 0–5 years in Mauritania's main referral hospital. These findings call for intensified efforts, and specific programs and policies, to improve vaccination coverage, access to resources of safe water, intensify health education, and improve access to and quality of healthcare, in order to control and reduce the morbidity and mortality caused by respiratory diseases and diarrhea in children. Clinicians should be alert to early diagnosis and to prevent complications and death. Future studies are needed to show the effectiveness of the introduction of vaccination programs for pneumococcal diseases and rotavirus infection in the child population, since 2013.

Author Contributions: M.L.C.B.A. and J.H. analyzed and interpreted the results, drafted the manuscript, and critically revised the manuscript. A.W., K.M., M.A.B. and M.S. contributed to the conceptualization of the study, obtained the data and interpreted the results. A.H.M., M.B. and A.F.-M. interpreted the results and critically revised the manuscript. All authors read and approved the final manuscript.

Funding: This research received no external funding.

Acknowledgments: The authors thank all staff members of the pediatric service at the National Referral Hospital for their help with data abstraction. We appreciate the useful contribution of Hama Cheikh/Bellamachand JH for language editing. J.H. is a class 1 research fellow at the Brazilian National Council for Scientific and Technological Development (CNPq).

Conflicts of Interest: The authors declare no conflicts of interest.

References

1. Walker, C.L.F.; Rudan, I.; Liu, L.; Nair, H.; Theodoratou, E.; Bhutta, Z.A.; O'Brien, K.L.; Campbell, H.; Black, R.E. Global burden of childhood pneumonia and diarrhoea. *Lancet* **2013**, *381*, 1405–1416. [CrossRef]
2. Vinekar, K; Schaad, N.; Ber-Lucien, M.A.; Leshem, E.; Oboho, I.K.; Joseph, G.; Juin, S.; Dawood, F.S.; Parashar, U.; Katz, M.A.; et al. Hospitalizations and deaths because of respiratory and diarrheal diseases among Haitian children under five years of age, 2011–2013. *Pediatr. Infect. Dis. J.* **2015**, *34*, e238–e243. [CrossRef] [PubMed]
3. Global Burden of Disease Collaborative Network, Study 2016 Results (GBD 2016). Available online: http://ghdx.healthdata.org/gbd-results-tool/result/6be59e68f0af0a790a5560a10503a421 (accessed on 27 March 2018).
4. Bagherian, H.; Farahbaksh, M.; Rabiei, R.; Moghaddasi, H.; Asadi, F. National communicable disease surveillance system: A review on information and organizational structures in developed countries. *Acta Inform. Med.* **2017**, *25*, 271–276. [CrossRef] [PubMed]
5. Smok, B.; Zieniewicz-Cieślik, K.; Smukalska, E.; Pawłowska, M. Acute diarrhoea induced by rotavirus in children hospitalised in provincial hospital for infectious diseases in Bydgoszcz in 2014 year. *Przegl Epidemiol.* **2016**, *70*, 462–470. [PubMed]
6. UNICEF/WHO. Diarrhea: Why Children Are Still Dying and What Can Be Done. Available online: http://www.who.int/maternal_child_adolescent/documents/9789241598415/en/ (accessed on 25 February 2018).
7. Von Gottberg, A.; De Gouveia, L.; Tempia, S.; Quan, V.; Meiring, S.; Von Mollendorf, C.; Madhi, S.A.; Zell, E.R.; Verani, J.R.; O'Brien, K.L.; et al. Effects of vaccination on invasive pneumococcal disease in South Africa. *New Engl. J. Med.* **2014**, *371*, 1889–1899. [CrossRef] [PubMed]
8. Africa BBC. Mauritania Profile Timeline. Available online: https://www.bbc.co.uk/news/world-africa-13882166 (accessed on 19 February 2018).

9. UNICEF. Enquête par Grappes à Indicateurs Multiples (MICS). Available online: https://www.unicef.org/french/statistics/index_24302.html (accessed on 20 January 2018).

10. Akseer, N.; Kamali, M.; Husain, S.; Mirza, M.; Bakhache, N.; Bhutta, Z.A. Strategies to avert preventable mortality among mothers and children in the Eastern Mediterranean Region: New initiatives, new hope. *East. Mediterr. Health J.* **2015**, *21*, 361–373. [CrossRef] [PubMed]

11. Malek, M.A.; Teleb, N.; Abu-Elyazeed, R.; Riddle, M.S.; Sherif, M.E.; Steele, A.D.; Glass, R.I.; Bresee, J.S. The epidemiology of rotavirus diarrhea in countries in the Eastern Mediterranean Region. *J. Infect. Dis.* **2010**, *202*, S12–S22. [CrossRef] [PubMed]

12. Al-Badani, A.; Al-Areqi, L.; Majily, A.; AL-Sallami, S.; AL-Madhagi, A.; Amood, A.K. Rotavirus diarrhea among children in Taiz, Yemen: Prevalence—risk factors and detection of genotypes. *Int. J. Pediatr.* **2014**, *2014*, 928529. [CrossRef] [PubMed]

13. Nech, M.A.; Sejad, M.O.A.; Dahdi, S.A. Le cancer du poumon à Nouakchott. Expérience du service de pneumologie. *Rev. Mal. Respir.* **2012**, *29*, A145. [CrossRef]

14. Sy, I.; Traoré, D.; Diène, A.N.; Koné, B.; Lô, B.; Faye, O.; Utzinger, J.; Cissé, G.; Tanner, M. Eau potable, assainissement et risque de maladies diarrhéiques dans la Communauté Urbaine de Nouakchott, Mauritanie. *Santé Publique* **2017**, *29*, 741–750. [CrossRef] [PubMed]

15. WHO. OMS Stratégie de Coopération: Un Aperçu: Mauritanie. Available online: http://apps.who.int/iris/handle/10665/136942 (accessed on 26 July 2018).

16. Esparza-Aguilar, M.; Gastañaduy, P.A.; Sánchez-Uribe, E.; Desai, R.; Parashar, U.D.; Richardson, V.; Patel, M. Diarrhoea-related hospitalizations in children before and after implementation of monovalent rotavirus vaccination in Mexico. *Bull. World Health Organ.* **2013**, *92*, 117–125. [CrossRef] [PubMed]

17. Gastañaduy, P.A.; Sánchez-Uribe, E.; Esparza-Aguilar, M.; Desai, R.; Parashar, U.D.; Patel, M.; Richardson, V. Effect of rotavirus vaccine on diarrhea mortality in different socioeconomic regions of Mexico. *Pediatrics* **2013**, *131*, e1115–e1120. [CrossRef] [PubMed]

18. Andrews, J.R.; Leung, D.T.; Ahmed, S.; Malek, M.A.; Ahmed, D.; Begum, Y.A.; Qadri, F.; Ahmed, T.; Faruque, A.S.G.; Nelson, E.J. Determinants of severe dehydration from diarrheal disease at hospital presentation: Evidence from 22 years of admissions in Bangladesh. *PLoS Negl. Trop. Dis.* **2017**, *11*, e0005512. [CrossRef] [PubMed]

19. Khoury, H.; Ogilvie, I.; El-Khoury, A.C.; Duan, Y.; Goetghebeur, M.M. Burden of rotavirus gastroenteritis in the Middle Eastern and North African pediatric population. *BMC Infect. Dis.* **2011**, *11*, 9. [CrossRef] [PubMed]

20. Mitra, A.K.; Rahman, M.M.; Fuchs, G.J. Risk factors and gender differentials for death among children hospitalized with diarrhoea in Bangladesh. *J. Health Popul. Nutr.* **2000**, *18*, 151–156. [PubMed]

21. Nagayama, Y.; Tsubaki, T.; Nakayama, S.; Sawada, K.; Taguchi, K.; Tateno, N.; Toba, T. Gender analysis in acute bronchiolitis due to respiratory syncytial virus. *Pediatr. Allergy Immunol.* **2006**, *17*, 29–36. [CrossRef] [PubMed]

22. Falagas, M.E.; Mourtzoukou, E.G.; Vardakas, K.Z. Sex differences in the incidence and severity of respiratory tract infections. *Respir. Med.* **2007**, *101*, 1845–1863. [CrossRef] [PubMed]

23. Jensen-Fangel, S.; Mohey, R.; Johnsen, S.P.; Andersen, P.L.; Sørensen, H.T.; Østergaard, L. Gender differences in hospitalization rates for respiratory tract infections in Danish youth. *Scand. J. Infect. Dis.* **2004**, *36*, 31–36. [CrossRef] [PubMed]

24. Mauritanie: Des cas de Diarrhée Accompagnée de Vomissements, Recensés au Brakna. Available online: http://cridem.org/C_Info.php?article=647060 (accessed on 30 August 2018).

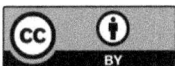

Tropical Medicine and
Infectious Disease

MDPI

Article

Diagnostic Performance of Kato Katz Technique and Point-of-Care Circulating Cathodic Antigen Rapid Test in Diagnosing *Schistosoma mansoni* Infection in HIV-1 Co-Infected Adults on the Shoreline of Lake Victoria, Tanzania

Humphrey D. Mazigo [1,*] and Jorg Heukelbach [2,3]

1   Department of Medical Parasitology, School of Medicine, Catholic University of Health and Allied Sciences, P.O. Box 1464, Mwanza, Tanzania
2   Department of Community Health, School of Medicine, Federal University of Ceará, Fortaleza CE 60430-140, Brazil; heukelbach@web.de
3   College of Public Health, Medical and Veterinary Sciences, Division of Tropical Health and Medicine, James Cook University, Townsville 4811, Queensland, Australia
*   Correspondence: humphreymazigo@gmail.com; Tel.: +255-78-606-0067

Received: 7 May 2018; Accepted: 22 May 2018; Published: 29 May 2018

Abstract: Background: The diagnostic performance of the Kato Katz (KK) technique and the point-of-care circulating cathodic antigen (POC-CCA) test in detecting *S. mansoni* infection in the presence of the human immunodeficiency virus-1 (HIV-1) infection has remained inconclusive. The present cross-sectional survey compared the diagnostic performance of the KK technique and the POC-CCA test in diagnosing *S. mansoni* infection in an adult population co-infected with HIV-1 in northwestern Tanzania. Methods: Single urine and stool samples from 979 adults were screened for *S. mansoni* infection using both the KK technique and POC-CCA tests. To compare the performance of the two diagnostic tests a combined artificial gold standard was created, based on either an egg-positive KK technique or a POC-CCA-positive test. Results: Based on the KK technique, the prevalence of *S. mansoni* was 47.3% (463/979, 95% CI: 44.2–50.4), as compared to 60.5% by the POC-CCA test (592/979; 95% CI: 57.4–63.5). The overall sensitivity and specificity of the POC-CCA test were 92.5% (95% CI: 89.4–94.9) and 73.3% (95% CI: 69.6–76.8), respectively. In the HIV-1 seropositive group, the sensitivity and specificity of the POC-CCA test were 78.1% (95% CI: 60.0–90.7) and 45.9% (95% CI: 35.8–56.3). Using a combined gold standard, the sensitivity of the POC-CCA test increased to >90% in both subgroups whereas that of the KK technique in the HIV-1 seropositive group was low (49.5%; 95% CI: 39.6–59.5). Conclusion: In the presence of HIV-1 co-infection, the KK technique attained a very low sensitivity. The POC-CCA test offers the best option for the rapid screening of *S. mansoni* infection in communities with a high prevalence of HIV-1 infection.

Keywords: *Schistosoma mansoni*; HIV-1; point-of-care circulating cathodic antigen; sensitivity; specificity; adult; Tanzania

---

1. Introduction

Intestinal schistosomiasis caused by *Schistosoma mansoni* remains one of the Neglected Tropical Diseases that is highly endemic in communities living along the shorelines of Lake Victoria in northwestern Tanzania [1,2]. The disease affects individuals of all age groups in these communities, with extremely high infection intensity [3–5].

Traditionally, the estimation of prevalence and intensity of *S. mansoni* infection in endemic areas is done using the Kato Katz (KK) technique [6]. The KK technique is regarded as a gold standard for diagnosis [6]. In addition, the KK technique provides quantitative information on egg intensity as an indicator of host helminth burden [6]. The technique is highly sensitive in areas with high endemicity levels, but less sensitive in areas where communities have light to moderate intensity of infection [7]. KK technique sensitivity can be increased by repeating stool samples to be collected and tested over consecutive days [7]. This adds more cost to the control programs and may also result in the withdrawal of study participants [7]. Moreover, the use of this technique for post-praziquantel treatment monitoring can lead to an overestimation of the effects of treatment [7].

In the past two decades, human immunodeficiency virus-1 (HIV-1) infection has been recognized as an important confounding factor in the parasitological diagnosis of *S. mansoni* infection using the KK technique [8–11]. In HIV-1/*S. mansoni* co-infected individuals, the excretion efficiency of *S. mansoni* eggs is reduced, with more eggs retained in the body [8,12]. Excretion of *S. mansoni* eggs from an infected individual is a function of the immune system determined by $CD4^+$ Th_2 type levels [11]. HIV-1 kills $CD4^+$ Th_2 cells, which may affect the excretion efficiencies of *S. mansoni* eggs; this in turn affects the sensitivity of the KK technique [11]. One study reported reduced *S. mansoni* egg excretion in HIV/*S. mansoni* co-infected individuals in western Kenya [11]. This has significant implications on the parasitological diagnosis of *S. mansoni* infection using the KK technique [11,13], especially in adult individuals likely to be co-infected with HIV-1 [10]. This can lead to a misclassification or missed diagnosis in individuals with light to moderate intensity. In addition, individuals co-infected with HIV-1 infection are likely to retain *S. mansoni* eggs in their bodies, which can lead to development of severe hepatosplenic morbidities [14].

To overcome these challenges, a point-of-care circulating cathodic antigen (POC-CCA) test that detects *S. mansoni* antigen released by live adult worms in the urine samples of infected individuals has been developed [15,16]. The test has been widely scrutinized [17] and has shown to have a higher sensitivity than the KK technique [7,16–21]. A single POC-CCA test has been shown to be more sensitive than six KK thick smears [7]. However, the performance of the KK technique and POC-CCA test in detecting *S. mansoni* infection in the presence of HIV-1 infection has remained inconclusive. The present survey was designed to compare the performance (sensitivity and specificity) of the KK technique and the POC-CCA test in diagnosing *S. mansoni* infection in the adult population either co-infected or not with HIV-1 in northwestern Tanzania.

2. Materials and Methods

2.1. Study Area

The study was performed at Sangabuye, Kayenze, Igalagala, and Igombe, four villages located at the southern shore of Lake Victoria, in the Ilemela district (32–34° E and 2–4° S), Mwanza region, northwestern Tanzania [10,22]. These are fishing villages highly endemic for *S. mansoni* infection [4]. A high proportion of adult individuals is co-infected with HIV-1 [10]. In these communities, Lake Victoria is the main source of water for domestic and economic use, such as washing, cooking, and fishing. Mass drug administration of praziquantel is focused on schoolchildren [1].

2.2. Study Design, Sample Size, Sampling Procedure, and Inclusion Criteria

This was a nested data analysis based on a cross-sectional study conducted between September and December 2012 [10,14,22]. It included all individuals aged 15–55 years living in the selected villages, with no history of praziquantel use in the past six months and no antiretroviral therapy for those who were diagnosed with HIV-1 infection. Participants were randomly selected from randomly-selected households. The sample included in the study and the selection criteria for the study participants have previously been described by Mazigo et al. (2014) [10].

If selected individuals declined to participate or were not present at the household after multiple attempts, a new member of the household was randomly selected. For households that remained vacant after multiple visits, a neighboring household was selected.

2.3. Data Collection

2.3.1. Questionnaire

A pre-tested questionnaire was used to collect the participant's demographic information, history of praziquantel drug use, previous HIV-1 testing, and the outcome and history of the antiretroviral treatment.

2.3.2. Human Immunodeficiency Virus-1 Screening

Testing for HIV-1 infection followed national guidelines, which require participants to be counselled by a qualified nurse. By the time of this study, the Tanzanian algorithm for HIV testing recommended the use of the qualitative rapid tests, Determine® and UN-Gold® [23]. In all identified HIV-1-positive participants, venous blood samples were obtained for CD4⁺ analysis by FACSCalibur machine.

2.3.3. Parasitological Screening for *Schistosoma mansoni* Infection

A single stool sample was collected in a labeled container from each participant. Four thick KK smears were prepared following standard procedures [6] using a template of 41.7 mg (Vestergaard Frandsen, Lausanne, Switzerland). The prepared KK slides were independently examined after 24 h for the presence of *S. mansoni* eggs, and the eggs were counted and recorded. To avoid inter-observer bias, all the slides were examined by one experienced microscopist. For quality control, 10% of the negative and positive slides were re-examined by a reference technician.

2.3.4. Circulating Cathodic Antigen Test

A single urine sample was collected in a labeled container from each participant and examined for the presence of the circulating cathodic antigen (CCA) using the POC-CCA tests following the manufacturer's instructions (Rapid Medical Diagnostic- http://www.rapid-diagnostics.com/) [16]. Trace results were considered as positive. All laboratory technicians involved in CCA testing were blinded for the KK parasitological and HIV-1 results of the study participants.

2.4. Data Analysis

A Microsoft Excel spreadsheet was used for double data entry, and data analysis was performed using Stata Version 15 (StataCorp, 2017, Stata statistical software: release 15. StataCorp LP, College Station, TX, USA). Numbers and percentages were used to describe categorical variables. A comparison of either proportions or categorical variables was done using chi-squared (χ^2) or Fisher exact tests, where appropriate. For continuous variables, descriptive statistics were reported as means with standard deviation for normally distributed variables and medians with interquartile ranges (IQR) for variables that were not normally distributed.

The prevalences of *S. mansoni* infection based on KK technique and POC-CCA test and their 95% confidence intervals (CI) were calculated using binomial regression, controlling for the village of residence. The arithmetic mean of the *S. mansoni* egg counts for each participant was calculated from the counts of four KK thick smears and multiplied by 24 to obtain individual eggs per gram of feces. *S. mansoni* egg counts were logarithmically transformed to check for normality but only non-transformed means are presented. Mean egg counts for *S. mansoni* between sex and age were compared using Student t-test (two groups) or ANOVA (more than two groups). The intensity of infection was categorized according to WHO criteria, with 1–99 eggs per gram of feces (epg), 100–399 epg, ≥400 epg defined as low, moderate, and heavy intensities of infection, respectively [24].

Understanding the limitation of the KK technique in diagnosing *S. mansoni* infection [25], we constructed an artificial gold standard based on either the KK technique or POC-CCA positivity [26]. Thus, sensitivity, specificity, positive and negative predictive values of the POC-CCA test were calculated using two gold standards: (1) egg-positive by KK technique (as a reference standard for the diagnosis of *S. mansoni* infection); and (2) combined gold standard (infection-positive by either KK technique or POC-CCA-positivity [26]. The sensitivity of the POC-CCA test was calculated using egg-detection (KK technique) as reference standard for diagnosis of *S. mansoni* infection. Specificity, i.e., the percentage of negative individuals correctly identified as such, was calculated as described in [27] and sensitivity was calculated as a percentage of positive individuals correctly identified by the test [27]. In addition, a positive predictive value (PPV = proportion of positive test results that are truly positive) and negative predictive value (NPV = proportion of negative test results that are truly negative) are presented [27].

The sensitivity, specificity, positive and negative predictive values, positive and negative likelihood ratios of the KK and POC-CCA tests using a combined gold standard with their 95% CI were determined using the *diagt* or *diagti* command in Stata 15 (StataCorp, 2017, Stata statistical software: release 15. StataCorp LP, College Station, TX, USA), against the gold standard as described above [27]. The performance agreement between the two diagnostic tests was evaluated using Kappa statistics with their 95% CI for each of the sub-study population (i.e., general population, HIV-1 negative, HIV-1 positive). The Kappa values were interpreted according to previous classifications by Landis and Koch [28].

2.5. Ethical Considerations

Ethical approval was sought from the joint Ethical and Review Committee of Bugando Medical Centre and Catholic University of Health and Allied Sciences. The study received further ethical approval from the National Ethical Review Committee, National Institute for Medical Research, Tanzania. The study received further permission from the district administrative and division authorities. Kiswahili translated informed consent forms were used to obtain participants' consent to participate in the study and assent for those who were aged 15–<18 years. Written informed consent was obtained from guardians/parents of all participants aged 15–<18 years. For illiterate participants, a thumb print was used to sign the consent/assent forms after a clear description of the study objectives was given to them. To maintain confidentiality, all the demographic and other clinical data of the study participants were kept in a closed cabinet and whenever the data were accessed no participant names were disclosed; only the identification number was used to identify a participant. All study participants infected with *S. mansoni* were treated with praziquantel (40 mg/kg) according to WHO guidelines [24].

3. Results

3.1. Characterization of Study Population

A total of 979 study participants aged 15–55 years was included in the study. Of these, 45.8% and 54.2% were male and female, respectively (Table 1). The overall mean age was 33.2 ± 10.7 years. Age categories and sex of the study participants are shown in Table 1. Other characteristics of the study participants have been described in detail previously [10,14].

Table 1. Demographic characteristics of the study participants from four villages, Ilemela district, north-western Tanzania.

Sex	Age Groups (Years)					Total
	15–20 N (%)	21–30 N (%)	31–40 N (%)	41–50 N (%)	51–55 N (%)	
Female	82 (63.1)	179(54.4)	146(50.7)	86(57.7)	38(45.8)	531(54.2)
Male	48(36.9)	150(45.6)	142(49.3)	63(42.3)	45(54.2)	448(45.8)
Total	130	329	288	149	83	979

3.2. Prevalence of HIV-1 Infection

The overall prevalence of HIV-1 infection was 13.3% (130/979, 95% CI: 11.3–15.6). Female participants had the higher prevalence, as compared to male participants (16% vs. 10%, $p < 0.01$). The age groups >20 years had the highest HIV-1 seropositivity, as compared to the youngest age groups ($p < 0.01$); 31–40 year-olds had the highest prevalence (16.7%).

3.3. Prevalence and Intensity of Schistosoma mansoni Infection

Table 2 shows the prevalence of *S. mansoni* infection in relation to the demographic characteristics of the study participants and HIV-1 serostatus, and by the diagnostic method. Based on the KK technique, the overall prevalence of *S. mansoni* was 47.3% (463/979, 95% CI: 44.2–50.4), as compared to 60.5% by POC-CCA test (592/979; 95% CI: 57.4–63.5).

In both the KK technique and POC-CCA test, males had a significantly higher prevalence than females (Table 2). Similarly, significant age differences in the prevalence of *S. mansoni* infections were noted, with the youngest age group (15–20 years) having the highest prevalence (Table 2).

The overall geometrical mean eggs per gram (GMepg) of feces was 173.75 epg (95% CI: 151.5–199.3). Male participants had the highest GMepg as compared to female participants (219.1 GMepg vs. 132.1 GMepg, $t = 5.3349$, $p < 0.0001$). There was a significant difference in GMepg between age groups ($p = 0.001$), with the youngest age group having the highest GMepg (277.2, 95% CI: 196.4–391.3).

Of the 130 HIV-1-seropositive individuals, 40% (52/130) had detectable *S. mansoni* eggs in their stool samples, whereas 75.4% (98/130) were identified as infected, based on the POC-CCA test (Table 2). On the other side, in the HIV-1-negative population, the prevalences were 48.4% and 58.2%, based on the KK technique and POC-CCA test, respectively.

Table 2. Prevalence of *S.mansoni* infection based on Kato Katz technique and point-of-care circulating cathodic antigen test, stratified by sex, age and HIV-1 infection status.

Variable		N	KK Technique n (%)	*p*-Value	POC-CCA Test n (%)	*p*-Value
Sex	Female	531	212(39.9)	$p < 0.01$	293(55.2)	$p < 0.01$
	Male	448	251(56.1)		299(66.7)	
Age group (years)	15–20	130	81 (62.3)	$p < 0.01$	99(79.1)	$p < 0.01$
	21–30	329	171(51.9)		217(65.9)	
	31–40	288	122(42.4)		161(55.9)	
	41–50	149	56(37.6)		68(45.6)	
	51–60	83	33(39.8)		47(56.6)	
HIV-1 serostatus	Positive	130	52(40.0)	0.07	98(75.4)	$p < 0.01$
	Negative	849	411(48.4)		494(58.2)	
Intensity of *S. mansoni* infection (epg)	1–99	195	195(42.1)	n/a	174(89.2)	$p < 0.02$
	100–399	126	126(27.2)		122(96.8)	
	≥400	142	142(40.7)		138(97.2)	
Overall		979				

3.4. Diagnostic Performance of Kato Katz Technique and Point-of-Care Circulating Cathodic Antigen Test

In the general population, among 621 individuals diagnosed positive with either diagnostic method, 158 (25.4%) individuals were missed by the KK technique, whereas only 29 (4.7%) individuals were missed by the POC-CCA technique (Table 3). In the HIV-1-seronegative group, 105 (20.3%) of 516 individuals that tested positive in either test were missed by the KK technique and only 22 (4.3%) by POC-CCA test (Table 3). In the HIV-seropositive group, the relative frequency of missed diagnosis by the KK technique was highest—53/105 (50.5%) individuals were missed by the KK technique, as compared to 7/105 (6.7%) by the POC-CCA test (Table 3). Considering the intensity of infection in Table 2, the POC-CCA test missed 10.8%, 3.2% and 2.8% of individuals who had low, moderate, and heavy intensity of infection.

Table 3. Diagnostic performance of the point-of-care circulating cathodic antigen and the Kato-Katz technique for the diagnosis of *Schistosoma mansoni* infection in an adult population co-infected or not with HIV-1 infection.

Sub-Population	Diagnostic Test		KK Technique		Total
			Positive	Negative	
General population	POC-CCA	Positive	434	158	592
		Negative	29	358	387
	Total		463	516	979
HIV-1-seronegative	POC-CCA	Positive	389	105	494
		Negative	22	333	355
	Total		411	438	849
HIV-1-seropositive	POC-CCA	Positive	45	53	98
		Negative	7	25	32
	Total		52	78	130

KK-Kato Katz technique, POC-CCA-Point-of-care circulating cathodic antigen test.

3.5. Sensitivity and Specificity of Point-of-Care Circulating Cathodic Antigen Test

3.5.1. Using Kato Katz as a Gold Standard Technique

The overall sensitivity and specificity of the POC-CCA test using the KK technique as a gold standard technique in the general population were 92.5% and 73.3%, respectively (Table 4). In relation to HV-1 serostatus, for the HIV-1-seronegative group, the sensitivity of POC-CCA test was 93.8% and specificity was 78.7% (Table 4). For the HIV-1-seropositive group, the sensitivity and specificity were 78.1% and 45.9%, respectively (Table 4). There was a significant substantial agreement between the two tests in the general population (Kappa = 0.62, agreement = 80.9%, $p < 0.001$) and in the HIV-1-seronegative group (Kappa = 0.70, agreement = 85%, $p < 0.001$). However, a significant poor agreement between the two tests was observed in the HIV-1-seropositive group (Kappa = 0.16, agreement = 53.9%, $p < 0.001$).

3.5.2. Using Combined Gold Standard

In the general population, the sensitivity of the POC-CCA test using a combined gold standard was 95.3% (95% CI: 93.4–96.9). For the HIV-1-seronegative group, the sensitivity of POC-CCA test was 95.7%. In the HIV-1-seropositive group, the sensitivity was 93.3%. The positive and negative predictive values for the general population and HIV-1-seropositive group are shown in Table 4.

3.5.3. Sensitivity of the Kato Katz Technique Using Combined Gold Standard

The sensitivity of the KK technique using the combined gold standard was 74.6% (95% CI: 70.9–77.9) in the general population, Table 5. In relation to HIV-1 serostatus, for the HIV-1-seronegative and -seropositive groups, the sensitivities were 79.7% and 49.5%. For the HIV-1-infected group, sensitivity was 49.5% (95% CI: 39.6–59.5). The positive and negative predictive values of the KK technique both in the general and HIV-1 seropositive group are shown in Table 5.

Table 4. Sensitivity and specificity of point-of-care circulating cathodic antigen test using the Kato Katz technique and a combined gold standard in sub-populations of study participants.

Sub-Population	Sensitivity % (95% CI)	Specificity % (95% CI)	Positive Predictive Values % (95% CI)	Negative Predictive Values % (95% CI)	Kappa Statistics
		Using Kato Katz technique as a gold standard			
General population	92.5% (89.4–94.9)	73.3% (69.6–76.8)	69.4% (65.2–73.3)	93.7% (91.1–95.8)	0.62
HIV-1-seronegative	93.8% (90.8–96.1)	78.7% (74.9–82.3)	76% (71.7–80.0)	94.6% (92.0–96.6)	0.70
HIV-1-seropositive	78.1% (60.0–90.7)	45.9% (35.8–56.3)	32.1% (21.9–43.6)	86.5% (74.2–94.4)	0.16
		Using combined gold standard			
In general population	95.3% (93.4–96.9)	100% (99.0–100.0)	100% (99.4–100.0)	92.5% (89.4–94.9)	—
HIV-1-seronegative	95.7%	100%	100% (99.3–100.0)	93.8% (90.8–96.1)	—
HIV-1-seropositive	93.3% (86.7–97.3)	100% (86.3–100.0)	100% (96.3–100.0)	78.1% (60.0–90.7)	—

Table 5. Sensitivity and specificity of the Kato Katz technique using a combined gold standard in a sub-population of study participants.

Sub-Population	Sensitivity % (95% CI)	Specificity % (95% CI)	Positive Predictive Values % (95% CI)	Negative Predictive Values % (95% CI)
General population	74.6% (70.9–77.9)	100% (99.0–100.0)	100% (99.2–100.0)	69.4% (65.2–73.3)
HIV-1-seronegative	79.7% (75.9–83.0)	100% (98.9–100.0)	100% (99.1–100.0)	76% (71.7–80.0)
HIV-1-seropositive	49.5% (39.6–59.5)	100% (93.2–100.0)	100% (93.2–100.0)	32.1% (21.9–43.6)

4. Discussion

The main findings from this study indicate that the POC-CCA test is more sensitive than the parasitological KK technique in detecting *S. mansoni* infection among the general study population, specifically in the HIV-1/*S. mansoni* co-infected population. The sensitivity of the KK technique is relatively low, especially in the HIV-positive subpopulation, and the number of adult individuals detected with *S. mansoni* infection by the POC-CCA test was considerably higher than those detected using four KK thick smears. These results have implications for diagnostic methods to be used in mass screening programs in similar settings, especially among adult individuals.

Many studies in sub-Saharan Africa have recorded similar findings [17,19–21]. The performance of the POC-CCA test is influenced by the baseline intensity of *S. mansoni* infection [7]. The high sensitivity of the test is achieved in areas with a high intensity of infection [7] and in areas with a low intensity of *S. mansoni* infection, low test sensitivity has been reported [29]. In our study, the performance of the POC-CCA test was mainly influenced by the intensity of *S. mansoni* infection, and the majority of individuals with a low intensity of infection were missed by the test. The test missed very few individuals who had a moderate or heavy intensity of infection. Previous studies have demonstrated a positive relationship between the intensity of *S. mansoni* infection and positivity of the POC-CCA test [30,31]. We noted a low specificity of POC-CCA test and this partly is explained by the low sensitivities of the KK technique [7].

The use of the KK technique as a gold standard in evaluating the performance of other diagnostic tests has its limitations [6,25]. Thus, we developed an artificial gold standard, as previously described by Midzi et al. (2009) [26], to compare the diagnostic performance of the KK technique and POC-CCA test. Using the combined gold standard, the sensitivity of the POC-CCA test both in general and in the HIV-1 seropositive group improved markedly to >90%. The observed sensitivity was higher than that of the KK technique both in the general population and in the HIV-1-seropositive subgroup. Given the fact that adult individuals in *S. mansoni*-endemic areas are likely to carry a low intensity of infection and co-infections with HIV-1 affect the performance of the parasitological technique [9,11], the use of alternative diagnostic tests such as the POC-CCA test is highly recommended in the adult population.

Using the combined gold standard, the KK technique recorded very low sensitivity in the HIV-seropositive subpopulation, which was below 50%. Partly, reduced egg excretion efficiencies caused by the HIV-1 infection may explain the poor performance of the KK technique in the co-infected adult individuals [9–11,32]. Other authors have recorded a low sensitivity of the KK technique in pre-school children populations likely to have a low intensity of infection [18,29,33]. The performance of the KK technique appears to be influenced by the prevalence and *S. mansoni* intensity of infection or transmission intensity [34]. In areas were *S. mansoni* prevalence exceeds 50%, the performance of the KK technique yields results relatively similar to the POC-CCA test [34]. However, in areas with a lower prevalence of *S. mansoni* infection, the performance of the KK technique decreases whereas that of the POC-CCA test is increased [34]. If control programs adapt selective treatments based on parasitological results, a proportion of individuals would miss the treatment, especially in settings with a high HIV prevalence. This proportion will maintain transmission of the disease in that particular setting. Thus, employment of multiple diagnostic tests is highly recommended in epidemiological surveys to increase the chances of detecting targeted infection, especially in adult individuals likely to be have low infection intensity and to be co-infected with HIV-1. The use of multiple diagnostic tests (use of both tests in screening, or in case of limited funding, POC-CCA for screening, and KK for confirmation of diagnosis) allows a more accurate determination of disease burden when planning intervention programs [35]. However, POC-CCA is more expensive, and the control programs need to consider refunding. The cost of the POC-CCA test is about 5.00 USD under field conditions, whereas the cost for the KK technique is only about 1.50 USD per person.

In general, the KK technique has remained the diagnostic test of choice for epidemiological surveys aiming at estimating the prevalence and intensity of infection [6,18,29]. However, the sensitivity and specificity of the KK technique has remained a topic of discussion for many years [18,34,36]. Authors have documented its low sensitivity in detecting infection in individuals carrying low intensity of infections, especially young children and adult individuals likely to be co-infected with HIV-1 [18,34,36]. This makes the KK technique less useful in areas with low rates of transmission characterized by populations carrying low intensities of infection [18,34]. Partly, the low sensitivity of the KK technique is explained by the day-to-day variability in eggs output and the heterogeneous distribution of the *S. mansoni* eggs within the fecal samples [25].

Our study is subject to limitations. Considering the day-to-day variability of *S. mansoni* egg output [25], the use of a single stool sample to examine for *S. mansoni* infection may have led to an underestimation of the prevalence of *S. mansoni* using the KK technique. In addition, the low number of HIV-1/*S. mansoni*-co-infected individuals may have affected the power in assessing the sensitivity and specificity of the two tests. Considering the absence of a diagnostic standard, we combined both diagnostic tests to create an artificial gold standard. We are aware that this method is limited, as the tests—to some degree—are evaluated against their own results, and thus have taken care in the interpretation of respective study results. False-positive detection results can be considered as low, as the KK technique detects eggs of *S. mansoni*, and the POC-CCA specific antigens. Nevertheless, the data shows that a high number of diagnostic cases are missed by the use of only one method.

5. Conclusions

Considering the better diagnostic performance of POC-CCA, especially regarding the sensitivity in the HIV-positive population, and the high number of schistosomiasis cases missed by the KK technique in this group, POC-CCA should be used in screening programs in communities with a high prevalence of HIV infection. An approach using multiple testing techniques for the detection of schistosomiasis cases is recommended.

Author Contributions: H.D.M. conceived and designed the study, performed data collection, analyzed the data, and drafted the first version of the manuscript. J.H. analyzed the data, interpreted the results, and wrote the paper. Both authors read and approved the final manuscript, contributed to the critical review and contributed substantially to the work reported.

Funding: This work was supported by Training Health Researchers into Vocational Excellence in East Africa (THRiVE), grant number 087540, funded by the Wellcome Trust to H.D.M. Its contents are solely the responsibility of the authors and do not necessarily represent the official views of the supporting offices.

Acknowledgments: We thank the study participants from the study villages. We are grateful to the National Institute for Medical Research for laboratory work, logistical and financial management support. H.D.M. is a Senior Lecturer at School of Medicine, Catholic University of Health and Allied Sciences and Research Fellow at the National Institute for Medical Research, Mwanza, Tanzania. J.H. is a class 1 research fellow at Conselho Nacional de DesenvolvimentoCientífico e Tecnológico (CNPq/Brazil).

Conflicts of Interest: The authors declare no conflict of interest.

References

1. Mazigo, H.D.; Nuwaha, F.; Kinung'hi, S.M.; Morona, D.; Pinot de Moira, A.; Wilson, S.; Heukelbach, J.; Dunne, D.W. Epidemiology and control of human schistosomiasis in Tanzania. *Parasites Vectors* **2012**, *5*, 274. [CrossRef] [PubMed]
2. Rollinson, D.; Knopp, S.; Levitz, S.; Stothard, J.R.; Tchuem Tchuente, L.A.; Garba, A.; Mohammed, K.A.; Schur, N.; Person, B.; Colley, D.G.; et al. Time to set the agenda for schistosomiasis elimination. *Acta Trop.* **2013**, *128*, 423–440. [CrossRef] [PubMed]
3. Mugono, M.; Konje, E.; Kuhn, S.; Mpogoro, F.J.; Morona, D.; Mazigo, H.D. Intestinal schistosomiasis and geohelminths of Ukara Island, north-western Tanzania: Prevalence, intensity of infection and associated risk factors among school children. *Parasites Vectors* **2014**, *7*, 612. [CrossRef] [PubMed]
4. Malenganisho, W.L.; Magnussen, P.; Friis, H.; Siza, J.; Kaatano, G.; Temu, M.; Vennervald, B.J. *Schistosoma mansoni* morbidity among adults in two villages along Lake Victoria shores in Mwanza District, Tanzania. *Trans. R. Soc. Trop. Med. Hyg.* **2008**, *102*, 532–541. [CrossRef] [PubMed]
5. Kardorff, R.; Gabone, R.M.; Mugashe, C.; Obiga, D.; Ramarokoto, C.E.; Mahlert, C.; Spannbrucker, N.; Lang, A.; Gunzler, V.; Gryseels, B.; et al. *Schistosoma mansoni*-related morbidity on Ukerewe Island, Tanzania:

Clinical, ultrasonographical and biochemical parameters. *Trop. Med. Intern. Health* **1997**, *2*, 230–239. [CrossRef]

6. Katz, N.; Chaves, A.; Pellegrino, J. A simple device for quantitative stool thick-smear technique in *Schistosomiasis mansoni*. *Rev. Inst. Med. Trop. Sao Paulo* **1972**, *14*, 397–400. [PubMed]

7. Lamberton, P.H.; Kabatereine, N.B.; Oguttu, D.W.; Fenwick, A.; Webster, J.P. Sensitivity and specificity of multiple Kato-Katz thick smears and a circulating cathodic antigen test for *Schistosoma mansoni* diagnosis pre- and post-repeated-praziquantel treatment. *PLoS Negl. Trop. Dis.* **2014**, *8*, e3139. [CrossRef] [PubMed]

8. Karanja, D.M.; Boyer, A.E.; Strand, M.; Colley, D.G.; Nahlen, B.L.; Ouma, J.H.; Secor, W.E. Studies on schistosomiasis in western Kenya: II. Efficacy of praziquantel for treatment of schistosomiasis in persons coinfected with human immunodeficiency virus-1. *Am. J. Trop. Med. Hyg.* **1998**, *59*, 307–311. [CrossRef] [PubMed]

9. Kallestrup, P.; Zinyama, R.; Gomo, E.; Butterworth, A.E.; van Dam, G.J.; Erikstrup, C.; Ullum, H. Schistosomiasis and HIV-1 infection in rural Zimbabwe: Implications of coinfection for excretion of eggs. *J. Infect. Dis.* **2005**, *191*, 1311–1320. [CrossRef] [PubMed]

10. Mazigo, H.D.; Dunne, D.W.; Wilson, S.; Kinung'hi, S.M.; Pinot de Moira, A.; Jones, F.M.; Morona, D.; Nuwaha, F. Co-infection with *Schistosoma mansoni* and human immunodeficiency virus-1 (HIV-1) among residents of fishing villages of north-western Tanzania. *Parasites Vectors* **2014**, *7*, 587. [CrossRef] [PubMed]

11. Karanja, D.M.; Colley, D.G.; Nahlen, B.L.; Ouma, J.H.; Secor, W.E. Studies on schistosomiasis in western Kenya: I. Evidence for immune-facilitated excretion of schistosome eggs from patients with *Schistosoma mansoni* and human immunodeficiency virus coinfections. *Am. J. Trop. Med. Hyg.* **1997**, *56*, 515–521. [CrossRef] [PubMed]

12. Dunne, D.W.; Hassounah, O.; Musallam, R.; Lucas, S.; Pepys, M.B.; Baltz, M.; Doenhoff, M. Mechanisms of *Schistosoma mansoni* egg excretion: Parasitological observations in immunosuppressed mice reconstituted with immune serum. *Parasites Immunol.* **1983**, *5*, 47–60. [CrossRef]

13. Mazigo, H.D.; Nuwaha, F.; Wilson, S.; Kinung'hi, S.M.; Morona, D.; Waihenya, R.; Heukelbach, J.; Dunne, D.W. Epidemiology and interactions of human immunodeficiency virus-1 and *Schistosoma mansoni* in sub-Saharan Africa. *Infect. Dis. Poverty* **2013**, *2*, 2. [CrossRef] [PubMed]

14. Mazigo, H.D.; Dunne, D.W.; Morona, D.; Lutufyo, T.E.; Kinung'hi, S.M.; Kaatano, G.; Nuwaha, F. Periportal fibrosis, liver and spleen sizes among *S. mansoni* mono- or co-infected individuals with human immunodeficiency virus-1 in fishing villages along Lake Victoria shores, north-western Tanzania. *Parasites Vectors* **2015**, *8*, 260. [CrossRef] [PubMed]

15. Van Dam, G.; Wichers, J.; Ferreira, T.F.; Ghati, D.; Van Amerongen, A.; Deelder, A. Diagnosis of schistosomiasis by reagent strip test for detection of circulating cathodic antigen. *J. Clin. Microbiol.* **2004**, *42*, 5458–5461. [CrossRef] [PubMed]

16. Stothard, J.R.; Kabatereine, N.B.; Tukahebwa, E.M.; Kazibwe, F.; Rollinson, D.; Mathieson, W.; Webster, J.P.; Fenwick, A. Use of circulating cathodic antigen (CCA) dipsticks for detection of intestinal and urinary schistosomiasis. *Acta Trop.* **2006**, *97*, 219–228. [CrossRef] [PubMed]

17. Danso-Appiah, A.; Minton, J.; Boamah, D.; Otchere, J.; Asmah, R.H.; Rodgers, M.; Bosompem, K.M.; Eusebi, P.; De Vlas, S.J. Accuracy of point-of-care testing for circulatory cathodic antigen in the detection of schistosome infection: Systematic review and meta-analysis. *Bull. World Health Organ.* **2016**, *94*, 522A–533A. [CrossRef] [PubMed]

18. Okoyo, C.; Simiyu, E.; Njenga, S.M.; Mwandawiro, C. Comparing the performance of circulating cathodic antigen and Kato-Katz techniques in evaluating *Schistosoma mansoni* infection in areas with low prevalence in selected counties of Kenya: A cross-sectional study. *BMC Public Health* **2018**, *18*, 478. [CrossRef] [PubMed]

19. Lindholz, C.G.; Favero, V.; Verissimo, C.M.; Candido, R.R.F.; de Souza, R.P.; Dos Santos, R.R.; Morassutti, A.L.; Bittencourt, H.R.; Jones, M.K.; St Pierre, T.G.; et al. Study of diagnostic accuracy of Helmintex, Kato-Katz, and POC-CCA methods for diagnosing intestinal schistosomiasis in Candeal, a low intensity transmission area in northeastern Brazil. *PLoS Negl. Trop. Dis.* **2018**, *12*, e0006274. [CrossRef] [PubMed]

20. Clements, M.N.; Corstjens, P.; Binder, S.; Campbell, C.H., Jr.; de Dood, C.J.; Fenwick, A.; Harrison, W.; Kayugi, D.; King, C.H.; Kornelis, D.; et al. Latent class analysis to evaluate performance of point-of-care CCA for low-intensity *Schistosoma mansoni* infections in Burundi. *Parasites Vectors* **2018**, *11*, 111. [CrossRef] [PubMed]

21. Ferreira, F.T.; Fidelis, T.A.; Pereira, T.A.; Otoni, A.; Queiroz, L.C.; Amancio, F.F.; Antunes, C.M.; Lambertucci, J.R. Sensitivity and specificity of the circulating cathodic antigen rapid urine test in the diagnosis of *Schistosomiasis mansoni* infection and evaluation of morbidity in a low-endemic area in Brazil. *Rev. Soc. Bras. Med. Trop.* **2017**, *50*, 358–364. [CrossRef] [PubMed]

22. Mazigo, H.; Dunne, D.W.; Kinung'hi, S.M.; Fred, N. Praziquantel efficacy against *Schistosoma mansoni* among HIV-1 infected and uninfected adults living in fishing villages along Lake Victoria, northwest Tanzania. *Infect. Dis. Poverty* **2014**, *3*, 47. [CrossRef] [PubMed]

23. Lyamuya, E.F.; Aboud, S.; Urassa, W.K.; Sufi, J.; Mbwana, J.; Ndugulile, F.; Massambu, C. Evaluation of simple rapid HIV assays and development of national rapid HIV test algorithms in Dar es Salaam, Tanzania. *BMC Infect. Dis.* **2009**, *9*, 19. [CrossRef] [PubMed]

24. World Health Organization. Prevention and control of schistosomiasis and soil-transmitted helminthiasis. In *World Health Organization Technical Report Series*; World Health Organization: Geneva, Switzerland, 2002; Volume 912.

25. Berhe, N.; Medhin, G.; Erko, B.; Smith, T.; Gedamu, S.; Bereded, D.; Moore, R.; Habte, E.; Redda, A.; Gebre-Michael, T. Variations in helminth faecal egg counts in Kato–Katz thick smears and their implications in assessing infection status with *Schistosoma mansoni*. *Acta Trop.* **2004**, *92*, 205–212. [CrossRef] [PubMed]

26. Midzi, N.; Butterworth, A.E.; Mduluza, T.; Munyati, S.; Deelder, A.M.; van Dam, G.J. Use of circulating cathodic antigen strips for the diagnosis of urinary schistosomiasis. *Trans. R. Soc. Trop. Med. Hyg.* **2009**, *103*, 45–51. [CrossRef] [PubMed]

27. Nausch, N.; Dawson, E.M.; Midzi, N.; Mduluza, T.; Mutapi, F.; Doenhoff, M. Field evaluation of a new antibody-based diagnostic for *Schistosoma haematobium* and *S. mansoni* at the point-of-care in northeast Zimbabwe. *BMC Infect. Dis.* **2014**, *14*, 165. [CrossRef] [PubMed]

28. Landis, J.R.K.G. An application of hierarchical kappa-type statistics in the assessment of majority agreement among multiple observers. *Biometrics* **1977**, *33*, 363–374. [CrossRef] [PubMed]

29. Coulibaly, J.T.; Knopp, S.; N'Guessan, N.A.; Silue, K.D.; Furst, T.; Lohourignon, L.K.; Brou, J.K.; N'Gbesso, Y.K.; Vounatsou, P.; N'Goran, E.K.; et al. Accuracy of urine circulating cathodic antigen (CCA) test for *Schistosoma mansoni* diagnosis in different settings of Cote d'Ivoire. *PLoS Negl. Trop. Dis.* **2011**, *5*, 1384. [CrossRef] [PubMed]

30. Silveira, A.M.; Costa, E.G.; Ray, D.; Suzuki, B.M.; Hsieh, M.H.; Fraga, L.A.; Caffrey, C.R. Evaluation of the CCA immuno-chromatographic test to diagnose *Schistosoma mansoni* in Minas Gerais State, Brazil. *PLoS Negl. Trop. Dis.* **2016**, *10*, e0004357. [CrossRef] [PubMed]

31. Mwinzi, P.N.; Kittur, N.; Ochola, E.; Cooper, P.J.; Campbell, C.H., Jr.; King, C.H.; Colley, D.G. Additional evaluation of the point-of-contact circulating cathodic antigen assay for *Schistosoma mansoni* infection. *Front. Public Health* **2015**, *3*, 48. [CrossRef] [PubMed]

32. Fontanet, A.L.; Woldemichael, T.; Sahlu, T.; van Dam, G.J.; Messele, T.; Rinke de Wit, T.; Masho, W.; Yeneneh, H.; Coutinho, R.A.; van Lieshout, L. Epidemiology of HIV and *Schistosoma mansoni* infections among sugar-estate residents in Ethiopia. *Ann. Trop. Med. Parasitol.* **2000**, *94*, 145–155. [CrossRef] [PubMed]

33. Coulibaly, J.T.; N'Gbesso, Y.K.; Knopp, S.; N'Guessan, N.A.; Silue, K.D.; van Dam, G.J.; N'Goran, E.K.; Utzinger, J. Accuracy of urine circulating cathodic antigen test for the diagnosis of *Schistosoma mansoni* in preschool-aged children before and after treatment. *PLoS Negl. Trop. Dis.* **2013**, *7*, e2109. [CrossRef] [PubMed]

34. Kittur, N.; Castleman, J.D.; Campbell, C.H., Jr.; King, C.H.; Colley, D.G. Comparison of *Schistosoma mansoni* Prevalence and intensity of infection, as determined by the circulating cathodic antigen urine assay or by the Kato-Katz fecal assay: A systematic review. *Am. J. Trop. Med. Hyg.* **2016**, *94*, 605–610. [CrossRef] [PubMed]

35. Lodh, N.; Mwansa, J.C.; Mutengo, M.M.; Shiff, C.J. Diagnosis of *Schistosoma mansoni* without the stool: Comparison of three diagnostic tests to detect *Schistosoma* [corrected] *mansoni* infection from filtered urine in Zambia. *Am. J. Trop. Med. Hyg.* **2013**, *89*, 46–50. [CrossRef] [PubMed]

36. De Vlas, S.J.; Gryseels, B. Underestimation of *Schistosoma mansoni* prevalences. *Parasitol. Today* **1992**, *8*, 274–277. [CrossRef]

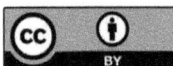

Tropical Medicine and Infectious Disease

MDPI

Article

Epidemiology and Spatiotemporal Patterns of Leprosy Detection in the State of Bahia, Brazilian Northeast Region, 2001–2014

Eliana Amorim de Souza [1,*], Anderson Fuentes Ferreira [2], Jorg Heukelbach [2,3], Reagan Nzundu Boigny [2], Carlos Henrique Alencar [2] and Alberto Novaes Ramos, Jr. [2]

[1] Multidisciplinary Institute for Health, Campus Anísio Teixeira, Federal University of Bahia, Vitória da Conquista BA 45.029-094, Brazil
[2] Department of Community Health, School of Medicine, Federal University of Ceará, Fortaleza CE 60430-140, Brazil; anderson_deco.f2@hotmail.com (A.F.F.); heukelbach@web.de (J.H.); reagan.nzundu@gmail.com (R.N.B.); carllosalencar@hotmail.com (C.H.A.); novaes@ufc.br (A.N.R.J.)
[3] College of Public Health, Medical and Veterinary Sciences, Division of Tropical Health and Medicine, James Cook University, Townsville 4811, Australia
* Correspondence: amorim_eliana@yahoo.com.br

Received: 29 April 2018; Accepted: 25 July 2018; Published: 31 July 2018

Abstract: The detection of leprosy cases is distributed unequally in Brazil, with high-risk clusters mainly in the North and Northeast regions. Knowledge on epidemiology and spatiotemporal patterns of leprosy occurrence and late diagnosis in these areas is critical to improve control measures. We performed a study including all leprosy cases notified in the 417 municipalities of Bahia state, from 2001 to 2014. New case detection (overall and pediatric <15 years) and grade 2 disability (G2D) rates were calculated and stratified according to socio-demographic variables. Spatial analyses were performed to detect high-risk areas for occurrence and late diagnosis. A total of 40,060 new leprosy cases was reported in the period (mean = 2861 cases/year), 3296 (8.2%) in <15-year-olds, and 1921 (4.8%) with G2D. The new case detection rate was 20.41 cases/100,000 inhabitants (95% CI: 19.68–21.17). A higher risk was identified in older age groups (RR = 8.45, 95% CI: 7.08–10.09) and in residents living in the state capital (RR = 5.30, 95% CI: 4.13–6.79), in medium-sized cities (RR = 2.80; 95% CI: 2.50–3.13), and in the west (RR = 6.56, 95% CI: 5.13–8.39) and far south regions of the state (RR = 6.56, 95% CI: 5.13–8.39). A higher risk of G2D was associated with male gender (RR = 2.43, 95% CI: 2.20–2.67), older age (RR = 44.08, 95% CI: 33.21–58.51), Afro-Brazilian ethnicity (RR = 1.59; 95% CI: 1.37–1.85), living in medium-sized cities (RR = 2.60; 95% CI: 2.27–2.96) and residency in the north (RR = 5.02; 95% CI: 3.74–6.73) and far south (RR = 7.46; 95% CI: 5.58–9.98) regions. Heterogeneous space–time patterns of leprosy distribution were identified, indicating high endemicity, recent transmission, and late diagnosis. This heterogeneous distribution of the disease was observed throughout the study period. Leprosy remains a relevant public health problem in Bahia state. The disease has a focal distribution. We reinforce the importance of integrating surveillance, prevention and control actions in regions of higher risk of leprosy detection and late diagnosis, and in the most vulnerable populations.

Keywords: leprosy; epidemiology; spatial analysis; prevention and control; Brazil

---

1. Introduction

Leprosy is a Neglected Tropical Disease (NTD), mainly affecting highly vulnerable populations [1,2]. Brazil reported a total of 25,218 leprosy cases in 2016, representing 12% of global cases, and 92% of cases in Latin America [3].

The Brazilian Ministry of Health (MoH) established different control strategies aiming for the reduction of the leprosy burden in the country [4]. The Brazilian guidelines for surveillance, attention and elimination of leprosy define measures focusing on primary health care, within the realm of the nationwide Unified Health System (*Sistema Único de Saúde* [SUS]). Primary health care is defined to be responsible for diagnosis, treatment, prevention of disabilities and surveillance. Cases with complex clinical presentations, such as relapses, children <15 years of age and leprosy reactions should be referred to specialized secondary clinics and tertiary care [4].

The early detection of new cases relies on spontaneous presentation of patients to the health system, active case finding and contact tracing (including clinical examination and Bacillus Calmette-Guérin (BCG) vaccination of contacts) [4]. However, due to operational difficulties within the SUS, there are still shortcomings regarding coverage and quality of control and prevention measures [5,6].

As a result of nationwide implementation of these systematic measures, the detection rate of new cases of leprosy cases increased on a first run, but then decreased steadily during the past years. Despite these achievements, leprosy continues being endemic in Brazil, with an overall detection rate of 12.2 cases per 100,000 inhabitants in 2016 [7].

The main targets of the Global Leprosy Strategy of the World Health Organization (WHO) include G2D and leprosy in <15-year-olds, with reduction of new cases with G2D to <1 case per million population [1]. The occurrence of leprosy in children <15 years indicates active transmission of *Mycobacterium leprae*, while the diagnosis of cases with G2D is considered a strong indicator for late diagnosis [4]. The analysis of both epidemiological indicators reveals operational problems in Brazil's health services network, indicated by 8.40 G2D cases per million population and 3.63 new cases per 100,000 inhabitants in <15-year-olds [7].

The analysis of leprosy detection patterns in space and time is essential for the description of transmission dynamics, considering the focal epidemiological pattern of leprosy [8]. In Brazil, leprosy shows a heterogeneous spatial distribution, with persistence of areas with different levels of endemicity. Higher detection rates are observed mainly in socioeconomically deprived regions [9]. The North, Northeast and Central West regions present the highest disease burden [7]. In this context, the identification of areas of high endemicity is also an important tool to monitor and evaluate the effectiveness of control measures on a nationwide level [1,4,8,10,11]. However, there are only few systematic studies on spatial patterns of leprosy in Brazil's Northeast region.

The present study aims to fill this gap by describing the main epidemiological indicators for leprosy, and by characterizing the spatial and temporal patterns of leprosy detection in the state of Bahia, from 2001 to 2014.

2. Methods

2.1. Study Area, Population and Design

Bahia state has a population of about 15 million and is one of the Brazilian states with the highest poverty rates [12,13]. It is the largest state in Brazil's Northeast (Figure 1). Socio-economic indicators have improved recently (e.g., the Human Development Index [HDI] improved from 0.512 in 2000 to 0.660 in 2010), but social inequality remains at high levels [14]. SUS healthcare coverage, indicated by population coverage of the primary healthcare-based Family Health Strategy (a priority service for development of leprosy control actions) increased from 15.4% in 2001 to 68.9% in 2014 [15].

The study population consisted of all confirmed leprosy cases notified 2001–2014 in inhabitants of Bahia state. We performed an epidemiological analysis of these cases, and spatial analyses in two temporal sections using the 417 municipalities of the state as units [12].

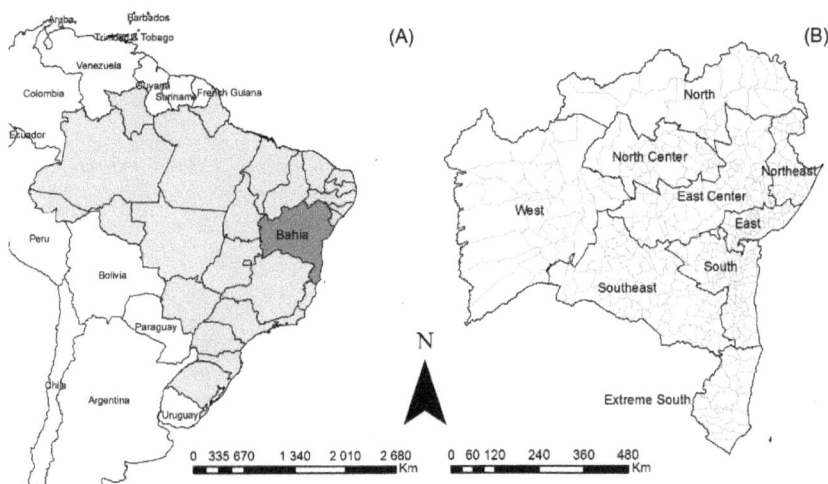

Figure 1. Study area: (**A**) location of the Bahia state; (**B**) Bahia state with its nine regions and 417 municipalities.

2.2. Data Sources and Variables

We used the database of the National Disease Notification System of the MoH (SINAN), formally obtained from the Health Secretariat of Bahia state. SINAN is a standardized software-based system for the compulsory notification of diseases, including leprosy. Information on socio-demographic and clinical data are also available. Only confirmed cases, based on clinical and epidemiological criteria, are reported. For monitoring of cases during treatment, a follow-up report is used by the health services to be completed at the time of discharge [4]. This follow-up report improves quality of SINAN data. In this study, the cases that were defined as 'diagnostic error' during follow-up were excluded.

For the calculation of epidemiological indicators, population data were obtained from the Brazilian Institute of Geography and Statistics (IBGE), based on the population censuses of the State (2000 and 2010), and on population estimates for inter-census years (2001–2009; 2011–2014).

2.3. Statistical Analyses

2.3.1. Epidemiological Analysis

The following indicators were calculated from secondary SINAN data: (1) annual case detection rate per 100,000 inhabitants, indicating frequency and magnitude; (2) detection rate in <15-year-olds per 100,000 inhabitants, indicating active transmission; and (3) new cases with G2D per 1,000,000 population at the time of diagnosis, indicating under-notification and late diagnosis [4].

Crude rates were calculated per year and the mean rates for the periods 2001–2007 and 2008–2014, as well as the mean for the entire period (2001–2014), smoothing differences over time. The two periods were used considering the first as an initial period of decentralization of control actions for primary health care services and the second, as a phase of consolidation of this process. We used the standardized populations of each period under analysis as the denominator. For all indicators, we calculated their respective binomial 95% confidence intervals (95% CI) [16].

We then stratified the indicators by sociodemographic characteristics: gender, ethnicity (Caucasian, Afro-Brazilian, Asian, Mixed/Pardo-Brazilian, Amerindian), age group (<15, 15–29, 30–39, 40–49, 50–59, 60–69, ≥70 years), residence in the state capital, and size of municipality (small, <100,000 inhabitants; medium size with 100,000–500,000 inhabitants; and large, >500,000 inhabitants). Relative risks (RR) and their 95% CI were calculated to determine the differences between the groups. The statistical significance of differences was evaluated by the chi-square test.

We used the classification of endemicity levels of municipalities, as defined by the Brazilian MoH: the general detection rate was considered hyperendemic when there were >40.00 cases per 100,000 inhabitants; very high >20.00 to 39.99 cases per 100,000 inhabitants; high >10.00 to 19.99 cases per 100,000 inhabitants; medium >2.00 to 9.99 cases per 100,000 inhabitants; and low <2.00 cases per 100,000 inhabitants. Similarly, the detection rate in cases <15 years was classified as low (<0.50/100,000 inhabitants); intermediate (0.5–2.49/100,000 inhabitants); high (2.5–4.99/100,000 inhabitants); very high (5.0–9.99/100,000 inhabitants) and hyperendemic (>10.0/100,000 inhabitants) [4].

2.3.2. Spatial Analyses in the Temporal Sections

Spatial analyses were performed to identify spatial aggregates for the abovementioned leprosy indicators. To reduce random fluctuations (esp. in the case of rare events and small populations) and to minimize the influence of operational factors, the abovementioned indicators were smoothed by applying the local empirical Bayesian method (a procedure for statistical inference in which the prior distribution is estimated from the data). Smoothing is based on information from surrounding municipalities.

The identification of possible areas of spatial autocorrelation was based on Local Moran's method (Local Indicators of Spatial Association; LISA), which compares the value of the rate of each municipality and its neighbors, verifying spatial dependence and identifying patterns of spatial autocorrelation. The generated scatter diagram recognizes four situations: municipalities with high or low detection rates, surrounded by municipalities with high or low detection rates (Q1—High-High and Q2—Low-Low) and municipalities with high or low detection rates, surrounded by municipalities with low or high detection rates (Q3—High-Low and Q4—Low-High). For spatial representation, we applied Moran Maps, considering municipalities with a statistically significant difference. The definition of risk areas for the detection of leprosy cases, active transmission and late diagnosis was based on the identification of municipalities with high values of the respective epidemiological indicators.

We also used the Gi* index ('Gi star') of Getis-Ord, for the analysis of spatial dependence. The analyses assume that a high value of the Z score and small p value of a parameter indicate spatial agglomeration of high values. A low negative Z score and small p value indicate spatial grouping of low values [17]. These indices identify the presence of aggregates of high-values or low-values within the aggregate of municipalities.

Statistical analyses were performed with Stata version 11.2 (StataCorp LP, College Station, TX, USA). ArcGIS version 9.3 (Environmental Systems Research Institute—ESRI, Redlands, CA, USA) and Terra View version 4.1 (INPE, São José dos Campos, SP, Brazil) were used for spatial analyses, including processing, analysis, presentation of cartographic data and calculations of the indicators of spatial autocorrelation, as well as construction of thematic maps.

The study was conducted in accordance with the Declaration of Helsinki, and the protocol was approved by the Ethical Review Board of the Federal University of Ceará (protocol number: 544,962 28/02/2014).

3. Results

3.1. Epidemiological Analysis

A total of 40,060 new leprosy cases was notified during the study period, with an average of 2861 cases per year, and an overall detection rate of 20.41 cases per 100,000 inhabitants (Table 1). Socio-demographic characteristics of cases are depicted in Table 1. Crude case detection rates were significantly higher among the older age groups, as compared to <15-year-olds, and among Asian ethnic group, residents in medium-sized cities and those living outside the state capital. With the exception of the Southwest, all regions had significantly higher detection rates as compared to the Northeast region of the State (Table 1).

There was a total of 3219 (8.0%) cases in <15-year-olds, an average of 230 cases per year, with a mean case detection rate of 5.71 cases per 100,000 inhabitants. Socio-demographic characteristics of cases in children are depicted in Table 2. Case detection was significantly higher among children of all ethnicities other than Caucasian. Children living in medium-sized cities presented higher risk. With the exception of the Southwest of the State, all regions showed significantly higher detection rates as compared to the Northeast (Table 2).

The proportion of new cases with G2D was 4.80% (1921/40,054), and G2D per million people was 9.80. Details of new cases diagnosed with G2D are presented in Table 3. The detection of new cases with G2D at diagnosis was significantly higher among males, ≥70-year-olds and among Afro-Brazilians (Table 3). Residency in medium and small-sized cities and outside the state capital was associated with a higher risk of new cases with G2D. In the far south region, the G2D detection rates were highest (Table 3).

3.2. Spatiotemporal Analyses

The spatial distribution of overall crude detection rates showed that in the first observation period (2001–2007), most municipalities reported cases (93.5%, 390); 172 (44.1%) of these were classified as medium endemic, 90 (23.1%) as highly endemic and 52 (13.3%) as hyperendemic (Figure 2A). In the State's North, West and Far South regions we identified the highest proportions of highly endemic and hyperendemic municipalities. In the following period (2008–2014), the number of municipalities with medium endemicity (48.5%, 193) increased and those with hyperendemicity (8.3%, 33) reduced. After smoothing, the distribution patterns remained similar, but spatial high-risk areas became more obvious (Figure 2B). Spatial association using Getis-Ord Gi* identified high-risk clusters for leprosy detection in the North, West and Far South regions of Bahia, over the entire observation period. Clusters of low risk were identified in the South, East and Central-East regions (Figure 2C). Spatial presentation using local Moran's index recognized areas of spatial autocorrelation in the North, West and Far South regions (Figure 2D). These areas occurred throughout the entire observation period.

Table 1. Sociodemographic characteristics of leprosy cases and associated factors in Bahia state, 2001–2014.

Variables	Cases (Total)	Average Cases Annually (2001–2014) n (%)	Detection Rate [a]	95% CI	RR	95% CI	p Value
Gender [b]							
Male	20,132	1438 (50.3)	20.75	19.70–21.85	1.03	0.96–1.11	0.3900
Female	19,922	1423 (49.7)	20.08	19.07–21.15	Ref	-	-
Age group (years) [b]							
<15	3219	230 (8.0)	5.44	4.78–6.19	Ref	-	-
15–29	9330	666 (23.3)	15.87	14.70–17.12	2.91	2.51–3.39	<0.0001
30–39	7092	507 (17.7)	26.15	23.99–28.55	4.81	4.11–5.62	<0.0001
40–49	6706	479 (16.7)	32.85	30.04–35.93	6.03	5.16–7.06	<0.0001
50–59	6052	432 (15.1)	43.86	39.89–48.16	8.05	6.86–9.45	<0.0001
60–69	4015	287 (10.0)	44.30	39.49–49.76	8.14	6.85–9.68	<0.0001
≥70	3640	260 (9.1)	46.03	40.76–51.97	8.45	7.08–10.09	<0.0001
Ethnicity [b]							
Caucasian	6914	494 (20.1)	16.10	14.74–17.58	Ref	-	-
Afro-Brazilian	6188	442 (18.0)	22.22	20.24–24.39	1.38	1.33–1.43	<0.0001
Asian	345	25 (1.0)	26.97	18.50–40.40	1.68	1.50–1.87	<0.0001
Mixed/Pardo-Brazilian	20,799	1486 (60.5)	19.15	18.20–20.20	1.19	1.16–1.22	<0.0001
Amerindian	156	11 (0.5)	18.48	10.20–32.70	1.15	1.00–1.35	0.0881
City size (by inhabitants)							
Small (<100,000)	21,348	1525 (53.3)	18.10	17.21–19.03	1.34	1.21–1.49	<0.0001
Medium (100,000–500,000)	12,279	877 (30.7)	37.66	35.25–40.23	2.80	2.50–3.13	<0.0001
Large (>500,000)	6433	460 (16.1)	13.45	12.29–14.75	Ref	-	-
Residing in the state capital							
Yes	4962	354 (12.4)	12.96	11.66–14.36	Ref	-	-
No	35,098	2507 (87.6)	22.22	21.37–23.11	1.72	1.54–1.92	<0.0001
Region [b]							
North	7916	565 (19.8)	55.65	51.21–60.38	6.18	4.85–7.88	<0.0001
Northeast	1030	74 (2.6)	8.93	7.16–11.28	Ref	-	-
South	2791	199 (7.0)	11.87	10.31–13.62	1.32	1.01–1.72	0.0422
South-west	2635	188 (6.6)	10.76	9.32–12.40	1.20	0.91–1.57	0.1912
East	7677	548 (19.2)	12.27	11.28–13.33	1.36	1.07–1.74	0.0121
Central East	4457	318 (11.1)	15.37	13.76–17.13	1.71	1.33–2.20	<0.0001
West	5576	398 (13.9)	47.67	43.18–52.55	5.30	4.13–6.79	<0.0001
Far south	6252	447 (15.6)	58.91	53.75–64.69	6.56	5.13–8.39	<0.0001
Central North	1725	123 (4.3)	15.98	13.40–19.00	1.78	1.33–2.37	0.0001
Total	40,060	2861 (100.0)	20.41	19.68–21.17	-	-	-

CI: confidence intervals; RR: relative risk; -: not calculated; [a] The average annual detection rate (per 100,000 inhabitants), based on the calculation of the average number of new cases in the period of fourteen years as the numerator and the size of the population in the middle of the study period, as the denominator. Population data on ethnicity were obtained from the Brazilian national census (2000 and 2010). The number of the population in relation to ethnicity, for the middle of the period, was derived from the Continuous National Household Sample Survey (PNAD) estimates; [b] Data not available in all cases (Gender: 6 cases, Age group: 6 cases, Ethnicity: 5658 cases, Health Regions: 1 case).

Table 2. Sociodemographic characteristics of leprosy cases in <15 year-olds and associated factors in Bahia state, 2001–2014.

Variables	Cases	Average Annual (2001–2014) n (%)	Detection Rate in Children [a]	95% CI	RR	95% CI	p Value
Gender							
Male	1585	113 (49.2)	5.51	4.59–6.63	Ref	–	–
Female	1634	117 (50.8)	5.90	4.92–7.07	1.35	1.22–1.50	<0.0001
Ethnicity [b]							
Caucasian	448	32 (16.4)	3.51	2.49–4.95	Ref	–	–
Afro-Brazilian	475	34 (17.4)	7.25	5.19–10.12	2.06	1.81–2.35	<0.0001
Asian	25	2 (0.9)	8.05	2.21–29.34	2.05	1.37–3.06	0.0005
Mixed/Pardo-Brazilian	1767	126 (64.6)	5.15	4.33–6.14	1.47	1.33–1.63	<0.0001
Amerindian	21	2 (0.8)	12.38	3.40–45.13	2.65	1.71–4.10	<0.0001
City size (inhabitants)							
Small (<100,000)	1735	124 (53.9)	4.89	4.10–5.83	1.76	1.36–2.28	<0.0001
Medium (100,000–500,000)	970	69 (30.1)	10.42	8.24–13.19	4.70	3.65–6.06	<0.0001
Large (>500,000)	514	37 (16.0)	4.43	3.22–6.11	9.85	7.71–12.59	<0.0001
Residing in the state capital							
Yes	422	30 (13.1)	4.39	3.08–6.27	Ref	–	–
No	2797	200 (86.9)	5.97	5.20–6.86	1.35	1.22–1.50	<0.0001
Region							
North	731	52 (22.7)	16.70	12.74–21.89	8.25	6.47–10.53	<0.0001
Northeast	71	5 (2.2)	2.00	0.86–4.69	Ref	–	–
South	197	14 (6.1)	2.84	1.69–4.77	1.40	1.07–1.84	0.0141
South-west	120	9 (3.7)	1.85	0.97–3.52	0.87	0.65–1.16	0.3442
East	683	49 (21.2)	4.30	3.25–5.68	2.11	1.65–2.69	<0.0001
Central East	308	22 (9.6)	3.58	2.36–5.41	1.76	1.36–2.28	<0.0001
West	362	26 (11.2)	9.60	6.56–14.07	4.70	3.65–6.06	<0.0001
Far south	659	47 (20.5)	19.99	15.03–26.58	9.85	7.72–12.59	<0.0001
Central North	88	6 (2.7)	2.59	1.19–5.65	1.33	0.98–1.82	0.0706
Total	3219	230 (100.0)	5.71	5.02–6.49	–	–	–

CI: confidence intervals; RR: relative risk; -: not calculated; [a] Average annual detection rate (per 100,000 inhabitants), based on the calculation of the average number of new cases in the period of fourteen years as the numerator and the size of the population in the middle of the study period, as the denominator. Population data on ethnicity were obtained from the Brazilian national census (2000 and 2010). The number of the population in relation to ethnicity, for the middle of the period, was derived from PNAD estimates; [b] Data not available in all cases (Ethnicity: n = 483).

Table 3. Sociodemographic characteristics of leprosy cases with G2D at diagnosis and factors in Bahia state, 2001–2014.

Variables	Cases	Average Annual (2001–2014) n (%)	Detection Rate [a]	95% CI	RR	95% CI	p Value
Gender							
Male	1351	97 (70.3)	14.00	11.48–17.08	2.43	2.20–2.67	<0.0001
Female	570	41 (29.7)	5.80	4.28–7.87	Ref	-	-
Age group (years)							
<15	56	4 (2.9)	0.98	0.38–2.52	Ref	-	-
15–29	300	21 (15.6)	5.00	3.27–7.64	5.39	4.05–7.17	<0.0001
30–39	310	22 (16.1)	11.40	7.53–17.26	12.07	9.08–16.05	<0.0001
40–49	316	23 (16.4)	15.80	10.53–23.71	16.35	12.31–21.73	<0.0001
50–59	323	23 (16.8)	23.30	15.53–34.96	24.73	18.62–32.84	<0.0001
60–69	286	20 (14.9)	30.90	20.00–47.73	33.33	25.03–44.39	<0.0001
≥70	330	24 (17.2)	42.50	28.56–63.24	44.08	33.21–58.51	<0.0001
Ethnicity [b]							
Caucasian	342	24 (20.0)	7.80	5.24–11.61	Ref	-	-
Afro-Brazilian	353	25 (20.7)	12.60	8.54–18.60	1.59	1.37–1.85	<0.0001
Asian	15	1 (0.9)	10.90	1.92–61.74	1.47	0.88–2.47	0.1420
Mixed/Pardo-Brazilian	986	70 (57.7)	9.00	7.12–11.37	1.14	1.00–1.29	0.0364
Amerindian	13	1 (0.8)	16.60	2.93–94.02	1.93	1.11–3.37	0.0196
City size (inhabitants)							
Small (<100,000)	974	70 (50.7)	8.30	6.57–10.49	1.16	1.02–1.31	0.0222
Medium (100,000–500,000)	605	43 (31.5)	18.50	13.74–24.92	2.60	2.27–2.96	<0.0001
Large (>500,000)	342	24 (17.8)	7.00	4.70–10.42	Ref	-	-
Residing in the state capital							
Yes	254	18 (13.2)	6.60	4.18–10.43	Ref	-	-
No	1667	119 (86.8)	10.50	8.78–12.56	1.59	1.39–1.82	<0.0001
Region							
North	322	23 (16.8)	22.60	15.06–32.91	5.02	3.74–6.73	<0.0001
Northeast	52	4 (2.7)	4.90	1.91–12.60	Ref	-	-
South	174	12 (9.1)	7.10	4.06–12.41	1.64	1.20–2.24	0.0017
South-west	187	13 (9.7)	7.40	4.33–12.66	1.69	1.25–2.30	0.0008
East	387	28 (20.1)	6.30	4.36–9.11	1.37	1.03–1.83	0.0324
Central East	220	16 (11.5)	7.70	4.74–12.51	1.68	1.24–2.28	0.0007
West	121	9 (6.3)	10.80	5.68–20.53	2.29	1.66–3.17	<0.0001
Far south	357	26 (18.6)	34.30	23.41–50.26	7.46	5.58–9.98	<0.0001
Central North	101	7 (5.3)	9.10	4.41–18.78	2.07	1.49–2.90	<0.0001
Total	1921	137 (100.0)	9.80	8.29–11.58	-	-	-

CI: confidence intervals; RR: relative risk; -: not calculated; [a] The average annual detection rate (per million people), based on the calculation of the average number of new cases in the period of fourteen years as the numerator and the size of the population in the middle of the study period, as the denominator. Population data on ethnicity were obtained from the Brazilian national census (2000 and 2010). The number of the population in relation to ethnicity, for the middle of the period, was derived from PNAD estimates; [b] Data not available in all cases (Ethnicity: n = 212).

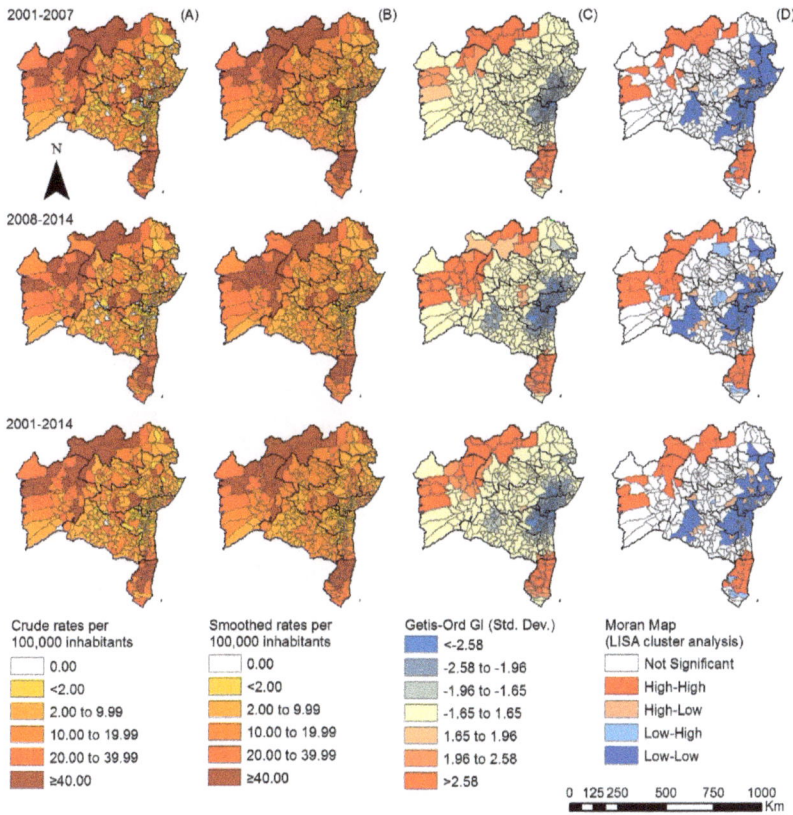

Figure 2. Spatiotemporal distribution of the overall new case detection rate of leprosy by municipality, Bahia state, 2001–2014: (**A**) crude detection rates (per 100,000 inhabitants); (**B**) Bayesian-smoothed detection rate (per 100,000 inhabitants); (**C**) hot-spot analysis (Getis-Ord Gi*) and (**D**) LISA cluster analysis (Moran Map).

For the population <15 years of age, the spatial analysis of crude detection rates revealed a high number of municipalities with high endemicity (Figure 3A). In the first period analyzed (2001–2007), among the 225 (53.9%) municipalities that registered cases in this age group, 54 (28.1%) presented high endemicity. During 2008–2014, the number of highly-endemic municipalities (31.5%, 57) increased (Figure 3A). These patterns were similar after smoothing (Figure 3B). Getis-Ord Gi* analysis (Figure 3C) indicated the existence of high-risk clusters, initially in the North and Far South regions (2001–2008) which persisted during the second period (Figure 3C). A new high-risk cluster appeared in the western part of the State. The local Moran's index confirmed high detection clusters in the previously described regions and indicated the emergence of a cluster in the Far South region with low detection (Figure 3D).

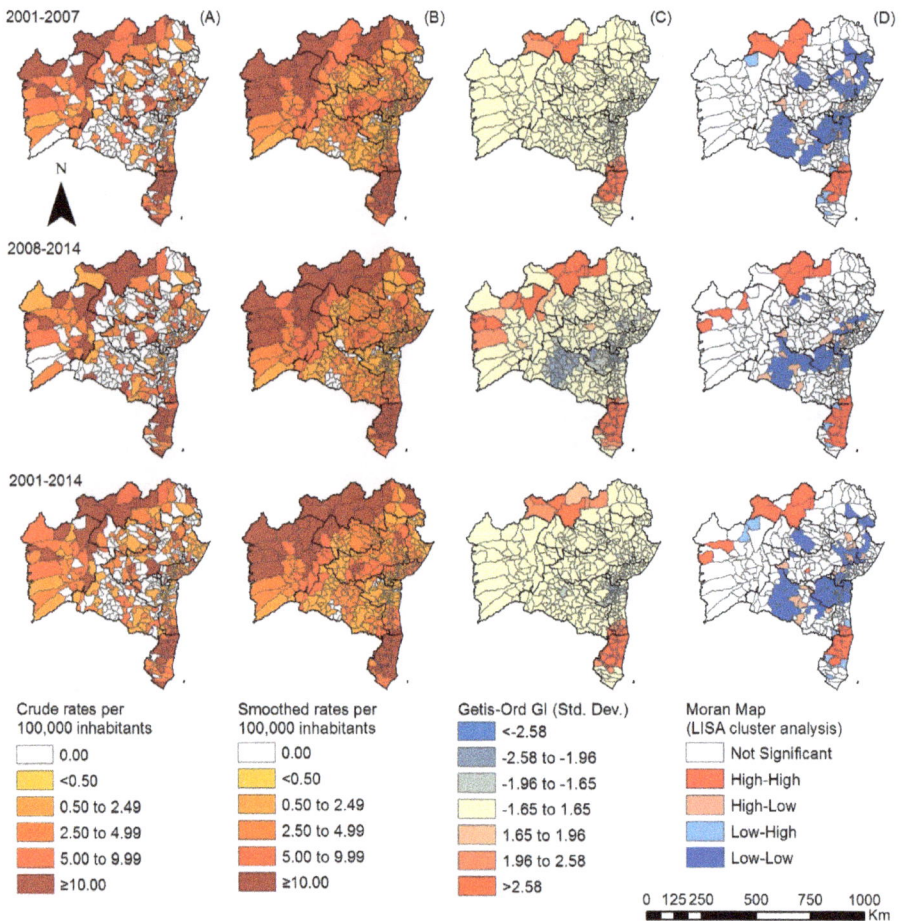

Figure 3. Spatiotemporal distribution of the overall new case detection rate of leprosy in <15 year-olds by municipality, Bahia state, 2001–2014: (**A**) crude detection rates of new cases of leprosy (per 100,000 inhabitants); (**B**) Bayesian-smoothed detection rate (per 100,000 inhabitants); (**C**) hot-spot analysis (Getis-Ord Gi*) and (**D**) LISA cluster analysis (Moran Map).

During the first period, new cases with G2D at the time of diagnosis were recorded in 189 (54.6%) municipalities (Figure 4A), most with less than 1 case with G2D per million people; 8.0% of all municipalities had a rate of more than 4 cases per million people, mainly in the North, West and Far South regions. The Getis-Ord Gi* analysis indicated agglomeration in the North, West and Far South regions, the latter being larger in extent (Figure 4C). During the second period, there was a general increase of the number of municipalities composing the main clusters. The local Moran's index also indicated the existence of clusters, with high rates in the North and Far South, in addition to low rates, in a small area in the South of the State (Figure 4D).

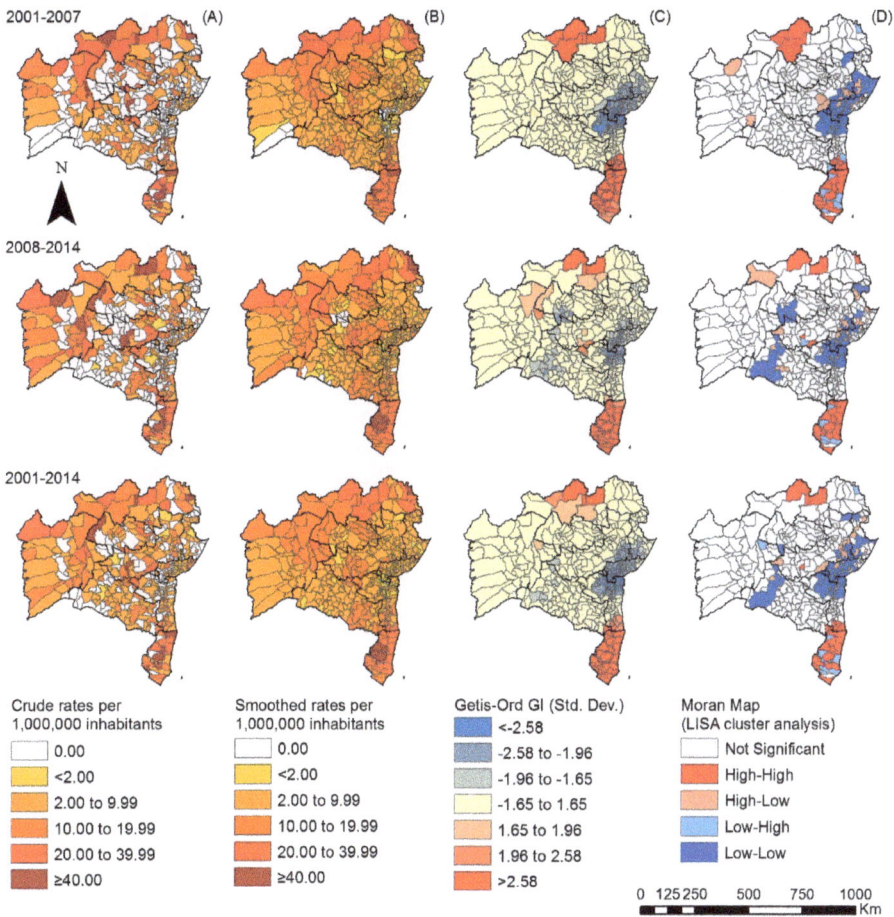

Figure 4. Spatiotemporal distribution of G2D per million people by municipality, Bahia state, 2001–2014: (**A**) crude detection rate of new cases of leprosy (per 1,000,000 inhabitants); (**B**) Bayesian-smoothed detection rate (per 1,000,000 inhabitants); (**C**) hot-spot analysis (Getis-Ord Gi*) and (**D**) LISA cluster analysis (Moran Map).

4. Discussion

This is the first study assessing systematically the epidemiology and distribution of leprosy in the state of Bahia in northeast Brazil. Despite intensive control programs, the State has sustained high levels of endemicity over a period of 14 years, including a significant proportion of children and people with G2D at the time of diagnosis. Among the new cases, people aged ≥50 years were most heavily affected, with no significant gender differences. Most municipalities were defined as medium, highly endemic or hyperendemic, according to definitions of the Brazilian MoH [4].

Medium-sized cities and the extreme south of the State showed a higher leprosy risk than the other areas. Spatiotemporal patterns were heterogeneous, but in general the different indicators and analytical tools applied revealed similar high-risk areas for detection, recent transmission and late diagnosis. In fact, the occurrence of well-defined clusters was confirmed for the three Brazilian MoH/WHO indicators, using different spatial analysis techniques, mainly in the North, West and South regions of the State.

Males had a strikingly higher risk for G2D at diagnosis than females. In fact, healthcare-seeking behavior is known to be different in males, and this group usually presents less commonly and later to the health system than the female population. The reasons for this are multiple and include a historically-built way of living masculinity, which renders men negligent regarding their own health [13], a higher stigmatization, but also simply practical issues such as opening hours which often are not practical for the working population. Consequently, late diagnosis of leprosy is more common in males, reaffirming the social aspects of the disease from a gender perspective [7,18,19].

Another study conducted in Brazil from 2001 to 2013 revealed a significantly higher number of cases in men than in women, and the likelihood of presenting multibacillary cases and G2D at diagnosis was twice as high among men [20]. Another possible explanation relates to physiological risk factors [21].

However, the way that health services are organized and develop their actions can improve access to healthcare, especially prevention activities in primary health care [18,19]. A special focus should be given to the male population regarding prevention and early detection of the disease [4,6]. We suggest further the integration of specific actions of leprosy health surveillance to the National Policy of Comprehensive Attention to Men's Health in Brazil, and to the National Policy of Workers' Health. However, issues related to leprosy stigma should be considered for the development of these measures [22].

We observed that the risk of leprosy increased with age, which may be related to the aging population in Brazil, as well as humoral factors and possible functional impairments, which may affect social engagement, including access to health services [23]. Other studies also revealed an immunological deregulation with aging [20,24]. The changes in the immune system of the elderly may contribute to the increase of susceptibility to infectious and degenerative diseases, including leprosy [25].

The Brazilian MoH already highlighted the higher incidence, more common late diagnosis and higher risk for multibacillary disease among older age groups. Consequently, the elderly population should be a focus of specific strategies directed not only at early diagnosis, but at the systematic follow-up during and after treatment as a chronic disease, in view of the high occurrence of comorbidities, leprosy reactions, drug interactions and progression of functional limitations [19,24–27]. Specific strategies are important, such as active case finding at the residence, and measures to avoid lost opportunities for diagnosis at health centers. The Family Health Strategy should be understood as crucial in this context, as it counts on guidelines for comprehensive and longitudinal care to families, especially to those with high vulnerability [27,28].

A previous study revealed that among the elderly in Brazil the development of illnesses and disabilities causing dependence have been more frequent in the lower income strata. Therefore, in addition to expanding access to health services and actions, measures aimed at improving living conditions are necessary, reducing social inequities [23,26].

In our study, Afro-Brazilian, Asian and Amerindian ethnic groups showed a significantly higher risk for leprosy detection, and/or late diagnosis. These results indicate possible inequalities in access to health services related to ethnicity [29]. Considering the scars produced by a society where Afro-Brazilians and Amerindians historically suffered from slavery and systematic oppression, until today the social position occupied by many keeps them in a condition of higher vulnerability to diseases, especially infectious diseases and more specifically neglected tropical diseases such as leprosy, schistosomiasis, Chagas' disease, and leishmaniasis [30]. Interventions should be made prioritizing this population, since both ethnicities are very common in the state of Bahia [12], implying a priority attention, promoting equity of care and attention in the health network. In the context of social vulnerability, the control of leprosy should be based on broad social reforms considering the social determinants of health [29], contrary to the current political and social reality of the country based on fiscal austerity measures.

The highest relative risk of occurrence of cases was observed in medium-sized cities, but more than half of the cases were registered in small cities. In the state of Bahia, in small-sized municipalities, there are usually no specialized services for leprosy available [31]. Therefore, in these areas, diagnosis and treatment also of complicated cases are strongly linked to primary health care [4]. Consequently, health professionals should be trained systematically to perform diagnosis, treatment and psychosocial rehabilitation of cases. However, several studies revealed operational difficulties of primary health services in the development of leprosy control measures [5,6,32], such as contact tracing [6]. Therefore, municipalities of medium and small size should be prioritized and must receive attention from State and Federal governments in order to strengthen regional support networks. A previous study from the state of Bahia revealed that from 2003 to 2014, only 47% of leprosy contacts were examined [5]. The proportion of cases diagnosed by contact tracing reduced from 18% in 2004 to 8% in 2014. It is important to focus on contact surveillance as a priority strategy for the control of leprosy, following the recommendation of the Brazilian Ministry of Health [1,4,5]. More than 80 municipalities of Bahia maintained high or very high detection rates in children, evidencing considerable ongoing transmission [4]. There are clear difficulties for timely diagnosis also in this age group. Diagnosis often requires the performance of specialists, given its clinical complexity especially in children. Similar scenarios have been identified in municipalities in other states and regions of Brazil [10]. A study carried out in the urban area of the capital city of Salvador, Bahia, recognized an increased risk of occurrence in children <15 years in 22 neighborhoods, with an average occurrence of at least 10 cases per 100,000 inhabitants [33]. Another longitudinal study in the state of Bahia revealed that although the general detection showed a tendency of reduction, in children <15 years, there was maintenance of detection rates for more than a decade [34].

The WHO global strategy for the period 2016–2020 defined one of the main targets as the reduction in the number of children diagnosed with leprosy, and zero visible deformities [1]. A joint effort of health services, universities, and social movements is required in order to provide quality access for children [35].

The spatial analyses of new cases with G2D revealed late diagnosis in the great majority of the municipalities of Bahia, enhancing transmission [1,4]. A previous study from the State evidenced a significant increase of people with G2D [35] over time. An ecological study involving the states of Mato Grosso, Tocantins, Pará, Maranhão and Rondônia, between 2001 and 2012, recognized that the rate of new cases with G2D was stable, varying from 3.62 cases per 100,000 inhabitants in 2001 to 3.41 cases per 100,000 inhabitants in 2012. [36]. The physical disabilities caused by leprosy pervert the conditions of poverty and leprosy-related stigma [22]. In addition to efficient rehabilitation services, it is necessary to establish community-based rehabilitation strategies, promote social inclusion, empower the population and enhance social participation [37]. These strategies are fundamental to break the cycles of vulnerability, demanding intersectoral and sustainable measures [9].

Local autocorrelation methods emphasized the existence of clusters with statistical significance among the epidemiological indicators analyzed. The clusters indicate an increased risk of transmission, active circulation of *M. leprae* and a high number of cases with advanced disability. The results of the Local and Getis-Ord Gi* Moran parameters confirmed two significant clusters in the north and the south. Other studies of this nature revealed several municipality clusters for high leprosy transmission and late diagnosis in an endemic area using different statistical approaches [38].

Intensive monitoring of high risk areas is crucial in order to institute more comprehensive surveillance measures, and to provide comprehensive longitudinal care during and after specific treatment, including social rehabilitation measures and stigma coping [22,37]. In addition, the detection of under-notifications and hidden endemic scenarios in neighboring areas is important, as low endemicity levels in some areas may be related to the poor quality of health services in the realm of active case finding and early diagnosis, not due to the absence of transmission [5,6,32].

For sustainable control, the historical, social, economic and cultural contexts of endemic areas must be considered in an integrative manner [29]. It is necessary to carry out future studies, focusing on individual, social, and programmatic dimensions of vulnerability. The maintenance of high levels of leprosy endemicity reaffirms the need for interdisciplinary research and for constructing dynamic prevention measures and health promotion [39].

The study presents limitations regarding the use of secondary databases, considering non-completeness and inconsistencies for some variables. However, the incorporation of the state database in a historical series of 14 years, together with the need for studies with this approach in the state of Bahia, justifies its use. The definition of the clusters did not allow to delimit their borders with high accuracy, even with the high probability of their existence. A low-frequency area surrounded by areas with a higher number of cases was included in a cluster, although it may have different characteristics. The integration of different analytical techniques has increased consistency of the evidence provided in this study. Considering the large number of municipalities in the State with a small population, the incorporation of the local spatial smoothing method to the analysis was a useful tool for monitoring and surveillance of leprosy. This occurs not only because it is a rare event in some municipalities, but because they often have a small population. The analysis is thus a practical approach to estimate underreported cases, a common reality in different municipalities of Brazil [40].

We conclude that leprosy persists as a relevant public health problem in the state of Bahia. The identified spatiotemporal patterns revealed the maintenance of high-risk clusters for detection, transmission and late diagnosis. We reinforce the importance of integrating surveillance, prevention and control actions in regions of higher risk of leprosy detection and disabilities, and in the most vulnerable populations.

Author Contributions: E.A.S. and A.N.R.J. conceptualized the study. E.A.S., A.F.F., and A.N.R.J. performed the data analysis and interpretation. E.A.S., A.F.F., J.H., and A.N.R.J. contributed to writing. E.A.S., A.F.F., J.H., R.N.B., C.H.A., and A.N.R.J. critically reviewed the final version. All authors approved the final version of the manuscript.

Funding: The study was supported by the Brazilian National Council for Scientific and Technological Development (CNPq), process number 404505/2012-0, MCTI/CNPq/MS-SCTIE-Decit N°40/2012–Research on Neglected Diseases. E.A.S. was a doctoral fellow at the Coordination for the Improvement of Higher Education Personnel (CAPES). A.F.F. is a master fellow at CNPq/Brazil. R.N.B. was a master fellow at CNPq/Brazil. J.H. is class 1 research fellow at CNPq/Brazil.

Conflicts of Interest: The authors declare no conflict of interest.

References

1. World Health Organization, Regional Office for South-East Asia; Department of Control of Neglected Tropical Diseases, WHO. *Global Leprosy Strategy 2016–2020: Accelerating towards a Leprosy-Free World*; WHO SEARO: New Delhi, India, 2016; Available online: http://apps.who.int/iris/bitstream/handle/10665/208824/9789290225096_en.pdf?sequence=14&isAllowed=y (accessed on 8 July 2018).

2. Martins-Melo, F.R.; Carneiro, M.; Ramos, A.N., Jr.; Heukelbach, J.; Ribeiro, A.L.P.; Werneck, G.L. The burden of Neglected Tropical Diseases in Brazil, 1990–2016: A subnational analysis from the Global Burden of Disease Study 2016. *PLoS Negl. Trop. Dis.* **2018**, 12, e0006559. [CrossRef] [PubMed]

3. World Health Organization. Global leprosy update, 2016: Accelerating reduction of disease burden. *Wkly. Epidemiol. Rec.* **2017**, 92, 501–520.

4. Ministério da Saúde do Brasil, Secretaria de Vigilância em Saúde; Departamento de Vigilância das Doenças Transmissíveis. *Diretrizes Para Vigilância, Atenção e Eliminação da Hanseníase Como Problema de Saúde Pública: Manual Técnico-Operacional*; Ministério da Saúde: Brasília, Brazil, 2016. Available online: http://portalarquivos2.saude.gov.br/images/pdf/2016/fevereiro/04/diretrizes-eliminacao-hanseniase-4fev16-web.pdf (accessed on 8 July 2018).

5. Souza, E.A.; Boigny, R.N.; Ferreira, A.F.; Alencar, C.H.; Oliveira, M.L.W.; Ramos, A.N., Jr. Programmatic vulnerability in leprosy control: Gender-related patterns in Bahia State, Brazil. *Cad. Saúde Pública* **2018**, 34, e00196216. [PubMed]

6. Romanholo, H.S.B.; Souza, E.A.; Ramos, A.N., Jr.; Kaiser, A.C.G.C.B.; Silva, I.O.D.; Brito, A.L.; Vasconcellos, C. Surveillance of intradomiciliary contacts of leprosy cases: Perspective of the client in a hyperendemic municipality. *Rev. Bras. Enferm.* **2018**, *71*, 163–169. [CrossRef] [PubMed]
7. Ministério da Saúde do Brasil, Secretaria de Vigilância em Saúde. *Boletim Epidemiológico—Hanseníase*; Ministério da Saúde: Brasília, Brazil, 2018; Volume 49. Available online: http://portalarquivos2.saude.gov.br/images/pdf/2018/janeiro/31/2018-004-Hanseniase-publicacao.pdf (accessed on 8 July 2018).
8. Silva, L.J.D. The concept of space in infectious disease epidemiology. *Cad. Saúde Pública* **1997**, *13*, 585–593. [CrossRef] [PubMed]
9. Pescarini, J.M.; Strina, A.; Nery, J.S.; Skalinski, L.M.; Andrade, K.V.F.; Penna, M.L.F.; Brickley, E.B.; Rodrigues, L.C.; Barreto, M.L.; Penna, G.O. Socioeconomic risk markers of leprosy in high-burden countries: A systematic review and meta-analysis. *PLoS Negl. Trop. Dis.* **2018**, *12*, e0006622. [CrossRef] [PubMed]
10. Lana, F.C.F.; Pinheiro Amaral, E.; Moura Lanza, F.; Lamounier Lima, P.; Nascimento de Carvalho, A.C.; Gonçalves Diniz, L. [Hansen's Disease in children under fifteen years-old in Jequitinhonha Valley, Minas Gerais, Brazil]. *Rev. Bras. Enferm.* **2007**, *60*, 696–700. [CrossRef] [PubMed]
11. Barbosa, C.C.; Bonfim, C.V.D.; Brito, C.M.G.; Ferreira, A.T.; Gregório, V.R.D.N.; Oliveira, A.L.S.; Portugal, J.L.; Medeiros, Z.M. Spatial analysis of reported new cases and local risk of leprosy in hyper-endemic situation in Northeastern Brazil. *Trop. Med. Int. Health.* **2018**, *23*, 748–757. [CrossRef] [PubMed]
12. Instituto Brasileiro de Geografia e Estatística, IBGE. *Dados Populacionais*; IBGE: Brasília, Brazil, 2014. Available online: https://www.ibge.gov.br/ (accessed on 8 July 2018).
13. Alves, R.F.; Silva, R.P.; Ernesto, M.V.; Lima, A.G.B.; Souza, F.M. Gender and health: Men's care in debate. *Psicol. Teor. Prát.* **2011**, *13*, 152–166.
14. Instituto de Pesquisa Econômica Aplicada. IPEA. *Programa das Nações Unidas para o Desenvolvimento, PNUD; Fundação João Pinheiro, FJP. IPEA Data*; IPEA: Brasília, Brazil, 2013. Available online: http://www.ipeadata.gov.br/Default.aspx (accessed on 8 July 2018).
15. Ministério da Saúde. Histórico de Cobertura da Saúde da Família. Available online: http://dab.saude.gov.br/portaldab/historico_cobertura_sf.php (accessed on 2 September 2016).
16. Altman, D.G. Confidence intervals for the number needed to treat. *BMJ* **1998**, *317*, 1309–1312. [CrossRef] [PubMed]
17. Environmental Systems Research Institute, ESRI. *ArcGIS Desktop: Release 10*; ESRI: Redlands, CA, USA, 2011.
18. Machin, R.; Couto, M.T.; Sibele Nogueira da Silva, G.; Schraiber, L.B.; Gomes, R.; Santos Figueiredo, W.D.; Valença, O.A.; Pinheiro, T.F. Concepts of gender, masculinity and healthcare: A study of primary healthcare professionals. *Ciênc. Saúde Coletiva* **2011**, *16*, 4503–4512. [CrossRef]
19. Ministério da Saúde, Secretaria de Vigilância em Saúde. *Alerta Para o Exame Sistemático de Hanseníase na População Masculina e em Idosos*; Ministério da Saúde: Brasília, Brasil, 2016. Available online: http://portalarquivos.saude.gov.br/images/pdf/2016/setembro/06/Nota-Informativa-Conjunta-n---01--SAS-e-SVS--para-publica----o.pdf (accessed on 15 April 2018).
20. Nobre, M.L.; Illarramendi, X.; Dupnik, K.M.; Hacker, M.D.A.; Nery, J.A.D.C.; Jerônimo, S.M.B.; Sarno, E.N. Multibacillary leprosy by population groups in Brazil: Lessons from an observational study. *PLoS Negl. Trop. Dis.* **2017**, *11*, e0005364. [CrossRef] [PubMed]
21. Guerra-Silveira, F.; Abad-Franch, F. Sex bias in infectious disease epidemiology: Patterns and processes. *PLoS ONE* **2013**, *8*, e62390. [CrossRef] [PubMed]
22. Van Brakel, W.H.; Sihombing, B.; Djarir, H.; Beise, K.; Kusumawardhani, L.; Yulihane, R.; Kurniasari, I.; Kasim, M.; Kesumaningsih, K.I.; Wilder-Smith, A. Disability in people affected by leprosy: The role of impairment, activity, social participation, stigma and discrimination. *Glob. Health Action* **2012**, *5*, e18394. [CrossRef] [PubMed]
23. Lima-Costa, M.F.; Barreto, S.; Giatti, L.; Uchôa, E. Socioeconomic circumstances and health among the Brazilian elderly: A study using data from a National Household Survey. *Cad. Saúde Pública* **2003**, *19*, 745–757. [CrossRef] [PubMed]
24. Assis, I.S.; Arcoverde, M.A.M.; Ramos, A.C.V.; Alves, L.S.; Berra, T.Z.; Arroyo, L.H.; Queiroz, A.A.R.; Santos, D.T.D.; Belchior, A.S.; Alves, J.D.; et al. Social determinants, their relationship with leprosy risk and temporal trends in a tri-border region in Latin America. *PLoS Negl. Trop. Dis.* **2018**, *12*, e0006407.
25. Agondi, R.C.; Rizzo, L.V.; Kalil, J.; Barros, M.T. Immunosenescence. *Rev. Bras. Alerg. Imunopatol.* **2012**, *35*, 167–168.

26. Nogueira, P.S.F.; Marques, M.B.; Coutinho, J.F.V.; Maia, J.C.; Silva, M.J.D.; Moura, E.R.F. Factors associated with the functional capacity of older adults with leprosy. *Rev. Bras. Enferm.* **2017**, *70*, 711–718. [CrossRef] [PubMed]
27. Pelarigo, J.G.T.; Prado, R.B.R.; Nardi, S.M.T.; Quaggio, C.M.D.P.; Camargo, L.H.S.; Marciano, L.H.S.C. Cognitive impairment, functional independence and depressive symptoms in elderly people with prior history of leprosy. *Hansen. Int.* **2014**, *39*, 30–39.
28. Motta, L.B.D.; Aguiar, A.C.D.; Caldas, C.P. The Family Health Strategy and healthcare for the elderly: Experiences in three Brazilian cities. *Cad. Saúde Pública* **2011**, *27*, 779–786. [CrossRef] [PubMed]
29. Buss, P.M.; Pellegrini Filho, A. Health and its social determinants. *Phys. Rev. Saúde Coletiva* **2007**, *17*, 77–93. [CrossRef]
30. Chor, D.; Lima, C.R.D.A. Epidemiologic aspects of racial inequalities in health in Brazil. *Cad. Saúde Pública* **2005**, *21*, 1586–1594. [CrossRef] [PubMed]
31. Instituto Brasileiro de Geografia e Estatística, IBGE. *Unidade da Federação: Bahia*; IBGE: Brasília, Brasil, 2014. Available online: https://cidades.ibge.gov.br/brasil/ba (accessed on 8 July 2018).
32. Arantes, C.K.; Garcia, M.L.R.; Filipe, M.S.; Nardi, S.M.T.; Paschoal, V.D.A. Health services assessment of early leprosy diagnosis. *Epidemiol. Serv.Saúde* **2010**, *19*, 155–164.
33. Souza, C.; Rodrigues, M. Magnitude, trend and spatialization of leprosy on minors of fifteen years in the state of Bahia, with focus on risk areas: An ecological study. *Hygeia* **2015**, *11*, 201–212.
34. Souza, E.A.; Ferreira, A.F.; Boigny, R.N.; Alencar, C.H.; Heukelbach, J.; Martins-Melo, F.R.; Barbosa, J.C.; Ramos, A.N., Jr. Leprosy and gender in Brazil: Trends in an endemic area of the Northeast region, 2001–2014. *Rev. Saúde Pública* **2018**, *52*, 20. [CrossRef] [PubMed]
35. Cabral-Miranda, W.; Chiaravalloti Neto, F.; Barrozo, L.V. Socio-economic and environmental effects influencing the development of leprosy in Bahia, north-eastern Brazil. *Trop. Med. Int. Health* **2014**, *19*, 1504–1514. [CrossRef] [PubMed]
36. Freitas, L.R.; Duarte, E.C.; Garcia, L.P. Trends of main indicators of leprosy in Brazilian municipalities with high risk of leprosy transmission, 2001–2012. *BMC Infect. Dis.* **2016**, *16*, 472. [CrossRef] [PubMed]
37. Mauro, V.; Biggeri, M.; Deepak, S.; Trani, J.-F. The effectiveness of community-based rehabilitation programmes: An impact evaluation of a quasi-randomised trial. *J. Epidemiol. Community Health* **2014**, *68*, 1102–1108. [CrossRef] [PubMed]
38. Alencar, C.H.; Ramos, A.N., Jr.; dos Santos, E.S.; Richter, J.; Heukelbach, J. Clusters of leprosy transmission and of late diagnosis in a highly endemic area in Brazil: Focus on different spatial analysis approaches. *Trop. Med. Int. Health* **2012**, *17*, 518–525. [CrossRef] [PubMed]
39. Ayres, J.; França Júnior, I.; Calazans, G.J.; Saletti Filho, H.C.; Czeresnia, D.; Freitas, C. The vulnerability concept and the practices of health: New perspectives and challenges. In *Promoção da Saúde: Conceitos, Reflexões, Tendências*, 2nd ed.; Czeresnia, D., Freitas, C.M., Eds.; Editora Fiocruz: Rio de Janeiro, Brazil, 2003; pp. 117–139. ISBN 9788575411834.
40. Assunção, R.M.; Schmertmann, C.P.; Potter, J.E.; Cavenaghi, S.M. Empirical Bayes' estimation of demographic schedules for small areas. *Demography* **2005**, *42*, 537–558. [CrossRef] [PubMed]

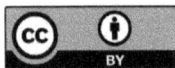

MDPI

St. Alban-Anlage 66

4052 Basel

Switzerland

Tel. +41 61 683 77 34

Fax +41 61 302 89 18

www.mdpi.com

Tropical Medicine and Infectious Disease Editorial Office

E-mail: tropicalmed@mdpi.com

www.mdpi.com/journal/tropicalmed

www.ingramcontent.com/pod-product-compliance
Lightning Source LLC
Chambersburg PA
CBHW051841210326

41597CB00033B/5737